LATERALITY IN SPORTS

LATERALITY IN SPORTS

THEORIES AND APPLICATIONS

Edited by

FLORIAN LOFFING

NORBERT HAGEMANN

BERND STRAUSS

CLARE MACMAHON

ELSEVIER

AMSTERDAM • BOSTON • HEIDELBERG • LONDON
NEW YORK • OXFORD • PARIS • SAN DIEGO
SAN FRANCISCO • SINGAPORE • SYDNEY • TOKYO

Academic Press is an imprint of Elsevier

Academic Press is an imprint of Elsevier
125 London Wall, London EC2Y 5AS, United Kingdom
525 B Street, Suite 1800, San Diego, CA 92101-4495, United States
50 Hampshire Street, 5th Floor, Cambridge, MA 02139, United States
The Boulevard, Langford Lane, Kidlington, Oxford OX5 1GB, United Kingdom

Notices
Knowledge and best practice in this field are constantly changing. As new research and experience broaden our understanding, changes in research methods, professional practices, or medical treatment may become necessary.

Practitioners and researchers must always rely on their own experience and knowledge in evaluating and using any information, methods, compounds, or experiments described herein. In using such information or methods they should be mindful of their own safety and the safety of others, including parties for whom they have a professional responsibility.

To the fullest extent of the law, neither the Publisher nor the authors, contributors, or editors, assume any liability for any injury and/or damage to persons or property as a matter of products liability, negligence or otherwise, or from any use or operation of any methods, products, instructions, or ideas contained in the material herein.

Library of Congress Cataloging-in-Publication Data
A catalog record for this book is available from the Library of Congress

British Library Cataloguing-in-Publication Data
A catalogue record for this book is available from the British Library

ISBN: 978-0-12-801426-4

For information on all Academic Press publications
visit our website at https://www.elsevier.com/

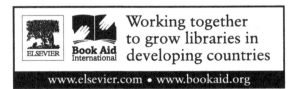

Working together
to grow libraries in
developing countries

www.elsevier.com • www.bookaid.org

Publisher: Nikki Levy
Acquisition Editor: Nikki Levy
Editorial Project Manager: Barbara Makinster
Production Project Manager: Julie-Ann Stansfield
Designer: Matthew Limbert

Typeset by TNQ Books and Journals

Contents

A

LATERALITY – AN IMPORTANT AND OFTEN DISREGARDED TOPIC

B

MOTOR CONTROL AND LEARNING

8. Laterality of Basic Motor Control Mechanisms: Different Roles of the Right and Left Brain Hemispheres

ROBERT L. SAINBURG

9. Effector Transfer

CHARLES H. SHEA, STEFAN PANZER AND DEANNA M. KENNEDY

10. Near Misses and the Effect of Attentional Asymmetries on Sporting Performance

OWEN CHURCHES AND MICHAEL E.R. NICHOLLS

C

PERFORMANCE IN SPORTS

14. Laterality Effects on Performance in Team Sports: Insights From Soccer and Basketball

TINO STÖCKEL AND DAVID P. CAREY

15. Skill Acquisition in Left- and Right-Dominant Athletes: Insights From Elite Coaching

DAVE WHITESIDE, TIM BUSZARD, GEORGIA GIBLIN AND MACHAR REID

List of Contributors

Joseph Baker York University, Toronto, ON, Canada

Kevin Ball Victoria University, Melbourne, VIC, Australia

Christina Bermeitinger University of Hildesheim, Hildesheim, Germany

Dirk Büsch University of Health and Sport, Technique and Art, Berlin, Germany

Tim Buszard Innovation and Insights Group, Tennis Australia, Melbourne, VIC, Australia; Victoria University, Footscray, VIC, Australia

David P. Carey Bangor University, Bangor, United Kingdom

Owen Churches Flinders University, Adelaide, SA, Australia

Jacqueline A. de Nooijer Erasmus University Rotterdam, Rotterdam, The Netherlands

Todd S. Ellenbecker Physiotherapy Associates Scottsdale Sports Clinic, Scottsdale, AZ, United States; Medical Services ATP World Tour, FL, United States

Charlotte Faurie University of Montpellier, Montpellier, France

Georgia Giblin Innovation and Insights Group, Tennis Australia, Melbourne, VIC, Australia; Queensland Academy of Sport, Brisbane, QLD, Australia

Norbert Hagemann University of Kassel, Kassel, Germany

Lauren Julius Harris Michigan State University, East Lansing, MI, United States

Thomas Heinen University of Hildesheim, Hildesheim, Germany

Deanna M. Kennedy Texas A&M University, TX, United States

Florian Loffing University of Kassel, Kassel, Germany

Clare MacMahon Swinburne University of Technology, Melbourne, VIC, Australia

Stijn Valentijn Mentzel University of Münster, Münster, Germany

Michael E.R. Nicholls Flinders University, Adelaide, SA, Australia

Stefan Panzer Saarland University, Saarbrücken, Germany

Lucy Parrington Swinburne University of Technology, Melbourne, VIC, Australia

Michel Raymond University of Montpellier, Montpellier, France

Machar Reid Innovation and Insights Group, Tennis Australia, Melbourne, VIC, Australia; University of Western Australia, Crawley, WA, Australia

Robert L. Sainburg Penn State College of Medicine, Hershey, PA, United States; Pennsylvania State University, University Park, PA, United States

Jörg Schorer University of Oldenburg, Oldenburg, Germany

Charles H. Shea Texas A&M University, TX, United States

Christina Steingröver   University of Oldenburg, Oldenburg, Germany

Tino Stöckel   University of Rostock, Rostock, Germany

Bernd Strauss   University of Münster, Münster, Germany

Judith Tirp   University of Oldenburg, Oldenburg, Germany

Natalie Uomini   Max Planck Institute for the Science of Human History, Jena, Germany

Till Utesch   University of Münster, Münster, Germany

Christoph von Laßberg   University of Tübingen, Tübingen, Germany

Dave Whiteside   Innovation and Insights Group, Tennis Australia, Melbourne, VIC, Australia; Victoria University, Footscray, VIC, Australia

Roel M. Willems   Radboud University Nijmegen, Nijmegen, The Netherlands; Max Planck Institute for Psycholinguistics, Nijmegen, The Netherlands

Editor Biographies

Florian Loffing, PhD

Florian Loffing is a postdoctoral fellow at the Institute of Sports and Sports Sciences of the University of Kassel (Germany). He obtained his PhD from the University of Münster (Germany), Department of Sport Psychology, for his dissertation on performance in left- and right-handed professional tennis players. Florian's research interests focus upon the perceptual-cognitive processes and mechanisms that underlie skilled performance in sports. This specifically includes the examination of laterality effects on visual anticipation, decision-making, and high achievement in the elite domain of sports. Florian's work has been published in several peer-reviewed journals including *PLoS One*, *Journal of Sport & Exercise Psychology*, *Human Movement Science*, *Acta Psychologica*, and *Journal of Sports Sciences*.

Norbert Hagemann, PhD

Norbert Hagemann is currently full professor for sport psychology at the University of Kassel (Germany). He received his PhD from the University of Münster for his thesis "Heuristic problem solving strategies of team coaches." Prof. Hagemann is studying the cognitive processes underlying how athletes perform in training and competitive situations. The focus is particularly on their perception and attention processes. Prof. Hagemann has been working on the topic of laterality for several years. This research has been supported by several research grants from the German Research Foundation. He regularly publishes and reviews papers in high-impact international peer-reviewed journals.

Bernd Strauss, PhD

Bernd Strauss, born in 1959, is currently full professor for sport psychology at the University of Münster, Germany (since 1998). He obtained his PhD from the University of Kiel (Germany) in 1992 with a thesis about complex problem solving. He had been the former president of the German Society of Sport Sciences (2003–2009). Currently he is president of the German Sport Psychology association. Bernd Strauss has published more than 20 books and more than 80 peer-reviewed papers. Currently he is editor-in-chief (in collaboration with Nikos Ntoumanis, AUS) of the journal

Psychology of Sport and Exercise published by Elsevier. His main research interests are focused on expertise in sports (perception, attention, laterality), social psychology (self-concept, influence of audiences on performances, sports spectators), and research methodology.

Clare MacMahon, PhD

Clare MacMahon is a senior lecturer and head of sports science at Swinburne University of Technology in Melbourne, Australia. She has an undergraduate degree in psychology from McGill University and post graduate degrees in human kinetics and human biodynamics from the University of Ottawa and McMaster University. In her work on sport expertise, with an interest in decision-making and the cognitive components of performance, Clare has conducted research in labs in Canada, the United States, Belgium, Germany, and Australia, working alongside world leaders in the area. Her work has been funded by the Social Sciences and Humanities Research Council of Canada and the Australian Research Council.

Preface

Why a book about laterality in sports? Like others, we are fascinated by sporting athletes' performances. Specifically, we are amazed at the ease and proficiency with which athletes perform sport-specific actions, sometimes with little difference between whether they are using the left or right side of their bodies. Our interest in laterality in sports is also deeply rooted in our personal experiences as sportspeople. We all have our own experiences of laterality in sports, which we believe blazed the trail for this book. While reading our anecdotes on laterality in sports below, you might catch yourself reminiscing about your own "laterality in sports" experiences.

As a right-handed player in youth tennis, Florian always lost against a particular left-hander who seemed to have a somewhat unorthodox style of play. As a right-foot dominant midfielder in soccer, he deliberately trained his left foot as he believed that mixed-footedness might provide an advantage for his play.

Norbert has been a goalkeeper in team handball and found it particularly difficult to defend against left-handed attackers. He had the impression that lefties throw in a strange, unpredictable manner. Based on this experience, he was driven to solve the mystery behind this phenomenon.

Forty years ago, as a right-hander, Bernd was playing team handball for several years, specializing in defense. However, although he trained very hard, he always found it extremely difficult to be successful against left-handed offense players.

Being right-handed and left-footed, Clare once realized that this mixing of laterality might cause her trouble in gymnastics. Specifically, while she cartwheeled with her left foot in front in a tumbling sequence, she tried to twist to her right, which was against the way her body was already moving from the roundoff.

Given these personal experiences and our general interest in the processes underlying sports performance, our group entered into a body of research in the area (e.g., Hagemann, 2009; Loffing & Hagemann, 2012, 2015; Loffing, Hagemann, Schorer, & Baker, 2015; Loffing, Hagemann, & Strauss, 2010, 2012; Loffing, Sölter, & Hagemann, 2014; Loffing, Sölter, Hagemann, & Strauss, 2015). In this regard, we are very grateful that the German Research Foundation (DFG) repeatedly funded most of this work (HA 4361/5-1, HA 4361/5-2, and STR 490/11-2), thereby also helping to bring all of the knowledge about laterality in sports together in this edition.

Delving into laterality in sports over the past years, we became more and more fascinated about this topic while, at the same time, realizing how much we can still learn about left and right sidedness in sports. The latter holds for rather general issues related to laterality (e.g., left vs right preference for sport tasks) but also for specific questions, for example, focusing on the perceptual, cognitive, or motor processes underlying athletes' skill acquisition and performance or coaches' or judges' decision-making and behavior. Given the diversity of topics related to laterality in sports and the fascinating research already done in this area by different groups worldwide, we thought the time was right to bring together different perspectives on laterality in sports.

When Nikki Levy, the publisher responsible for the psychology book series at Elsevier, then approached us in 2012 asking about "hot topics" that might make a good book, laterality immediately came to mind. The prospect of inviting top researchers from a variety of perspectives to write on this topic was exciting. With their outstanding work, we feel we have created a unique and outstanding contribution.

This book is the first publication to thoroughly address laterality in sports. The diversity of primarily sport-related laterality research is reflected in the selection of book chapters. Chapters cover a wide range of topics and perspectives, not only from sports sciences, but also from evolutionary biology and psychology, neuroscience, and cognitive psychology, and they are written by distinguished experts in their respective fields. Information on the book's structure, its sections, and its chapters are fully outlined in Chapter 1, Laterality in Sports: More Than Two Sides of the Same Coin.

A feature common to almost all chapters is that each of them gives a thorough and critical review of the topics at hand. Some chapters also deal with what are currently unexplored issues in sport-related laterality research to initiate new discussions and extend the current research agenda (e.g., skill acquisition). Furthermore, most chapters critically discuss potential implications for sport practice (e.g., performance enhancement, talent development, and identification) and highlight future perspectives. Collectively, this positions the book as a key resource in the area.

The diversity of topics and perspectives makes the book relevant for a broad audience. The primarily intended audience are researchers and (under)graduate students. Researchers from various fields (e.g., sports sciences, psychology, human movement sciences) who are interested in human lateralized behavior will benefit from the critical reviews, the elaboration on unexplored issues, and thorough discussions of future research perspectives. The book also helps upper-level undergraduates and graduate students to obtain comprehensive insights into research on laterality in sports. In this regard, the book will be a key basic reference for university classes on laterality issues in sports and related behavioral domains.

Last but not least, we anticipate that sports practitioners and upper-level coaches will also be interested in and benefit from reading the book.

There are a number of people to thank in bringing about this book. First, we would like to thank Nikki Levy very much for providing a great opportunity to publish this book with Elsevier. We also thank all contributors for their great effort, timely delivery of chapters, and excellent work and help in realizing this unique project. We are very happy that so many leading and well-known researchers in that particular field contribute to this edition and give deep insights in their work.

Our special thanks go to Barbara Makinster from Elsevier for her great support and abundance of patience throughout the whole book project.

We hope that you find some personal relevance in these pages and our colleagues help you to delve into a bit more understanding of your body and how it works. We hope you enjoy reading this book.

Kassel, Münster, Melbourne, August 2016
Florian, Norbert, Bernd, and Clare

References

Hagemann, N. (2009). The advantage of being left-handed in interactive sports. *Attention, Perception, & Psychophysics, 71*, 1641–1648.

Loffing, F., & Hagemann, N. (2012). Side bias in human performance: a review on the left-handers' advantage in sports. In T. Dutta, M. Mandal, & S. Kumar (Eds.), *Bias in human Behaviour* (pp. 163–182). Hauppauge, NY: Nova Science.

Loffing, F., & Hagemann, N. (2015). Pushing through evolution? Incidence and fight records of left-oriented fighters in professional boxing history. *Laterality: Asymmetries of Body, Brain and Cognition, 20*, 270–286.

Loffing, F., Hagemann, N., & Strauss, B. (2010). Automated processes in tennis: do left-handed players benefit from the tactical preferences of their opponents? *Journal of Sports Sciences, 28*, 435–443.

Loffing, F., Hagemann, N., & Strauss, B. (2012). Left-handedness in professional and amateur tennis. *PLoS ONE, 7*, e49325.

Loffing, F., Hagemann, N., Schorer, J., & Baker, J. (2015). Skilled players' and novices' difficulty anticipating left- vs. right-handed opponents' action intentions varies across different points in time. *Human Movement Science, 40*, 410–421.

Loffing, F., Sölter, F., Hagemann, N., & Strauss, B. (2015). Accuracy of outcome anticipation, but not gaze behavior, differs against left- and right-handed penalties in team-handball goalkeeping. *Frontiers in Psychology, 6*.

Loffing, F., Sölter, F., & Hagemann, N. (2014). Left preference for sport tasks does not necessarily indicate left-handedness: sport-specific lateral preferences, relationship with handedness and implications for laterality research in behavioural sciences. *PLoS One, 9*, e105800.

Laterality in Sports: More Than Two Sides of the Same Coin

Florian Loffing, Norbert Hagemann
University of Kassel, Kassel, Germany

Bernd Strauss
University of Münster, Münster, Germany

Clare MacMahon
Swinburne University of Technology, Melbourne, VIC, Australia

So, in the muscular exercises of tennis, racket, and fives, a man with an inert left hand would not score well in the game. Unless Esmeralda or La Sylphide could pirouette on the left tiptoe as well as on the right, she would be found wanting. Unless those really hard-working men who imperil their lives, day after day, in performing feats of rope dancing, rope swinging, trapèze performances, aerial leaping, globe climbing, and the like—unless such men could use the left arm and leg as rapidly and as firmly as the right, their lives would not be worth many months' purchase in the estimation of an insurance office actuary. And so the juggler, who tosses up his balls, cups, plates, and knives, does just as much work with the left hand as with the right. We therefore know that, whatever Nature did or did not intend, training will, to some extent, bring about equi-handedness and equal action in the two feet or legs. **Dickens, 1875, p. 137.**

Daily life is full of lateralized behavior. We choose between our left and right hands to use a key in a door, or grasp a cup of coffee, which direction to turn to see who is standing behind us, which eye to use when looking through the peep hole in a door, and which foot to use when kicking a stone while walking through the park. Lateralized behavior is well-researched, particularly in domains such as biology and psychology (e.g., McManus, 2002; Rogers, Vallortigara, & Andrew, 2013).

Also, the discussion of laterality in sports, with particular emphasis on left-handedness, has attracted sport practitioners and scientists for centuries (e.g., Dickens, 1875; Harris, 2010; Lundie, 1896). For example, in an essay on "left-handed people," Dickens (1875) reflected on the significance of bilateral competence in a variety of sporting tasks involving the hands or feet, suggesting that unilateral competence will unlikely be sufficient for attaining sporting excellence. Lundie (1896) focused on batting in cricket and highlighted the problems a left-handed batsman may impose on players of the opposing team. Even centuries before, fencing masters discussed the role of handedness and suggested a possible fighting advantage of relatively rare left-handed fencers (Harris, 2010; see also Harris, in this book). Throughout the chapters in this book, these and other fascinating aspects relating to laterality in sports will be addressed in more detail.

Sports are almost free of any restrictions specifying use of the left or right (Eastwood, 1972). Indeed, there are only a few exceptions, in sports like polo, where the rules dictate that the stick be held in the right hand, or in field or indoor hockey, where rules and the shape of a stick indicate how to hold a stick, or in athletics, where runners always move counterclockwise, as dictated by the running track. Apart from these or other rare occasions, athletes may vary the hand they use to play tennis, fence, throw and bat in baseball or cricket, hit the ball in golf, and shoot in ice hockey. Similarly, in boxing, wrestling, judo, or other combat sports, fighters differ in their preferred combat stance. In sports such as soccer, rugby, American football, or Australian rules football, players may prefer their left or right foot for kicking a ball. Some players may even be almost equally proficient in using both feet and one might ask if that may confer an advantage during match play and thus enables players to make more money with their sport (Bryson, Frick, & Simmons, 2013). Further variation in laterality is seen, for example, in gymnasts or figure skaters who turn left or right when performing a pirouette, in swimmers who turn left or right when performing a flip turn at the end of a lane, or in archers or biathletes who aim at targets using their left or right eyes.

While the above examples focus on choice of limb or lateralized performance in particular sports or in specific tasks within sports, symmetry is also important. In particular, sports that use both sides in cyclical movements, such as swimming, cycling, or running depend on symmetrical movement and strength. Injury is also a consideration, for both types of sports, but in particular for lateralized sports. Specifically, targeted training of both sides of the body may help counteract potentially harmful asymmetries in athletes' musculoskeletal systems which, for example, may evolve or become intensified from predominant unilateral control of movements in asymmetric sports (e.g., tennis, baseball).

Despite the obvious occurrence of lateralized behavior in sports, it has not been extensively studied and has only recently become a focus. Recent foci of exploration include effects of bilateral practice on motor skill acquisition, performance advantage of left-oriented athletes in interactive sports (e.g., fencing, boxing), or laterality effects on motor control in sports tasks. With this increase in focus and output in research on laterality in sports, we think the time is right to bring forward the underlying theories and to derive potential applications, to unite previously isolated studies.

This edition covers a wide range of topics and perspectives, theories, and applications not only from sports sciences, but also from evolutionary biology and psychology, neuroscience and cognitive psychology. All contributing authors from around the globe are distinguished and leading international experts in their respective fields.

THE STRUCTURE OF THE BOOK

This edition includes 15 chapters, with the following 14 chapters being divided up into three sections. The first section gathers together the basic knowledge from various disciplines that is necessary for an understanding of laterality phenomena in sports. The second section focuses on those motor control and motor learning processes that are important for lateralized behavior. When trying to explain laterality phenomena in sports, it is essential to understand how unilateral and bilateral movements are controlled along with the underlying learning mechanisms. The final section then discusses performance-related aspects in concrete sports situations.

Section A: Laterality—an Important and Often Disregarded Topic

In Chapter 2: Origins, Development and Persistence of Laterality in Humans, Charlotte Faurie, Natalie Uomini, and Michel Raymond elaborate on the complex interplay between the different factors that have an impact on the development and persistence of laterality in humans. The stable proportion of left- to right-handers since prehistoric times may result from mechanisms related to adaptation and natural selection. For example, the fighting hypothesis posits that negative frequency-dependent selection mechanisms could have provided the relatively rarer left-handers with a fitness advantage that may have helped them to overcome the potential costs associated with left-handedness. The authors discuss the fighting hypothesis as one possible explanation for the persistence of left-handedness from ancient to modern times.

Taking a sports context, negative frequency-dependent selection mechanisms may be illustrated nicely through the example of fencing. In Chapter 3: In Fencing, Are Left-Handers Trouble for Right-Handers? What Fencing Masters Said in the Past and What Scientists Say Today, Lauren Julius Harris gives a comprehensive overview of the relevance of handedness in fencing from both the scientist's theoretical and the fencing master's practical viewpoints. To this end, he adopts a historical perspective to also highlight the influence of cultural factors. By including well-researched quotes by former fencing masters, Harris illustrates how the discussion of the relevance of laterality in sports needs to be viewed as part of the classical nature versus nurture debate.

The majority of studies on asymmetry in human behavior use different tests or measures to differentiate various types of laterality, with handedness being the most prominent form. However, researchers interested in including laterality measures in their work may find it difficult to decide which of the many tests they should use. Till Utesch, Stijn Valentijn Mentzel, Bernd Strauss, and Dirk Büsch summarize different methods of assessing an individual's lateral preferences in Chapter 4: Measurement of Laterality and Its Relevance for Sports. They also describe how models based on item response theory may be used to test the construct validity of well-established laterality measures such as Oldfield's (1971) Edinburgh Handedness Inventory. The authors conclude by giving clear recommendations on the implementation of appropriate laterality measures in a sports context.

The interplay between the influences of nature or nurture is particularly important from the perspective of talent identification and development. The question is how much talent in sports is determined by endogenous or exogenous factors. This discussion is taken up in Chapter 5: Laterality And Its Role In Talent Identification And Athlete Development by Jörg Schorer, Judith Tirp, Christina Steingröver, and Joseph Baker, who clarify it with illustrations taken from the topic of laterality. The authors show very clearly that the success of left-handers in sports is not just due to endogenous factors, and they call for a stronger and more frequent emphasis on left-handed actions in both training and competitions.

Lateralized behavior is necessary in a variety of sport situations such as throwing a ball in baseball or cricket or hitting a forehand in tennis. The loads acting upon the limb that is predominantly carrying out such motor actions are heavier than those acting upon the nondominant limb. Consequently, asymmetries in muscular as well as skeletal structure may well evolve. In Chapter 6: Perspectives From Sports Medicine, Todd S. Ellenbecker adopts a sports medicine perspective and gives a comprehensive overview of the loads that may operate particularly on upper but also on lower extremities in sports such as tennis, which requires unilateral dominance. He discusses potential consequences for injury prevention, rehabilitation, or performance enhancement while highlighting recommendations for practitioners.

Section B: Motor Control and Learning

This section starts by emphasizing the close interplay between the motor system and cognition as proposed in the theories of embodied cognition. An interesting question in this context is how the different preferences for one side of the body have an impact on cognitive tasks. In Chapter 7: What Can We Learn About Cognition From Studying Handedness? Insights From Cognitive Neuroscience, Jacqueline A. de Nooijer and Roel M. Willems deliver comprehensive insights into this highly topical field of research and illustrate how handedness can influence basic cognitive functions such as memory, perception, and learning.

Any analysis of motor control processes requires an understanding of the two hemispheres of the brain. Building on an evolutionary approach, Robert L. Sainburg has developed an influential theory of motor control. His dynamic dominance theory assumes that handedness emerges through the interplay of different control mechanisms in the two hemispheres. The dominant hemisphere specializes in predictive control processes, whereas the nondominant hemisphere is responsible for impedance control processes. In Chapter 8: Laterality of Basic Motor Control Mechanisms: Different Roles of the Right and Left Brain Hemispheres, Sainburg also explains differences in the control processes of left- and right-handers and how these processes could contribute to left-handers being more successful in sports.

The human repertoire of movements is highly adaptable in order to cope with the greatest differences in demands imposed by individual courses of development. During new learning, neural codes are built up that are also applied in other situations or even in movements performed by another part of the body. In Chapter 9: Effector Transfer, Charles H. Shea, Stefan Panzer, and Deanna M. Kennedy do impressive work to show how studies on effector transfer can be used to gain a better understanding of how movement sequences are coded, structured, and executed. By including left- and right-handers in these studies, it also becomes possible to derive the role of lateral dominance and hemispherical asymmetry in the learning of movement skills.

Visual attention processes are essential when performing goal-directed actions. Nonetheless, paying attention to our surroundings seems to be distorted by a systematic leftward perceptual bias. In Chapter 10: Near Misses and the Effect of Attentional Asymmetries on Sporting Performance, Owen Churches and Michael E.R. Nicholls perform a thorough theoretical analysis from both a psychological and a neurological perspective of this bias known as pseudoneglect. Their analysis shows impressively how this bias can influence not only behavior in the laboratory and in everyday situations, but also the performance of athletes in various types of sports such as golf, Australian rules football, soccer, baseball, and archery.

Section C: Performance in Sports

When considering laterality in sport, most readers will probably think about carrying out movements with the left or right hand or with the left or right foot. However, in individual sports such as gymnastics, figure skating, or platform diving, the focus is on another form of laterality:

the preferred direction of rotation. In Chapter 11: Laterality in Individual Sports, Thomas Heinen, Christina Bermeitinger, and Christoph von Laßberg ask what constitutes an athlete's rotational preference. They review the theoretical and empirical findings on laterality and discuss the influence of perceptual-cognitive aspects. They close their chapter by presenting implications for sports practice.

Performing with the left-hand side may well be beneficial in so-called interactive sports in which athletes face each other in duel-like contests (e.g., playing tennis or fencing with the left hand, boxing from a "south-paw" stance). In Chapter 12: Performance Differences Between Left and Right-Sided Athletes in One-on-One Interactive Sports, Florian Loffing and Norbert Hagemann summarize evidence suggesting that "lefties" may have an advantage, and they analyze possible explanations for how or why this might occur. Alongside possible neuropsychological predispositions, the authors argue that left-sided athletes seem to benefit particularly from their opponents' lesser familiarity with the game-play behavior of relatively rare left-sided athletes. They give suggestions for additional explanatory approaches, research limitations, and directions for future research while also discussing practical implications.

In Chapter 13: Biomechanical Considerations of Laterality in Sport, Lucy Parrington and Kevin Ball analyze the biomechanical parameters involved in sport movements. They present an overview of the biomechanical differences between the dominant and the nondominant limb for unilateral and bilateral skills. Their overview of the literature on right/left limb kinematics and the underlying mechanisms reveals the advantages of having a technical similarity between the dominant and nondominant limb. Symmetry also seems to be important for repetitive tasks in order to prevent excessive strain and avoid injuries.

In team sports such as soccer and basketball, players are often under time pressure. This means that they may not have enough time available to choose to play a ball with their preferred or dominant foot or hand. Intuitively, we might expect that players therefore need to develop a high level of bilateral competence to become professional and/or to be successful at the professional level. In Chapter 14: Laterality Effects on Performance in Team Sports: Insights From Soccer and Basketball, Tino Stöckel and David P. Carey provide a scientific view on this issue by reviewing evidence on laterality distribution and proficiency. They review the evidence overall and also differentiate by sport-specific tasks (e.g., shooting, passing, and dribbling) in different competitive levels of soccer and basketball. Further, they ask whether bilateral training in these sports may alter athletes' preference and proficiency for sport-specific and everyday tasks. The authors conclude by inferring potential practical implications from the work reviewed and by suggesting research directions to further our theoretical understanding of bilateral competence in motor control.

Last but not least, based on what we have learned from the preceding chapters, we might ask whether it makes any difference to coaches if their athletes are left- or right-dominant (e.g., in tennis, cricket, or soccer) and if so, what coaches may need to consider for designing appropriate training interventions. When learning new skills or improving already acquired skills, coaches often ask their athletes to observe and to imitate a model's actions. Likewise, specific instructions and feedback are used to facilitate the learning of motor and tactical skills. In Chapter 15: Skill Acquisition in Left- and Right-Dominant Athletes: Insights From Elite Coaching, David Whiteside, Tim Buszard, Georgia Giblin, and Machar Reid review evidence of (the effectiveness of) these methods with a focus on practical applications and potential differences in coaching left- and right-dominant athletes.

When all of the chapters are considered together, this book provides a unique and impressive understanding of laterality in sports, what the underlying competing theories are, how they can be tested in the laboratory and in the field, and what scientists and practitioners can do for practice and application. We hope our book encourages readers entering the fascinating world of laterality in sports and related behavioral domains, thereby also stimulating concerted efforts in this area.

References

Bryson, A., Frick, B., & Simmons, R. (2013). The returns to scarce talent: footedness and player remuneration in European soccer. *Journal of Sports Economics, 14*, 606–628.

Dickens, C. (1875). Left-handed people. *All the year round, New Series (No. 336)*, 136–140.

Eastwood, P. (1972). Studies in games playing: laterality in a games context. In H. T. A. Whiting (Ed.), *Readings in sports psychology* (pp. 228–237). London: Lepus.

Harris, L. J. (2010). In fencing, what gives left-handers the edge? Views from the present and the distant past. *Laterality: Asymmetries of Body, Brain and Cognition, 15*, 15–55.

Lundie, R. A. (1896). Left-handedness. Chamber's Journal of popular literature. *Science and Arts, 73*, 9–12.

McManus, I. C. (2002). *Right hand, left hand: The origins of asymmetry in brains, bodies, atoms and culture*. London: Weidenfeld & Nicolson.

Oldfield, R. C. (1971). The assessment and analysis of handedness: the Edinburgh inventory. *Neuropsychologia, 9*, 97–113.

Rogers, L. J., Vallortigara, G., & Andrew, R. J. (2013). *Divided brains: The biology and behaviour of brain asymmetries*. New York, NY: Cambridge University Press.

LATERALITY – AN IMPORTANT AND OFTEN DISREGARDED TOPIC

2

Origins, Development, and Persistence of Laterality in Humans

Charlotte Faurie, Michel Raymond
University of Montpellier, Montpellier, France

Natalie Uomini
Max Planck Institute for the Science of Human History, Jena, Germany

THE COMPLEX MEASUREMENT OF HANDEDNESS

When asked whether they consider themselves right- or left-handed, many people respond according to the hand they use to write. However, consistency tests have revealed that people's responses do not always match their behavior (Annett, 1985). Moreover, there can be significant discrepancies between tasks (Salmaso & Longoni, 1985). This suggests that right- or left-handers are not general categories, but rather are defined as a function of the tasks. When the tasks considered are highly skilled and complex, and the individuals tested are specialized in these tasks, there is a very strong correlation between the different tasks (e.g., Connolly & Bishop, 1992; Marchant & McGrew, 1998). Measures of preference distributions in a population typically display a J-shaped curve, with most people strongly right-preferent, about 10–12% strongly left-preferent, and very few weakly preferent or ambidextrous (Annett, 1985; Corballis, 1997). In contrast, measures of relative proficiency show a normal distribution. Tested with tasks such as moving pegs, filling dots, or tapping, most people perform equally well with both hands and numbers decrease in both directions toward increasing differences between the hands (Corballis, 1997). However, it is shown that hand preference can be accurately predicted on the basis of relative proficiency level (difference in proficiency between the hands), in a theoretical case where hand preference is assessed for five different tasks (Bishop, 1989). Methods for assessing hand preference are varied: they include experimental manipulation tasks (such as reaching for food), which are used with infants and other animals, to self-report questionnaires for adult humans. These usually contain questions about habits like opening a bottle, sweeping the floor, picking up a coin, or holding a tennis racket. One commonly used questionnaire is the Edinburgh Handedness Inventory (Oldfield, 1971), where subjects rate their handedness preference for 10 activities.

Comparison studies can confirm the association between hand skill and hand preference. The Edinburgh Handedness Inventory was compared to a new computerized method of assessing handedness based on motor performance for drawing on a tablet (Henkel et al., 2001). This method distinguished between left-handers who had been forced to become right-handed in childhood and those who had not switched hands (Henkel et al., 2001).

Lattice analysis of responses to questionnaires (Doyen, Duquenne, Nuques, & Carlier, 2001) reveals that handedness is multidimensional, and that left-handers have more distinct patterns of handedness, while right-handers are globally more homogeneous in their reported behavior.

Questionnaires can be criticized because of their element of subjectivity. Moreover, they have mostly been standardized on North American or British populations, often on undergraduate students. For this reason, questionnaires lack cross-cultural applicability: since activities like holding a tennis racket, opening a beer can, or tooth brushing are not common to all cultures, the questionnaires that currently exist cannot be used to study the universality of human handedness. To study variations in hand preference in humans, it is important to choose typical tasks among human populations from different cultures. The measure of hand proficiency differences is not a relevant alternative, as handedness does not show the same patterns when assessed by preference or performance. Moreover, the tasks chosen to measure should be logically related to the hypothesis tested.

Although it seems that neither motor performance nor personal preference can give an accurate measure of overall "handedness," many different studies have converged on very similar figures and distributions of handedness. Frequencies of between 80% and 90% right-handers have been reported for the large Anglo-Saxon populations that have been assessed with questionnaires. Ellis, Ellis, and Marshall (1988) found 83% of self-reported right-handers in one British town of healthy people using the Edinburgh Handedness Inventory, and a population of Swedish university students was found to be consistently right-handed at 90% and left-handed at 9% for seven unimanual activities (Levander & Schalling, 1988).

Although the methods described above have mostly been applied to Western populations, other assessment techniques provide information about non-Western and past handedness prevalence.

HANDEDNESS IN THE PAST

In order to identify hand preferences in past species and our hominin ancestors, we can examine their fossil skeletons, fossil braincases, and the tools they made and used (Table 2.1). The skeleton can record asymmetrical muscle usage throughout a person's lifetime. This can occur in the form of greater bone density in the arm that is more used, as in professional tennis players today (Ireland et al., 2013). We infer that some prehistoric hominins—*Homo* species and Neanderthals—carried out extremely strenuous asymmetrical activities because their arm bones are up to 10 times more asymmetrical than those of modern professional sports players (Shaw & Stock, 2013; Stock, Shirley, Sarringhaus, Davies, & Shaw, 2013; Trinkaus, Churchill, & Ruff, 1994). However, the precise activity is not yet known. Neanderthals and their ancestors made spears (Wilkins, Schoville, Brown, & Chazan, 2012), presumably for hunting large game, but the body postures involved in that manner of spear use are still unknown. Experimental measures of muscle activity during the simulated task of underhand spear thrusting do not match that indicated by the fossil bone clues, which suggests that spear thrusting as currently proposed was not the cause of the fossil bone asymmetries in Neanderthals. Instead, the muscle activity of hide scraping is a better match (Shaw, Hofmann, Petraglia, Stock, & Gottschall, 2012).

In the endocast (fossil braincase), asymmetries can be measured in the patterns imprinted by the brain onto the inside of the skull (Bruner, De la Cuétara, Masters, Amano, & Ogihara, 2014). The brain asymmetries seen in living humans are also found among the majority of fossil hominins with preserved endocasts (Balzeau, Gilissen, & Grimaud-Hervé, 2012; Balzeau, Holloway, & Grimaud-Hervé, 2012; Holloway, 1981; Holloway & De La Coste-Lareymondie, 1982; Uomini, 2011, 2014). Since chimpanzees also show similar asymmetries, but to a lesser degree, it is likely that a slightly asymmetric brain was already present in the ancestor of chimpanzees and hominins (Balzeau, Gilissen, Holloway, Prima, & Grimaud-Hervé, 2014).

Diagonal cut-marks on teeth are thought to show the hand preference of fossil hominins. The current hypothesis is that these individuals ate strips of dried or cured meat by gripping the meat in the front teeth and cutting off bite-sized pieces near the mouth, similar to some groups of living humans (Semenov, 1964; Uomini, 2008). These cut-marks are found in many fossils of the genus *Homo* and are predominantly right-handed (Bruner & Lozano, 2014; Estalrrich & Rosas, 2013; Frayer et al., 2012;

TABLE 2.1   Summary of Fossil Hominin Data for Laterality

Species	Number of Individuals With Data	Types of Data	Number of Left-Handed Individuals (Percent)	Number of Right-Handed Individuals (Percent)	Sources
Neanderthals	50	Humeri, teeth, endocast	4 (8%)	39 (78%)	Bermúdez de Castro, Bromage, and Jalvo (1988), Bruner, Manzi, and Holloway (2006), Estalrrich and Rosas (2013), Fox and Frayer (1997), Fox and Pérez-Pérez (1994), Frayer et al. (2012), Grimaud-Hervud and de Lumley (1997), Holloway (1981), Holloway and Delacoste-Lareymondie (1982), Koby (1956), LeMay (1976), Trinkaus (1983), Trinkaus et al. (1994), Vandermeersch and Trinkaus (1995), and Volpato, Couture, Macchiarelli, and Vandermeersch (2011, 2012)
Homo heidelbergensis	21	Teeth	0	16 (76%)	Hillson, Parfitt, Bello, Roberts, and Stringer (2010), Lozano et al. (2009), and Pitts and Roberts (1997)
Homo erectus/ergaster	7	Humeri, endocast	1 (14%)	6 (86%)	Begun and Walker (1993), Holloway (1980), Macchiarelli et al. (2014), and Walker and Leakey (1993)
Australopithecus africanus	3	Endocast	0	3 (100%)	Beaudet et al. (2014)

Individuals are excluded from right/left determination if they show pathological asymmetry, mixed signals, or indeterminate data.
Results from Uomini, N. T. (2011). Handedness in Neanderthals. In N. J. Conard & J. Richter (Eds.), Neanderthal lifeways, subsistence and technology (pp. 139–154). Heidelberg: Springer; Uomini, N. T. (2014). Paleoneurology and behaviour. In E. Bruner (Ed.), Human Paleoneurology (pp. 121–144). Springer.

Lozano, Mosquera, de Castro, Arsuaga, & Carbonell, 2009; Uomini, 2011; Volpato et al., 2012).

An up-to-date review of the data for manual asymmetries in the course of human evolution (Table 2.1), from 3 million years ago to the present, suggests a pattern of increasing right-handedness starting from the common ancestor of *Homo sapiens* and Neanderthals (probably *Homo heidelbergensis*). Prior to *H. heidelbergensis*, there are not enough data points to determine species- or population-level handedness. Some individuals of prior species show a hand preference; however, this is expected for a primate that engages in complex skilled manipulations with its hands. Our Neanderthal cousins were 78% right-lateralized. This includes their brain asymmetries, skeletal asymmetries, and dental cut-mark hand preferences. The Neanderthals, who have sufficient data points, show a species-level right-handedness and a minority of left-handers for the first time in our hominin evolutionary tree.

GEOGRAPHICAL VARIATIONS

The cross-cultural comparison of handedness requires that the tasks selected to measure handedness have homologs in all ethnic groups (Raymond & Pontier, 2004). Thus several tasks commonly used in western countries to study handedness, such as writing or tooth brushing, are not eligible here. The handedness of the task should not be the subject of a rigorous social control for conformity, such as sometimes writing or eating (see e.g., Gilbert & Wysocki, 1992; Teng, Lee, Yang, & Chang, 1976). Also, the task should have some useful function, i.e., it could be observed without specific solicitation, in order to keep the interpretation of the results in an ecological meaningful frame. Thus several arbitrarily chosen tasks, such as the peg-moving task (the time taken by each hand to move all items from one slot to another), are not considered here (for a review, see Harris, 1992).

By standard measures of hand preference, lateralization increases with task skillfulness (Healey, Liederman, & Geschwind, 1986; Steenhuis & Bryden, 1989). Studying ethnographic video footage of the daily lives of people in three traditional cultures—the G/wi Bushmen from the Central Kalahari in Botswana, the Himba from northern Namibia, and the Yanomamö from the Orinoco forest in south Venezuela—Marchant, McGrew, and Eibl-Eibesfeldt (1995) found strong right-handedness as expected (individually and at the group level) for using tools, especially where a precision grip was involved, but ambipreference and a random distribution of laterality for other manual actions such as clapping, kicking, poking, and waving at insects. In these cases, the nontool-use hand actions were unlateralized both at the individual and the population level.

This finding directly challenges the accepted notion that humans are strongly lateralized for all activities; rather, there appear to be degrees of hand preference according to the type of task being tested (Annett, 1972; Bishop, 1989; Fagard & Corroyer, 2003; Healey et al., 1986).

As handedness is a specialization of one hand or arm for a particular function, we expect the function not to be easy to perform, in order for the specialization to be useful. Thus handedness is expected to be increased for those functions that are the most rewarding. When the manual activity is pivotal, ambidextrous individuals (i.e., with no hand specialization) are extremely rare—or even absent—as can be seen in surgeons, butchers, farmers, dentists, loggers, carpenters, etc. The same results hold for sport champions (fencers, pitchers, disc throwers, etc.), for the same reasons. Specialization for one hand or arm is then understandable, and the side chosen (right or left) should be randomly assigned. If this trait were neutral, the frequency of right-handers should change in each generation by drift alone, and the frequency of left-handers, at a given time, could take any value. However, in all known societies, left-handers have always been a minority compared to right-handers, suggesting that the neutral model does not adequately describe the evolution of handedness polymorphism. Handedness polymorphism has been found in all human groups studied, with the lowest frequency of left-handers being 3.4% among the Dioula and the highest 22.6% from the Yanomamö (Faurie, Schiefenhövel, Le Bomin, Billiard, & Raymond, 2005; Marchant et al., 1995). One robust result is sex difference, with a higher prevalence of left-handed men than women, across large samples and large number of studies, from many different places (Gilbert & Wysocki, 1992; Papadatou-Pastou, Martin, Munafò, & Jones, 2008). The sex difference suggests that a sex-dependent mechanism is involved (Billiard, Faurie, & Raymond, 2005).

HERITABILITY OF HAND PREFERENCE

The study of handedness in families allows the assessment of the transmission of this trait across generations. Table 2.2 shows a clear familial effect upon handedness: two right-handed parents produce fewer left-handed offspring than parents with any other handedness combination, and two left-handed parents produce the highest proportion of left-handed children, i.e., around 20–30% (see also McKeever, 2000). This suggests that hand preference is partly transmitted by parents to their children, either at a genetic or cultural level (learning, imitation), or both. Published heritability estimates for handedness range from 0.23 to 0.66 (review in Llaurens, Raymond, & Faurie, 2009). In addition, there is a higher prevalence of left-handedness in children of right-handed men and left-handed women (RxL mating) than left-handed men and right-handed women (LxR matings) (Annett, 1973; Ashton, 1982; Spiegler & Yeni-Komshian, 1983).

TABLE 2.2 Frequency of Left-Handers in Families, According to Maternal/Paternal Handedness and the Sex of the Offspring

Parental Handedness		Offspring	
Father	Mother	Sons	Daughters
R	R	10.4% (30,268)	8.5% (26,020)
R	L	22.1% (1815)	21.7% (1688)
L	R	18.2% (2308)	15.3% (2100)
L	L	27.0% (215)	21.4% (168)

Numbers in parentheses indicate sample sizes (total 64,582).
Combined results, adapted from McManus, I. C. (1991). The inheritance of left-handedness. In G. R. Bock &
J. Marsh (Eds.), Biological asymmetry and handedness *(pp. 251–281). Chichester: John Wiley & Sons.*

Such maternal effects could result from a sex-linked genetic effect, or from a greater social influence exerted by the mother on the child. Some sex-specific heritability estimates are presented in Table 2.3. The failure of simple genetic models (Annett, 1985; McKeever, 2000; McManus, 1991) to fit familial data indicates that the genetic determinism of handedness is not simple and may imply several genes or other unidentified factors (Armour, Davison, & McManus, 2014; Medland et al., 2009).

Genome-wide approaches have identified many regions that could possibly be implicated in handedness. Based on meta-analyses of genome-wide association studies, it was estimated that at least 40 loci are involved in determining handedness (McManus, Davison, & Armour, 2013), some of which also contribute to the determination of body left–right asymmetry (Brandler et al., 2013).

The transmission of genes could be distinguished from the transmission of environment by means of adoption studies: handedness of adopted children as a function of parental handedness was essentially random, whereas the handedness of a control group showed a significant correlation with their biological parents (Carter-Saltzman, 1980; Saudino & McManus, 1998). However, there have been few such studies, and the sample sizes are too small to distinguish properly between genetic and environmental components of variance. The study of twins could also clarify the relative contribution of genetic and environmental factors. Monozygotic twin pairs are significantly more likely to be concordant for handedness than dizygotic pairs (Sicotte, Woods, & Mazziotta, 1999) (Table 2.4). These data therefore suggest that there is a genetic contribution to handedness. However, despite identical genotypes, approximately 21.7% of monozygotic twins are discordant for handedness. Even if the genetic and cultural contributions to transmission of hand preference are not fully determined, these results provide convincing evidence for a significant heritability, allowing the action of natural selection on this trait.

TABLE 2.3   Sex-Specific Estimates of Handedness Heritability in Three Studies on UK University Students

Parent	Father						Mother					
	Male			Female			Male			Female		
Sex of Offspring												
Study	1	2	3	1	2	3	1	2	3	1	2	3
h²	17.4	16.8	–	3.5	31.9	–	56.6	42.3	79.2	51.1	58.3	46.5

Hull University (studies 1 and 2) and Open University (study 3). Left-handedness criterion: writing hand (studies 1 and 3) and left-hand preference for any one of 12 items (study 2).
Data from Annett, M. (1973). Handedness in families. Annals of Human Genetics, 37(1), 93–105; Annett, M. (1978). Genetic and nongenetic influences on handedness. Behavior Genetics, 8(3), 227–249.

TABLE 2.4 Number of Different Handedness Combinations in Monozygotic and Same Sex Dizygotic Twins

Handedness	Monozygotic	Dizygotic
R–R	2184	1951
R–L	629	585
L–L	87	53
Observed/expected discordant pairs	90.1%	99.3%

Dizygotic twins do not differ from binomial expectations in their hand preference, whereas monozygotic twins show more concordance than would be expected by chance.
Combined results, adapted from McManus, I. C. (1991). The inheritance of left-handedness. In G. R. Bock & J. Marsh (Eds.), Biological asymmetry and handedness *(pp. 251–281). Chichester: John Wiley & Sons.*

ENVIRONMENTAL FACTORS

Developmental Influence

There are several developmental factors implicated in handedness in humans. The existence of associations between left-handedness and various health problems has often led to a distinction being made between *pathological left-handedness*, which would arise from developmental stresses, and *familial left-handedness*, which would be due to genotype (Harris & Carlson, 1988). This hypothesis considered that some people are left-handed because they have suffered different types of pathology. The explanation of Satz, Orsini, Saslow, and Henry (1985) for the increased (often twofold) frequency of left-handers in clinical populations with central nervous system disorders (e.g., schizophrenia, epilepsy, mental retardation, or learning disabilities) was based on the claim that early brain insult may cause the individual to switch to the opposite hand for unimanual activities. Thereby, markers of any stressor or pathological factor disrupting normal development and inducing a switch in hand preference, regardless of mechanism, would be expected to show itself in higher percentages of left-handedness (Coren & Halpern, 1991). Several possible perinatal stressors have been proposed (e.g., premature birth, prolonged labor, Rhesus incompatibility, breech delivery, multiple birth, respiratory distress syndrome, primiparity, maternal age, low birth weight), although empirical data are inconclusive (see Llaurens et al., 2009 for a review), with the possible exception of ultrasound during pregnancy (Salvesen, 2011). Lateralized behaviors seem to be expressed in the early developmental stage (from 9–10 weeks) and are related with hand preference at a later age (10–12 years): handedness could thus be influenced by the in utero environment, although, according to Hepper (2013, p. 588), "the initial developmental emergence of lateralized behavior is under genetic control and is a fundamental feature of prenatal human development".

Cultural Influence

Cultural and environmental factors could change hand preference in three ways, which correspond to different degrees and types of pressure. (1) The first is by changing the hand used for some activities, with no change for other unimanual activities. This is frequent for the writing or eating hand, two tasks under cultural influence in several countries (Berdel-Martin & Barbosa-Freitas, 2002; De Agostini, Khamis, Ahui, & Dellatolas, 1997; Dellatolas et al., 1988; Salmaso & Longoni, 1985; Shimizu & Endo, 1983). For example, in school children in China and Taiwan, there are only 3.5% and 0.7% left-handed writers, respectively (Teng et al., 1976), in contrast with a 6.5% figure for Asian school children living in the United States, where cultural pressures have been reduced (Hardyck, Petrinovich, & Goldmann, 1976). (2) The second is by reducing the degree of hand preference, when weak pressure applies to all hand actions. Bryden, Ardila, and Ardila (1993) observed that positive reinforcement for right-hand use can modify patterns of handedness and alter the relations among different handedness tasks. (3) The third is by changing the overall preferred hand, when strong pressure applies to all hand actions. For example, Bryden et al. (1993) suggest that the Tucano of Amazonia successfully modify preference at an early age through positive reinforcement, and this switched preference is manifested in all unimanual activities.

EVOLUTIONARY FORCES ACTING ON THE POLYMORPHISM OF HANDEDNESS

The persistence of a polymorphism in all populations of a species is a rare case. If the trait is neutral, the polymorphism is eventually lost by genetic drift, at least in some populations. Directional selection, if acting alone, would lead to the fixation of the advantageous morph and eliminate the polymorphism as well. The ancient and ubiquitous polymorphism observed for handedness in human populations therefore suggests that handedness is not a neutral trait, and that some balancing selective forces are acting on it.

Left-Handedness as a Costly Trait

Whether or not left-handers display a reduced longevity has been a matter of a large debate (Llaurens et al., 2009), which is not yet settled. Two types of survival costs may explain a possible reduced longevity of left-handers: prenatal and perinatal birth stressors and brain damage, more probable in left-handers (as discussed earlier), and left-handers may have more lethal accidents (Aggleton, Kentridge, & Neave, 1993; Daniel & Yeo, 1994; Halpern & Coren, 1991). However, these negative selection pressures have not been directly quantified yet.

There is evidence for an excess of left-handedness among extremely low birth weight babies (O'Callaghan et al., 1987; Powls, Botting, Cooke, & Marlow, 1996). Low birth weight could play a key role in the health problems associated with left-handedness, particularly heart diseases (Yüksel, Arslan, & Dane, 2014). There is also some evidence that left-handedness is more common in a variety of disorders that presumably reflect developmental abnormality. These include autism (Dane & Balci, 2007), stuttering (Dellatolas, Annesi, Jallon, Chavance, & Lellouch, 1990), dyslexia (Leonard & Eckert, 2008), and schizophrenia (Dragovic & Hammond, 2005; Sommer, Ramsey, Kahn, Aleman, & Bouma, 2001). Moreover, left-handed children have been repeatedly found to have lower cognitive scores (reviewed in Faurie, Goldberg, Hercberg, Zins, & Raymond, 2008; see Johnston, Nicholls, Shah, & Shields, 2013 with a large sample size).

Another cost for left-handers resides in the lower body weight and size observed for left-handers (Coren, 1989; Fudin, Renninger, & Hirshon, 1994). This could have fitness consequences, as body size is an important component of selective value in humans (Guégan, Teriokhin, & Thomas, 2000; Mueller & Mazur, 2001; Nettle, 2002; Pawlowski, Dunbar, & Lipowicz, 2000; Silventoinen, Kaprio, Lahelma, Viken, & Rose, 2003). Some potential fitness costs are thus suggested by the literature, but a proper assessment of their actual evolutionary significance is still needed.

Left-Handedness as a Beneficial Trait

There is some evidence that left-handers could have greater inter-manual coordination (Gorynia & Egenter, 2000; Judge & Stirling, 2003). Left-handers have indeed smaller asymmetries in hand skills than right-handers (Curt, Maccario, & Dellatolas, 1992; Judge & Stirling, 2003; Peters & Servos, 1989) and are less lateralized in language dominance (Steinmetz, Volkmann, Jäncke, & Freund, 1991). Some studies point to better inter-hemispheric transfer in nonright-handers (Christman & Propper, 2001; Gorynia & Egenter, 2000). A larger *corpus callosum* has been detected in left-handers (Witelson, 1985), but the precise implications for interhemispheric interaction are unclear.

Creativity has also been reported to be linked with left-handedness (Newland, 1981), more specifically in men (Coren, 1995). A few studies have suggested that left-handers could have special talents such as enhanced musical (Aggleton, Kentridge, & Good, 1994; Kopiez, Galley,

& Lee, 2006) or mathematical capacities (Casey, Pezaris, & Nuttall, 1992; Crow, Crow, Done, & Leask, 1998). There is growing evidence, based on various large samples, that left-handers have, on average, a higher socioeconomic status (Denny & O'Sullivan, 2007; Faurie et al., 2008; Faurie, Llaurens, Hegay, & Raymond, 2012; Ruebeck, Harrington, & Moffitt, 2007). Such socioeconomic differences are likely to positively influence reproductive success (e.g., Cronk, 1991; Nettle & Pollet, 2008; Skjærvø, Bongard, Viken, Stokke, & Røskaft, 2011).

Frequency-Dependent Benefits

There are only a few possibilities to explain the maintenance of a polymorphism over a long time frame. Negative frequency dependence has been proposed as a possible mechanism acting on the polymorphism of handedness, according to the fighting hypothesis (Raymond, Pontier, Dufour, & Møller, 1996). In short, the relative rarity of left-handers compared to right-handers results in left-handers being unfamiliar to right-handers. This unfamiliarity provides two types of advantages for left-handers: they naturally perform actions that are unexpected, and whose outcomes are more difficult to predict. When the frequency of left-handers increases, they become more familiar to right-handers, and their advantage in fights decreases. Such negative frequency-dependent advantage for an inheritable trait is a sufficient condition to maintain a stable polymorphism. As the expected equilibrium value is 50%, well above the observed value, another type of selection must exist, such as an intrinsic cost associated with being a left-hander (as discussed earlier).

Many studies have been published to assess the relevance of the fighting hypothesis using sports data. The first prediction is a higher frequency of left-handers in interactive sports (where individuals are interacting, thus reflecting some fighting abilities), compared to noninteractive sports (Grouios, Tsorbatzoudis, Alexandris, & Barkoukis, 2000; Raymond et al., 1996). The second prediction is that left-hander frequencies are limited by the 50% threshold, above which right-handers have an advantage because they start to become uncommon. Overall, there is very strong support for these two predictions from various research teams, and for many interactive sports (Brooks, Bussière, Jennions, & Hunt, 2004; Goldstein & Young, 1996; Loffing & Hagemann, 2012; Loffing, Hagemann, & Strauss, 2012). Additionally, consistent with the fighting hypothesis, several experiments with videos have shown that it is more difficult to predict the outcome of an action performed by a left-hander than by a right-hander, and this difference is attenuated, or even reversed, by specific training (Hagemann, 2009; Loffing, Schorer, Hagemann, & Baker, 2012; Schorer, Loffing, Hagemann, & Baker, 2012). Sports data have their own limitations as a test of the fighting hypothesis, for example, when arbitrary conventions constrain the ritualized fight outside the ecological field of real fights (e.g., for some types of fencing, see Raymond et al., 1996) or when extensive training at the highest competition levels, including specific training against left-handers, necessarily decreases any frequency-dependent effect (e.g., Dochtermann, Gienger, & Zappettini, 2014).

In traditional societies, the level of violence is positively related to the frequency of left-handers (Faurie & Raymond, 2005), as predicted by theoretical models (Billiard et al., 2005), thus consistent with the frequency-dependence hypothesis. Additional data are needed, mostly from violent societies which are now dramatically disappearing. It is possible that the current massive westernization of the few remaining traditional societies, along with the expansion of the market economy, could change the ancestral relationships between fitness and fighting abilities and decrease or suppress any frequency-dependent advantage of left-handers (Faurie & Raymond, 2013). Data from modern societies are useless (except in situations where ability in sports influences mating success), as the level and type of violence has dramatically changed over the last two centuries (predominant use of long-range and powerful weapons, which probably do not offer a particular advantage to left-handers). The fighting hypothesis explaining the persistence of left-handers applies only to situations where fighting abilities are directly linked to success (as in sports) or to Darwinian fitness, as in most past societies or in the few remaining groups not yet affected by Western colonization and a market economy. How the handedness polymorphism will evolve under the new modern conditions remains an interesting issue.

CONCLUSION

For most manual tasks, especially those tasks involved in competitive activities, increasing performance by the specialization of one hand is certainly adaptive. For example, lateralized cats are faster at catching a virtual prey on a screen with one paw, compared to cats that have not specialized one of their paws (Fabre-Thorpe, Fagot, & Vauclair, 1991). In humans, hand or arm lateralization, whatever the side, is probably an adaptation for many activities, such as tool making and tool use (MacNeilage, Studdert-Kennedy, & Lindblom, 1987; Uomini, 2009) or stone throwing (Calvin, 1982, 1993; but see McCall & Whittaker, 2007). In fights, being lateralized certainly is an advantage. For example, many weapons are held with only one hand. Increasing the power, speed, and maneuverability of a particular arm or hand by specializing it is certainly pivotal. It is thus likely that hand specialization was largely selected for during the acquisition of complex tools or weapons, i.e., during the Paleolithic era. The higher prevalence of right-handedness might well be due to a previously existing cerebral bias (Corballis, 2003) or, in others words, to the cost associated with left-handedness. One of the observed costs is the smaller size and weight of left-handers (Coren, 1989; Fudin et al., 1994). Size is a component of the reproductive value, at least in males (Mueller & Mazur, 2001; Pawlowski et al., 2000). However, smaller size and weight are probably not a disadvantage in weapon fights. This is indicated by the fact that weapon fighting sports, such as fencing, do not have weight categories for competitions, as opposed to hand fighting sports, such as boxing. Generally, all sports using an object mediating an interaction between two opponents, such as a racket, sword, or ball, do not have weight categories, as opposed to all other interactive sports without such objects. This suggests that when weapons became prevalent among hominins, the weight (and or probably height) disadvantage of left-handers in fights was considerably reduced. In addition, a frequency-dependent advantage favors left-handers in interactive sports. The persistence of the polymorphism of handedness might well be partly explained by an advantage of left-handers in weapon manipulation and fights. This polymorphism, as well as handedness itself, needs to be understood in the view of adaptation and natural selection.

References

Aggleton, J. P., Kentridge, R. W., & Good, J. M. M. (1994). Handedness and musical ability: a study of professional orchestral players, composers, and choir members. *Psychology of Music, 22*(2), 148–156.

Aggleton, J. P., Kentridge, R. W., & Neave, N. J. (1993). Evidence for longevity differences between left handed and right handed men: an archival study of cricketers. *Journal of Epidemiology and Community Health, 47*(3), 206–209. http://www.ncbi.nlm.nih.gov/pmc/articles/PMC1059767/.

Annett, M. (1972). The distribution of manual asymmetry. *British Journal of Psychology, 63*(3), 343–358.

Annett, M. (1973). Handedness in families. *Annals of Human Genetics, 37*(1), 93–105.

Annett, M. (1978). Genetic and nongenetic influences on handedness. *Behavior Genetics, 8*(3), 227–249.

Annett, M. (1985). *Left, right, hand and brain: The right shift theory.* London, UK: LEA Publishers.

Armour, J. A., Davison, A., & McManus, I. C. (2014). Genome-wide association study of handedness excludes simple genetic models, *Heredity, 112*(3), 221–225.

Ashton, G. (1982). Handedness: an alternative hypothesis. *Behavior Genetics, 12*(2), 125–147.

Balzeau, A., Gilissen, E., & Grimaud-Hervé, D. (2012). Shared pattern of endocranial shape asymmetries among great apes, anatomically modern humans, and fossil hominins. *PLoS One, 7*(1), e29581.

Balzeau, A., Gilissen, E., Holloway, R. L., Prima, S., & Grimaud-Hervé, D. (2014). Variations in size, shape and asymmetries of the third frontal convolution in hominids: paleoneurological implications for hominin evolution and the origin of language. *Journal of Human Evolution, 76*(0), 116–128.

Balzeau, A., Holloway, R. L., & Grimaud-Hervé, D. (2012). Variations and asymmetries in regional brain surface in the genus *Homo. Journal of Human Evolution, 62*(6), 696–706.

Beaudet, A., Dumoncel, J., Thackeray, F., Durrleman, S., Subsol, G., Jessel, J.-P., … Braga, J. (2014). Identification of *Homo*-like features in virtually rendered South African Australopith endocasts. In *Poster presented at the African human fossil record conference, Toulouse, France, September 26–27, 2014.*

Begun, D. R., & Walker, A. C. (1993). The endocast. In A. C. Walker, & R. E. Leakey (Eds.), *The nariokotome Homo erectus skeleton* (pp. 326–358). Cambridge, MA: Harvard University Press.

Berdel-Martin, W. L., & Barbosa-Freitas, M. (2002). Mean mortality among Brazilian left- and right-handers: modification or selective elimination? *Laterality: Asymmetries of Body, Brain and Cognition, 7*(1), 31–44.

Bermúdez de Castro, J. M., Bromage, T. G., & Jalvo, Y. F. (1988). Buccal striations on fossil human anterior teeth: evidence of handedness in the middle and early Upper Pleistocene. *Journal of Human Evolution, 17*(4), 403–412.

Billiard, S., Faurie, C., & Raymond, M. (2005). Maintenance of handedness polymorphism in humans: a frequency-dependent selection model. *Journal of Theoretical Biology, 235*, 85–93.

Bishop, D. V. M. (1989). Does hand proficiency determine hand preference? *British Journal of Psychology, 80*(2), 191–199.

Brandler, W. M., Morris, A. P., Evans, D. M., Scerri, T. S., Kemp, J. P., Timpson, N. J., ... Paracchini, S. (2013). Common variants in Left/Right asymmetry genes and pathways are associated with relative hand skill. *PLoS Genetics, 9*(9), e1003751.

Brooks, R., Bussière, L. F., Jennions, M. D., & Hunt, J. (2004). Sinister strategies succeed at the cricket world cup. *Proceedings of the Royal Society B: Biological Sciences, 271*(Suppl. 3), S64–S66. http://www.jstor.org/stable/4142559.

Bruner, E., De la Cuétara, J. M., Masters, M., Amano, H., & Ogihara, N. (2014). Functional craniology and brain evolution: from paleontology to biomedicine. *Frontiers in Neuroanatomy, 8*.

Bruner, E., & Lozano, M. (2014). Extended mind and visuo-spatial integration: three hands for the Neandertal lineage. *Journal of Anthropological Sciences, 92*, 273–280.

Bruner, E., Manzi, G., & Holloway, R. (2006). Krapina and Saccopastore: endocranial morphology in the pre-Würmian Europeans. *Periodicum Biologorum, 108*(4), 433–441.

Bryden, M. P., Ardila, A., & Ardila, O. (1993). Handedness in native Amazonians. *Neuropsychologia, 31*, 301–308.

Calvin, W. H. (1982). Did throwing stones shape hominid brain evolution? *Ethology & Sociobiology, 3*(3), 115–124.

Calvin, W. H. (1993). The unitary hypothesis: a common neural circuitry for novel manipulations, language, plan-ahead, and throwing? In K. R. Gibson, & T. Ingold (Eds.), *Tools, language, and cognition in human evolution* (pp. 230–250). Cambridge, UK: Cambridge University Press. http://cogprints.org/3212/index.html.

Carter-Saltzman, L. (1980). Biological and sociocultural effects on handedness: comparison between biological and adoptive families. *Science, 209*(4462), 1263–1265.

Casey, M. B., Pezaris, E., & Nuttall, R. L. (1992). Spatial ability as a predictor of math achievement: the importance of sex and handedness patterns. *Neuropsychologia, 30*(1), 35–45.

Christman, S. D., & Propper, R. E. (2001). Superior episodic memory is associated with interhemispheric processing. *Neuropsychology, 15*(4), 607–616.

Connolly, K. J., & Bishop, D. V. M. (1992). The measurement of handedness: a cross-cultural comparison of samples from England and Papua New Guinea. *Neuropsychologia, 30*(1), 13–26.

Corballis, M. C. (1997). The genetics and evolution of handedness. *Psychological Review, 104*(4), 714–727.

Corballis, M. C. (2003). From mouth to hand: gesture, speech, and the evolution of right-handedness. *Behavioral & Brain Sciences, 26*(2), 199–260.

Coren, S. (1989). Southpaws—somewhat scrawnier. *JAMA: Journal of the American Medical Association, 262*(19), 2682–2683.

Coren, S. (1995). Differences in divergent thinking as a function of handedness and sex. *The American Journal of Psychology, 108*(3), 311–325.

Coren, S., & Halpern, D. F. (1991). Left-handedness: a marker for decreased survival fitness. *Psychological Bulletin, 109*, 90–106.

Cronk, L. (1991). Wealth, status, and reproductive success among the Mukogodo of Kenya. *American Anthropologist, 93*(2), 345–360.

Crow, T. J., Crow, L. R., Done, D. J., & Leask, S. (1998). Relative hand skill predicts academic ability: global deficits at the point of hemispheric indecision. *Neuropsychologia, 36*(12), 1275–1282.

Curt, F., Maccario, J., & Dellatolas, G. (1992). Distributions of hand preference and hand skill asymmetry in preschool children: theoretical implications. *Neuropsychologia, 30*(1), 27–34.

Dane, S., & Balci, N. (2007). Handedness, eyedness and nasal cycle in children with autism. *International Journal of Developmental Neuroscience, 25*(4), 223–226.

Daniel, W. F., & Yeo, R. A. (1994). Accident proneness and handedness. *Biological Psychiatry, 35*, 499.

De Agostini, M., Khamis, A. H., Ahui, A. M., & Dellatolas, G. (1997). Environmental influences in hand preference: an African point of view. *Brain and Cognition, 35*(2), 151–167.

Dellatolas, G., Annesi, I., Jallon, P., Chavance, M., & Lellouch, J. (1990). An epidemiological reconsideration of the Geschwind–Galaburda theory of cerebral lateralization. *Archives of Neurology, 47*(7), 778–782.

Dellatolas, G., De Agostini, M., Jallon, P., Poncet, M., Rey, M., & Lellouch, J. (1988). Mesure de la préférence manuelle par autoquestionnaire dans la population française adulte. *Revue de Psychologie Appliquée, 38*, 117–136.

Denny, K., & O'Sullivan, V. (2007). The economic consequences of being left-handed – some sinister results. *Journal of Human Resources, 42*, 353–374. http://www.jstor.org/stable/40057309.

Dochtermann, N. A., Gienger, C. M., & Zappettini, S. (2014). Born to win? Maybe, but perhaps only against inferior competition. *Animal Behaviour, 96*(0), e1–e3.

Doyen, A.-L., Duquenne, V., Nuques, S., & Carlier, M. (2001). What can be learned from a lattice analysis of a laterality questionnaire? *Behavior Genetics, 31*(2), 193–207.

Dragovic, M., & Hammond, G. (2005). Handedness in schizophrenia: a quantitative review of evidence. *Acta Psychiatrica Scandinavica, 111*(6), 410–419.

Ellis, S. J., Ellis, P. J., & Marshall, E. (1988). Hand preference in a Normal population. *Cortex, 24*(1), 157–163.

Estalrrich, A., & Rosas, A. (2013). Handedness in *Neandertals* from the El Sidrón (Asturias, Spain): evidence from instrumental striations with ontogenetic inferences. *PLoS One, 8*(5), e62797.

Fabre-Thorpe, M., Fagot, J., & Vauclair, J. (1991). Latéralisation chez le chat dans une tâche de pointage du membre antérieur en direction d'une cible mobile. *Comptes Rendus de l'Académie de Sciences de Paris, 313*(9), 427–433.

Fagard, J., & Corroyer, D. (2003). Using a continuous index of laterality to determine how laterality is related to interhemispheric transfer and bimanual coordination in children. *Developmental Psychobiology, 43*(1), 44–56.

Faurie, C., Goldberg, M., Hercberg, S., Zins, M., & Raymond, M. (2008). Socio-economic status and handedness in two large cohorts of French adults. *British Journal of Psychology, 99*, 533–554.

Faurie, C., Llaurens, V., Hegay, T., & Raymond, M. (2012). Handedness and socioeconomic status in an urban population in Uzbekistan. *Evolution and Human Behavior, 33*(1), 35–41.

Faurie, C., & Raymond, M. (2005). Handedness, homicide and negative frequency-dependent selection. *Proceedings of the Royal Society B: Biological Sciences, 272*(1558), 25–28.

Faurie, C., & Raymond, M. (2013). The fighting hypothesis as an evolutionary explanation for the handedness polymorphism in humans: where are we? *Annals of the New York Academy of Sciences, 1288*(1), 110–113.

Faurie, C., Schiefenhövel, W., Le Bomin, S., Billiard, S., & Raymond, M. (2005). Variation in the frequency of left-handedness in traditional societies. *Current Anthropology, 46*(1), 142–147.

Fox, C. L., & Frayer, D. W. (1997). Non-dietary marks in the anterior dentition of the Krapina Neanderthals. *International Journal of Osteoarchaeology, 7*(2), 133–149.

Fox, C. L., & Pérez-Pérez, A. (1994). Cutmarks and post-mortem striations in fossil human teeth. *Human Evolution, 9*(2), 165–172.

Frayer, D. W., Lozano, M., Bermúdez de Castro, J. M., Carbonell, E., Arsuaga, J. L., Radovčić, J., ... Bondioli, L. (2012). More than 500,000 years of right-handedness in Europe. *Laterality: Asymmetries of Body, Brain and Cognition, 17*(1), 51–69.

Fudin, R., Renninger, L., & Hirshon, J. (1994). Analysis of data from Reichler's (1979) The Baseball Encyclopedia: right-handed pitchers are taller and heavier than left-handed pitchers. *Perceptual and Motor Skills, 78*(3), 1043–1048.

Gilbert, A. N., & Wysocki, C. J. (1992). Hand preference and age in the United States. *Neuropsychologia, 30*(7), 601–608.

Goldstein, S. R., & Young, C. A. (1996). "Evolutionary" stable strategy of handedness in major league baseball. *Journal of Comparative Psychology, 110*(2), 164–169.

Gorynia, I., & Egenter, D. (2000). Intermanual coordination in relation to handedness, familial sinistrality and lateral preferences. *Cortex, 36*(1), 1–18.

Grimaud-Hervé, D., & de Lumley, M.-A. (1997). *L'évolution de l'enchéphale chez Homo erectus et Homo sapiens*. Paris: CNRS Editions.

Grouios, G., Tsorbatzoudis, H., Alexandris, K., & Barkoukis, V. (2000). Do left-handed competitors have an innate superiority in sports? *Perceptual and Motor Skills, 90*(3c), 1273–1282.

Guégan, J. F., Teriokhin, A. T., & Thomas, F. (2000). Human fertility variation, size-related obstetrical performance and the evolution of sexual stature dimorphism. *Proceedings of the Royal Society B: Biological Sciences, 267*(1461), 2529–2535.

Hagemann, N. (2009). The advantage of being left-handed in interactive sports. *Attention, Perception, & Psychophysics, 71*(7), 1641–1648.

Halpern, D. F., & Coren, S. (1991). Handedness and life span. *New England Journal of Medicine, 324*(14), 998.

Hardyck, C., Petrinovich, L. F., & Goldman, R. D. (1976). Left-handedness and cognitive deficit. *Cortex, 12*(3), 266–279.

Harris, L. J. (1992). Left-handedness. In I. Rapin, & S. J. Segalowitz (Eds.), *Handbook of neuropsychology* (pp. 145–208). Amsterdam: Elsevier.

Harris, L. J., & Carlson, D. F. (1988). Pathological left-handedness: an analysis of theories and evidence. In D. L. Molfese, & S. J. Segalowitz (Eds.), *Brain lateralization in children: Developmental implications* (pp. 289–372). New York, NY: Guilford Press.

Healey, J. M., Liederman, J., & Geschwind, N. (1986). Handedness is not a unidimensional trait. *Cortex, 22*(1), 33–53.

Henkel, V., Mergl, R., Juckel, G., Rujescu, D., Mavrogiorgou, P., Giegling, I., ... Hegerl, U. (2001). Assessment of handedness using a digitizing tablet: a new method. *Neuropsychologia, 39*(11), 1158–1166.

Hepper, P. G. (2013). The developmental origins of laterality: fetal handedness. *Developmental Psychobiology, 55*(6), 588–595.

Hillson, S. W., Parfitt, S. A., Bello, S. M., Roberts, M. B., & Stringer, C. B. (2010). Two hominin incisor teeth from the middle Pleistocene site of Boxgrove, Sussex, England. *Journal of Human Evolution, 59*(5), 493–503.

Holloway, R. L. (1980). The O.H. 7 (Olduvai Gorge, Tanzania) hominid partial brain endocast revisited. *American Journal of Physical Anthropology, 53*(2), 267–274.

Holloway, R. L. (1981). Volumetric and asymmetry determinations on recent hominid endocasts: spy I and II, Djebel Ihroud I, and the salé *Homo erectus* specimens, with some notes on Neandertal brain size. *American Journal of Physical Anthropology, 55*(3), 385–393.

Holloway, R. L., & De La Coste-Lareymondie, M. C. (1982). Brain endocast asymmetry in pongids and hominids: some preliminary findings on the paleontology of cerebral dominance. *American Journal of Physical Anthropology, 58*(1), 101–110.

Ireland, A., Maden-Wilkinson, T., McPhee, J., Cooke, K., Narici, M., Degens, H., & Rittweger, J. (2013). Upper limb muscle-bone asymmetries and bone adaptation in elite youth tennis players. *Medicine and Science in Sports and Exercise, 45*(9), 1749–1758.

Johnston, D. W., Nicholls, M. E. R., Shah, M., & Shields, M. A. (2013). Handedness, health and cognitive development: evidence from children in the National Longitudinal Survey of Youth. *Journal of the Royal Statistical Society: Series A (Statistics in Society)*, 176(4), 841–860.

Judge, J., & Stirling, J. (2003). Fine motor skill performance in left- and right-handers: evidence of an advantage for left-handers. *Laterality: Asymmetries of Body, Brain and Cognition*, 8(4), 297–306.

Koby, F.-E. (1956). Une incisive néandertalienne trouvée en Suisse. *Verhandlungen der Naturforschenden Gesellschaft Basel*, 67, 1–15.

Kopiez, R., Galley, N., & Lee, J. I. (2006). The advantage of a decreasing right-hand superiority: the influence of laterality on a selected musical skill (sight reading achievement). *Neuropsychologia*, 44(7), 1079–1087.

LeMay, M. (1976). Morphological cerebral asymmetries of modern man, fossil man, and nonhuman primates. *Annals of the New York Academy of Sciences*, 280, 349–366.

Leonard, C. M., & Eckert, M. A. (2008). Asymmetry and dyslexia. *Developmental Neuropsychology*, 33(6), 663–681.

Levander, M., & Schalling, D. (1988). Hand preference in a population of Swedish college students. *Cortex*, 24(1), 149–156.

Llaurens, V., Raymond, M., & Faurie, C. (2009). Why are some people left-handed? An evolutionary perspective. *Philosophical Transactions of the Royal Society B: Biological Sciences*, 364(1519), 881–894.

Loffing, F., & Hagemann, N. (2012). Side bias in human performance: a review on the left-handers' advantage in sports. In T. Dutta, M. K. Mandal, & S. Kumar (Eds.), *Bias in human behaviour* (pp. 163–182). Hauppage, NY: Nova Science.

Loffing, F., Hagemann, N., & Strauss, B. (2012). Left-handedness in professional and amateur tennis. *PLoS One*, 7(11), e49325.

Loffing, F., Schorer, J., Hagemann, N., & Baker, J. (2012). On the advantage of being left-handed in volleyball: further evidence of the specificity of skilled visual perception. *Attention, Perception, & Psychophysics*, 74(2), 446–453.

Lozano, M., Mosquera, M., de Castro, J. M. B., Arsuaga, J. L., & Carbonell, E. (2009). Right handedness of *Homo heidelbergensis* from sima de los huesos (Atapuerca, Spain) 500,000 years ago. *Evolution and Human Behavior*, 30(5), 369–376.

Macchiarelli, R., Bondioli, L., Bruner, E., Candilio, F., Coppa, A., Dean, M. C., ... Zanolli, C. (2014). The 1 Ma old human assemblage from the *Homo* site at Uadi Aalad, Buia (Danakil depression of Eritrea): an updated record. In *Poster presented at the African human fossil record conference, Toulouse, France, September 26–27*.

MacNeilage, P. F., Studdert-Kennedy, M. G., & Lindblom, B. (1987). Primate handedness reconsidered. *Behavioral & Brain Sciences*, 10(2), 247–303.

Marchant, L. F., & McGrew, W. C. (1998). Human handedness: an ethological perspective. *Human Evolution*, 13(3–4), 221–228.

Marchant, L. F., McGrew, W. C., & Eibl-Eibesfeldt, I. (1995). Is human handedness universal? Ethological analyses from three traditional cultures. *Ethology*, 101(3), 239–258.

McCall, G. S., & Whittaker, J. (2007). Handaxes still don't fly. *Lithic Technology*, 32, 195–202.

McKeever, W. F. (2000). A new family handedness sample with findings consistent with X-linked transmission. *British Journal of Psychology*, 91(1), 21–39.

McManus, I. C. (1991). The inheritance of left-handedness. In G. R. Bock, & J. Marsh (Eds.), *Biological asymmetry and handedness* (pp. 251–281). Chichester: John Wiley & Sons.

McManus, I. C., Davison, A., & Armour, J. A. L. (2013). Multilocus genetic models of handedness closely resemble single-locus models in explaining family data and are compatible with genome-wide association studies. *Annals of the New York Academy of Sciences*, 1288, 48–58.

Medland, S. E., Duffy, D. L., Wright, M. J., Geffen, G. M., Hay, D. A., Levy, F., ... Boomsma, D. I. (2009). Genetic influences on handedness: data from 25,732 Australian and Dutch twin families. *Neuropsychologia*, 47(2), 330–337.

Mueller, U., & Mazur, A. (2001). Evidence of unconstrained directional selection for male tallness. *Behavioral Ecology and Sociobiology*, *50*(4), 302–311.

Nettle, D. (2002). Height and reproductive success in a cohort of British men. *Human Nature*, *13*(4), 473–491.

Nettle, D., & Pollet, T. V. (2008). Natural selection on male wealth in humans. *The American Naturalist*, *172*(5), 658–666.

Newland, G. A. (1981). Differences between left- and right-handers on a measure of creativity. *Perceptual and Motor Skills*, *53*(3), 787–792.

O'Callaghan, M. J., Tudehope, D. I., Dugdale, A. E., Mohay, H., Burns, Y., & Cook, F. (1987). Handedness in children with birthweights below 1000 g. *The Lancet*, *329*(8542), 1155.

Oldfield, R. C. (1971). The assessment and analysis of handedness: the Edinburgh inventory. *Neuropsychologia*, *9*(1), 97–113.

Papadatou-Pastou, M., Martin, M., Munafò, M. R., & Jones, G. V. (2008). Sex differences in left-handedness: a meta-analysis of 144 studies. *Psychological Bulletin*, *134*(5), 677–699.

Pawlowski, B., Dunbar, R. I. M., & Lipowicz, A. (2000). Evolutionary fitness: tall men have more reproductive success. *Nature*, *403*(6766), 156.

Peters, M., & Servos, P. (1989). Performance of subgroups of left-handers and right-handers. *Canadian Journal of Psychology/Revue Canadienne de Psychologie*, *43*(3), 341–358.

Pitts, M., & Roberts, M. B. (1997). *Fairweather Eden: Life in Britain half a million years ago as revealed by the excavations at boxgrove*. London: Century.

Powls, A., Botting, N., Cooke, R. W. I., & Marlow, N. (1996). Handedness in very-low-birthweight (VLBW) children at 12 years of age: relation to perinatal and outcome variables. *Developmental Medicine & Child Neurology*, *38*(7), 594–602.

Raymond, M., & Pontier, D. (2004). Is there geographical variation in human handedness? *Laterality: Asymmetries of Body, Brain and Cognition*, *9*(1), 35–51.

Raymond, M., Pontier, D., Dufour, A.-B., & Møller, A. P. (1996). Frequency-dependent maintenance of left handedness in humans. *Proceedings of the Royal Society of London B: Biological Sciences*, *263*(1377), 1627–1633.

Ruebeck, C. S., Harrington, J. E., & Moffitt, R. (2007). Handedness and earnings. *Laterality: Asymmetries of Body, Brain and Cognition*, *12*(2), 101–120.

Salmaso, D., & Longoni, A. M. (1985). Problems in the assessment of hand preference. *Cortex*, *21*(4), 533–549.

Salvesen, K. Å. (2011). Ultrasound in pregnancy and non-right handedness: meta-analysis of randomized trials. *Ultrasound in Obstetrics & Gynecology*, *38*(3), 267–271.

Satz, P., Orsini, D. L., Saslow, E., & Henry, R. (1985). The pathological left-handedness syndrome. *Brain and Cognition*, *4*(1), 27–46.

Saudino, K., & McManus, I. C. (1998). Handedness, footedness, eyedness and earedness in the Colorado adoption project. *British Journal of Developmental Psychology*, *16*(2), 167–174.

Schorer, J., Loffing, F., Hagemann, N., & Baker, J. (2012). Human handedness in interactive situations: negative perceptual frequency effects can be reversed!. *Journal of Sports Sciences*, *30*(5), 507–513.

Semenov, S. A. (1964). *Prehistoric technology* (M. W. Thompson, Trans.). London: Cory, Adams & Mackay.

Shaw, C. N., Hofmann, C. L., Petraglia, M. D., Stock, J. T., & Gottschall, J. S. (2012). Neandertal humeri may reflect adaptation to scraping tasks, but not spear thrusting. *PLoS One*, *7*(7), e40349.

Shaw, C. N., & Stock, J. T. (2013). Extreme mobility in the late Pleistocene? Comparing limb biomechanics among fossil *Homo*, varsity athletes and Holocene foragers. *Journal of Human Evolution*, *64*(4), 242–249.

Shimizu, A., & Endo, M. (1983). Handedness and familial sinistrality in a Japanese student population. *Cortex*, *19*(2), 265–272.

Sicotte, N. L., Woods, R. P., & Mazziotta, J. C. (1999). Handedness in twins: a meta-analysis. *Laterality: Asymmetries of Body, Brain and Cognition*, *4*(3), 265–286.

Silventoinen, K., Kaprio, J., Lahelma, E., Viken, R. J., & Rose, R. J. (2003). Assortative mating by body height and BMI: Finnish twins and their spouses. *American Journal of Human Biology, 15*(5), 620–627.

Skjærvø, G. R., Bongard, T., Viken, Å., Stokke, B. G., & Røskaft, E. (2011). Wealth, status, and fitness: a historical study of Norwegians in variable environments. *Evolution and Human Behavior, 32*(5), 305–314.

Sommer, I., Ramsey, N., Kahn, R., Aleman, A., & Bouma, A. (2001). Handedness, language lateralisation and anatomical asymmetry in schizophrenia. *The British Journal of Psychiatry, 178*(4), 344–351.

Spiegler, B. J., & Yeni-Komshian, G. H. (1983). Incidence of left-handed writing in a college population with reference to family patterns of hand preference. *Neuropsychologia, 21*(6), 651–659.

Steenhuis, R. E., & Bryden, M. P. (1989). Different dimensions of hand preference that relate to skilled and unskilled activities. *Cortex, 25*(2), 289–304.

Steinmetz, H., Volkmann, J., Jäncke, L., & Freund, H.-J. (1991). Anatomical left-right asymmetry of language-related temporal cortex is different in left- and right-handers. *Annals of Neurology, 29*(3), 315–319.

Stock, J. T., Shirley, M. K., Sarringhaus, L. A., Davies, T. G., & Shaw, C. N. (2013). Skeletal evidence for variable patterns of handedness in chimpanzees, human hunter–gatherers, and recent British populations. *Annals of the New York Academy of Sciences, 1288*(1), 86–99.

Teng, E. L., Lee, P.-H., Yang, K.-S., & Chang, P. C. (1976). Handedness in a Chinese population: biological, social, and pathological factors. *Science, 193*(4258), 1148–1150.

Trinkaus, E. (1983). *The Shanidar Neandertals*. New York: Academic Press.

Trinkaus, E., Churchill, S. E., & Ruff, C. B. (1994). Postcranial robusticity in *Homo*. II: Humeral bilateral asymmetry and bone plasticity. *American Journal of Physical Anthropology, 93*(1), 1–34.

Uomini, N. T. (2008). In the knapper's hands: identifying handedness from lithic production and use. In L. Longo, & N. Skakun (Eds.). *"Prehistoric technology" 40 years later: Functional studies and the Russian legacy: Vol. 1783*. (pp. 51–62). Oxford: B.A.R. International Series.

Uomini, N. T. (2009). The prehistory of handedness: archaeological data and comparative ethology. *Journal of Human Evolution, 57*(4), 411–419.

Uomini, N. T. (2011). Handedness in Neanderthals. In N. J. Conard, & J. Richter (Eds.), *Neanderthal lifeways, subsistence and technology* (pp. 139–154). Heidelberg: Springer.

Uomini, N. T. (2014). Paleoneurology and behaviour. In E. Bruner (Ed.), *Human paleoneurology* (pp. 121–144). Springer.

Vandermeersch, B., & Trinkaus, E. (1995). The postcranial remains of the Régourdou 1 Neandertal: the shoulder and arm remains. *Journal of Human Evolution, 28*(5), 439–476.

Volpato, V., Couture, C., Macchiarelli, R., & Vandermeersch, B. (2011). Endostructural characterization of the Regourdou 1 Neandertal proximal arm: bilateral asymmetry and handedness. In S. Condemi, & G. Weniger (Eds.), *Continuity and discontinuity in the peopling of Europe: One hundred fifty years of Neanderthal study* (pp. 175–178). New York: Springer.

Volpato, V., Macchiarelli, R., Guatelli-Steinberg, D., Fiore, I., Bondioli, L., & Frayer, D. W. (2012). Hand to mouth in a Neandertal: right-handedness in Régourdou 1. *PLoS One, 7*(8), e43949.

Walker, A. C., & Leakey, R. E. (1993). The postcranial bones. In A. C. Walker, & R. E. Leakey (Eds.), *The nariokotome Homo erectus skeleton* (pp. 95–160). Berlin: Springer.

Wilkins, J., Schoville, B. J., Brown, K. S., & Chazan, M. (2012). Evidence for early hafted hunting technology. *Science, 338*(6109), 942–946.

Witelson, S. F. (1985). The brain connection: the corpus callosum is larger in left-handers. *Science, 229*(4714), 665–668.

Yüksel, R., Arslan, M., & Dane, Ş. (2014). Heart rate variability differs between right- and left-handed individuals. *Perceptual and Motor Skills, 118*(3), 890–896.

3

In Fencing, Are Left-Handers Trouble for Right-Handers? What Fencing Masters Said in the Past and What Scientists Say Today

Lauren Julius Harris

Michigan State University, East Lansing, MI, United States

INTRODUCTION

Gammy, scrammy, wack-handed, cack-handed, bawky, garpawed, and cow-pawed—just a few of the names the Scots and English have coined for left-handers. They don't sound nice, and they aren't. For example, "gammy" means clumsy, unable to function normally as from an injury; "wack" means crazy or eccentric, from being whacked too many times on the head; and "cack" is excrement, so "cack-handed" is, well, we get the idea. To be fair, two other more common left-hand names come from somewhere else: the French "gauche," which doubles for boorish or rude, and "sinister" from the Latin for left-hand side and coming to mean evil, unfavorable, and presaging trouble. There's also "awkward," from Old Norse, originally meaning "toward the left," or the "wrong way."

These names reflect centuries of animus against left-handers stemming from religion, prejudice against minorities, sanitary practices restricting the left hand to "unclean" acts, and the belief that left-handers lacked certain virtues and skills. Their reputed clumsiness inspired the psychologist Cyril Burt (1937, p. 287) to say:

> They squint, they stammer, they shuffle and shamble, they flounder about like seals out of water…they are fumblers and bunglers at whatever they do.

How remarkable, then, that in sports, where "grace," not "gammy," reigns, these "fumblers and bunglers" haven't just survived but thrived. Numbers alone tell the story. Ten to twelve percent of all adults are left-handed (Gilbert & Wysocki, 1992), but in major-league baseball it's about eighteen percent (e.g., Neft & Cohen, 1988). In baseball, they're called "southpaws" (*paw* in the sense of hand), a term now widely used for left-handers in general.[1] The figure is even higher for pitchers alone, 39% according to one report (Stewart, 2014). Left-handers are also over-represented in cricket (e.g., Brooks, Bussière, Jennions, & Hunt, 2004; Caesar, 2009; Edwards & Beaton, 1996), tennis (Holtzen, 2000), table tennis (Raymond, Pontier, Dufour, & Moller, 1996), and mixed martial arts (Baker & Schorer, 2013). In baseball, they also hit for more power (Grondin, Guiard, Ivry, & Koren, 1999) and in baseball and cricket for a higher average (Brooks et al., 2004; GitHub, 2014). And they bring wins. In cricket, left-handers accounted for nearly half of all batsmen on the most successful teams in the 2003 World Cup (Brooks et al., 2004; see also Robinson, 2012); in tennis, they were two to five times more common among top-ranked professionals from 1968 to 1999 (Holtzen, 2000); and among baseball pitchers surveyed from 1984 to 1989, they won more, lost less, and gave up fewer runs per game (Shaughnessy, 1989, p. 52). Left-handers also win more in wrestling (Ziyagil, Gursoy, Dane, & Yuksel, 2010) and boxing (Gursoy, 2009). In numbers, however, boxers may be a special case. Studies of current or recent cohorts show an overrepresentation of left-handers (Grouios, Tsorbatzoudis, Alexandris, & Barkoukis, 2000; Gursoy, 2009), whereas a study over a longer time span found, in early cohorts, an underrepresentation (Loffing & Hagemann, 2015). Where they agree is in finding more wins by left-handers for all time periods. The authors of the latter study suggest that, given left-handers' dangerous reputation, their early underrepresentation could reflect their difficulty getting bouts at a time when schedules were controlled by trainers and managers intent on protecting their right-handed fighters from defeats, while their more recent overrepresentation follows the waning of these practices and of prejudice against left-handers generally.

In baseball, scientists began examining left-handers' records in the 1950s (Lehman & Webb, 1951), but coaches and managers were already paying

---

[1]The term usually is said to come from the practice of arranging the baseball diamond with the batter facing east to avoid the afternoon sun and with the pitcher facing west; that way a left-hander's pitching arm would be toward the south (e.g., Southpaw, 2014). According to most accounts, the term was coined in the 1880s, but *The Oxford English Dictionary* (Southpaw, 2011) lists several earlier citations, the first in 1813, long before baseball existed in its modern form, and another in 1848 in the context of brawling, or fist-fighting. Perhaps its first use in baseball was in 1858 in a story in the *New York Atlas*: "Hallock, a 'south paw,' let fly a good ball into the right field."

attention, by one account (Uhrbrock, 1970, p. 285) starting in the 1920s when Babe Ruth, the New York Yankee slugger, ruled the roost. Ruth did more than blast towering home runs; before joining the Yankees, he was a stellar left-handed pitcher for the Boston Red Sox. By the 1880s, however, left-handers' numbers were already rising, presumably as their success was becoming known (James, 1988, pp. 112–123; see also Goldstein & Young, 1996). In cricket, they also were noticed early. For example, Charles Wordsworth (1891, p. 10), a classical scholar, teacher, and cricketer (and nephew of the poet), recalled a match in 1822 between his school Harrow and Eton (he was 16 at the time):

> ...my left-hand bowling (I batted right-handed) proved so successful, and was regarded by our opponents as so formidable, that in the following year, knowing that I was to be against them again, they endeavored to find a professional who could bowl left-handed, to give them the practice which they considered necessary to prevent their being defeated a second time.

Sports writers were taking notice as well. In 1835, a list of notable cricketers in *Fores's Sporting Notes and Sketches* included one Alfred J. Lowth, "left-handed" and the "best gentleman bowler in England" (p. 62).

Wordsworth bowled left but batted right. Had he batted left, he would have been a double threat, for as R.A. Lundie (1891, p. 9) remarked in an essay on handedness, published coincidentally the same year as Wordsworth's account:

> Any one who has watched a cricket-match...knows what trouble [a left-handed batsman] causes to his opponents; how the fielders have to change either their position or their functions every time he faces the bowler.

Cricket has two bases in the middle of the field, 66 feet apart, with all running between the two. For the left-handed batsman, Lundie supposed that the advantage comes from adjustments required by bowler and fielders alike, adjustments made harder, as both he and Wordsworth implied, by right-handers being less accustomed to competing against left-handers.

In baseball, with four bases in the shape of a diamond and run counterclockwise, the advantage for the left-handed batter is widely assumed to come from being closer to first base, or as someone remarked, "The southpaw has a start of six feet..." (Anon, quoted in Selzer, 1933, p. 77), implying that for ground balls, he can beat more throws to first. The problem, as Walsh (2007) pointed out, is that left-handers hit more grounders to the right side, which should nullify the benefits of being closer to first, since the ball will be fielded more often by the second baseman, who has a shorter throw to first than the shortstop or third baseman (direct outs to the first baseman contribute negligibly). If the left-hander's proximity advantage is further offset by the right-hander's advantage in hitting more *left*-side grounders, then there must be other reasons for the left-hander's higher batting average. At least one comes from facing right-handed pitchers. Outside pitches generally being harder to hit, the right-hander's curves and sliders don't break away (as they would for a right-handed batter), and even with the common practice of bringing in left-handers just to pitch to left-handers, left-handed batters still face many more right- than left-handed pitchers. It's why, for pitchers, as a reporter said about Major League Baseball's annual 50 round draft, "teams devote great amounts of time, energy, and stress into making sure they don't miss their share" [of left-handers] (Antonen, 2005).

For the sports listed here, there could be a variety of reasons for the southpaw advantage beyond the right-hander's being less accustomed to competing against them—the consensus is that this is true for all sports— but whatever the other reasons may be (some possibilities will be considered later), one thing is abundantly clear: in sports, left-handers can hardly be called *physically* clumsy or unbalanced. At least in baseball, however, that hasn't stopped questions about their *mental*, or *psychological*, balance. As a character said about "hooligans" in John Huston's (1950) film, *The Asphalt Jungle*, "They're like left-handed pitchers, they all have a screw loose." Or as a *New York Times* reporter said of Ruth after a game he pitched and won for the Red Sox against the Yankees (he scattered five hits and hit a home run), "All lefthanders are peculiar and Babe is no exception, because he can also bat" (Anonymous, 1915). More recently, John Hart, general manager of the Texas Rangers, put it this way: "Left-handers are different packages…[they] come at you in strange ways" (quoted in Antonen, 2005). In cricket, was Lundie (1896, p. 9) hinting at this in saying, "how odd [the left-hander] appears at the wrong, that is, the unusual, side of the wicket"?[2]

HANDEDNESS IN FENCING

The left-hander's record in baseball and other sports is undeniably impressive. It is no less so for fencing, the martial art of fighting with blades. For example, in a sample of 73 highly-skilled Greek fencers, 38% were left-handed (Groulos et al., 2000); in the 1981 World Championship, the figure for participants in the foil competition was 35%, with numbers

[2]In an illuminating essay on left and right in classical Greece and Italy, Michael Peters (1997, p. 6) noted that the term "left" has long been used in association with mind and to denote madness. For example, in Sophocles' *Ajax*, when Ajax goes mad and slaughters the cattle, mistaking them for his enemies, where the usual English translation of the chorus' lines reads, "Never were you in your right mind" as when you "fell upon the flocks," the original Greek reads "…when you went so far to the left."

rising for those advancing in the competition (Azémar, Ripoll, Simonet, & Stein, 1983); and in a survey of tournament champions, from 1979 to 1993, it was an astounding 44.5% (Azémar & Stein, 1994; cited in Raymond et al., 1996, Table 3), with left-handers taking the top eight places in the 1979 Pan American Games and the 1980 Olympics (Hécaen, 1984). It was the same with the 1996 Olympics included (Azémar, 2003, Table XI, p. 100). For épée, from the opening round to the round of 32 to the round of 8 to the medalist round of 4 to the championship round, the figures were 25.8%, 30.2%, 44.4%, 47.2%, and 66.7%, respectively. Worth special mention is Edoardo Mangiarotti (1919–2012), a right-hander who, after his father taught him to fence left-handed "to confuse opponents," went on to win 26 medals in the Olympic and World Championships, including 13 gold (Martin, 2012).

What Fencing Masters Have Long Known

Just as players and managers have long known about the left-hander's advantage in baseball, fencing masters have long known the same for fencing. They noted it in their instructional books and manuals and explained it the way most scientists do today. This essay presents examples from these works.

> A Man that cannot *Fence* will be more careful to keep out of Bullies and Gamesters Company, and will not be half so apt to stand upon Punctilio's [nice details of conduct], not to give Affronts…

So said John Locke in 1693 in *Some Thoughts Concerning Education*. He added that because "Fencing and Riding the great Horse" are "so generally looked upon as necessary Qualifications in the breeding of a Gentleman, it will be hard wholly to deny any one of that rank these Marks of Distinction" (p. 254, parag. 199). To achieve them for fencing (as for riding), young men sought instruction from former soldiers and other masters of arms. The more famous taught at schools and academies. One of the best known is depicted in Thomas Rowlandson's watercolor, "I shall conquer this," reproduced (in black and white for print versions of this book) in Fig. 3.1. It is Henry Angelo's Fencing Academy in London, established in 1755 by his illustrious father, the Italian-born Domenico, who after studying with fencing masters in Pisa and Paris and becoming a *maîtres d'armes*, came to London in 1750 and took the lead in changing fencing into a sport from its origins in military training. There, father and son taught generations of wealthy young. The lunging figure in the center of the scene is believed to be Henry himself. His opponent is unidentified but, if a student, is clearly no longer young. While they fence, Domenico, now headmaster, stands to the right, holding three foils in his arms, ready,

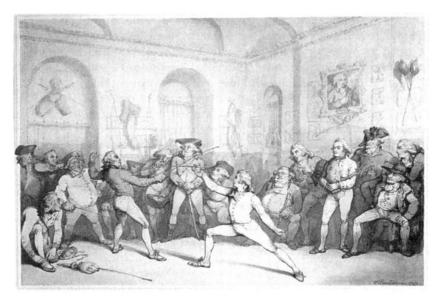

FIGURE 3.1 "I shall conquer this"; watercolor by Thomas Rowlandson (1787) of Henry Angelo's Fencing Academy in London.

as the British historian J.D. Aylward (1953, p. 149) supposed, to supply the combatants if a blade is broken. In 1787, when Rowlandson drew the scene, the academy had long been a gathering place for aristocrats as well as celebrities, including famed swordsmen who gave exhibitions there. One was the multitalented Joseph Bologne, Chevalier de Saint-Georges, a champion fencer as well as violinist, composer, and conductor (Czajkowski, 2005; Georgian Index, 2014). His portrait, by Mather Brown, is on the wall above Domenico. Among the spectators are said to be the Marquis of Buckingham and Dennis O'Kelly, owner of Eclipse, winner of the English Derby (see Aylward, 1953, p. 148).[3] To the left, on the wall between the two alcoves, there is an object resembling a hand and arm. According to Wolf (2001, 2002), it probably is a padded sleeve and glove for practice with "singlesticks," or wooden rods. On the floor to the left, there is another, now just a hand. Note that both are for the right hand.

Over the period I surveyed, a vast number of fencing manuals were produced. The antiquarian and Olympic fencer Egerton Castle (1885) estimated more than 400 from the fifteenth to the nineteenth century. I was fortunate that dozens of the most notable, along with newer works, were in the Michigan State University Library, gifts from Professor

[3]Judging from the ages of the spectators, including Henry's opponent, the occasion was not a regular class for "young scholars." The youngest would appear to be Henry himself (he was 31 at the time).

Charles Schmitter to mark his 45th and final year as fencing coach at Michigan State (Fiore, 1983). Now called the Charles and Ruth Schmitter Fencing Collection, its greatest of many jewels is Domenico Angelo's own manual, *L'École des Armes*, a large folio in the original French, published in 1763. Along with instructions for holding the weapon and for positioning the body and limbs, it features 47 richly-colored drawings illustrating positions and techniques, some showing Domenico himself, often with his friend, patron, and student Henry Herbert, the 10th Earl of Pembroke, as his opponent. Herbert perhaps also was Henry Angelo's opponent in the scene drawn by Rowlandson (in 1787, he would have been 51 years old).

The manuals are largely similar in format. Most start with accounts of the benefits of fencing and, as John Locke did, with explanations of its social rules. The Scottish master Sir William Hope (1707) was emphatic: "All Cursing and Swearing, and obscene Language, should be discharged [i.e., eliminated]" because a fencing school, "being a Place to which Persons of the best Quality do frequently resort, for their Exercise and Divertisement, all such Ungentlemanly, as well as Immoral Habits ought to be discountanced…" (p. 190). Along with written instructions, many manuals, like Angelo's, included illustrative drawings. Fig. 3.2 shows a drawing from a manual published in 1734, Monsieur L'Abbat's *The Art of Fencing*.[4]

Most manuals focused on a single weapon—the foil (or fleuret), épée, saber, rapier, small and back swords, and, for one manual, the Scotch broad sword. Only the first three are still used in competitive fencing.[5] Some manuals also included the dagger, a companion weapon used mainly to help parry the opponent's thrusts and held in the other hand, or *off-hand*, left for right-handers, right for left-handers. Held in the left, as the Italian master Giovanni de Grassi (1570) explained, it should protect the left side from the knee up,

---

[4]In London in 1787, Henry Angelo prepared an English-language version of his father's manual but reduced it "in size and price" to "render it of more general use" (p. vii). It was this version that he would have provided for his students (those of his father's students sufficiently skilled in French presumably used the original French version). Some of the English-language passages I have quoted are from the section in the translated edition under the heading, "Observations on left handed fencers" (pp. 80–81; originally "Observations sur le jeu de gaucher").

[5]The foil is a blunt weapon, resembling a small sword in the main, with a button at the point (originally developed in the mid-17th century as a training weapon for the court sword, a light one-handed sword designed almost wholly for thrusting); the épée is the heaviest (nearly the weight of an actual court sword) and has a sharp-pointed blade without a cutting edge, and a bowl-shaped guard for the hand; the saber has a curved guard and triangular blade and is used either as a cutting weapon or for both cutting and thrusting (descriptions from separate entries in *Webster's New International Dictionary of the English Language, Second Edition*, Unabridged (1957), and from Fencing (2014).

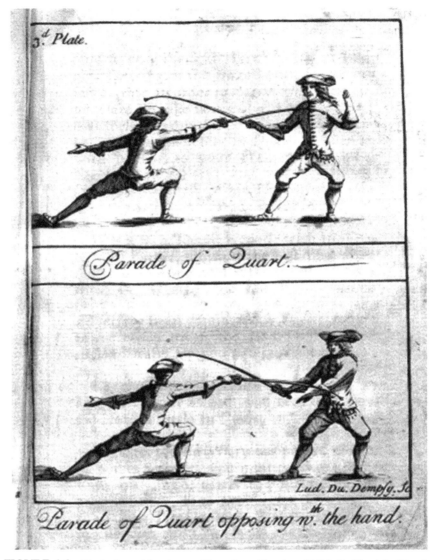

FIGURE 3.2 Illustration of fencing positions from Monsieur L'Abbat's *The Art of Fencing* (1734). *Reproduced with permission of Division of Special Collections, Michigan State University Library.*

while the sword beats off strikes to the right side and to the left below the knee (as described by Leonid Tarassuk, 1978; fn. 17, p. 41). As sword fighting evolved into the modern sport of fencing, with the introduction of lighter primary weapons such as the épée and foil, the use of daggers gradually fell out of favor because the new lighter weapons allowed for greater speed and

A. LATERALITY – AN IMPORTANT AND OFTEN DISREGARDED TOPIC

a stance that presented a smaller target (Anonymous, 2014). Where daggers were described, it therefore was primarily in the older manuals.

Hand Training: Right For All

The stranger greets thy hand with proffered left?/Accept not, 'tis of loyalty bereft./ Left-handed friends are underhanded foes./ True openness a swordless right hand shows.

Harvey. *Sheep in Wolves Clothing* (quoted in Burt, 1937, p. 314).

For most of recorded history, the right has been the favored hand, chosen for important public acts. The hand shake is among the most prominent. In the usual story of its origins, as told in the verse quoted above, an open right hand shows that the profferer intends no harm, since the right was the hand that held the sword. It also was the hand used for eating: as the author, said to be Plutarch (1533), remarked: "[We] do accustome our chyldren to take meate with the ryght hand, & if they do put forthe the lefte hande, we anone [at once] correct them" (trans. by T. Elyot, Chapter 4, p. 16; for other examples, see Harris, 2003). It was even the hand for gesturing. The author of a 19th century treatise on elocution declared: the right being the "hand of action," "principal gestures are to be made with the right arm" (Putnam, 1856, p. 48). As an earlier authority delicately explained, the left "communicates a great Awkwardness to the whole Deportment and Air; and though one does not see to what it is owing, yet it is strangely distasteful" (Hill, 1754, pp. 98–99).

Most especially, the right was the hand for writing, a practice increasingly required of all children with the expansion of formal schooling and literacy. With a drawing for guidance, Francis Clement's (1587) *The Petie Schole* showed how it should be done: "hold the pen in your right hande with your thombe, forefinger, & midfinger in this manner" (p. 55).

Certain objects, including eating utensils, presented no physical barriers to the left hand, so only custom determined hand use. Other objects were designed for the right, with their numbers increasing, as McManus (2009) noted, with the Industrial Revolution and the mass production of machines and tools: sewing machines, lathes, winches, vises, and the like. As someone said at the time, "many workmen's tools are fashioned in direct submission (so to speak) to right-handedness" (Anonymous, 1875, p. 136). As for writing, the left-handed child could follow custom and use the right or stay with the left and suffer the consequences: an ink-stained hand from being dragged through drying ink, a desk with inkwell on the right, and beatings from teachers like the one who, as one student recalled, would "walk about the school with a short stick" and "hit [me] on the knuckles when [I] had [my] pen in the left hand" (as told to Jackson, 1880, p. 637). Some teachers even bound the hand to prevent its use (Smith, 1903). Left-handers' reputed clumsiness may owe something to their problems writing with the right and using right-handed tools and implements. Some could not adjust and kept using their left, but most managed, more or less, so that at least by the mid-19th century, fewer than 5% of adults were estimated to write with the left hand. Among baseball players, in the first half of the twentieth century, we can suppose that this group included most left-handers, judging from those who can be seen in photographs using the right hand to sign contracts or autographs. Along with Ruth and Cobb, they include Ted Williams, the last 0.400 hitter (0.406 in 1941), and Vernon ("Lefty") Gomez, the Yankee pitcher. Some early scientists, however, among them Paul Broca (1865) and William Ogle (1871), recognized that left-handers, especially those with strong left-hand tendencies, still used their left for what Broca called untrained, "spontaneously-performed" acts (p. 382), such as lifting and carrying weights, throwing a ball or stone, striking with the fists, and waving a stick.

An Exception for Fencing

There is no reason to think that fencing masters endorsed right-hand customs less strictly than other teachers, so for them, to borrow John Locke's phrase, using the right for such acts as writing and eating presumably were no less "necessary Qualifications in the breeding of a Gentleman" than learning to fence and ride. For writing and eating, students of fence therefore should have been as right-handed as students anywhere. Fencing was different because students evidently were allowed to use their preferred hand, right or left, just as they would have done as children waving sticks and wooden swords. Like play swords, real swords were symmetric except for the hand guard for épée and sabre, which could be designed for either hand. There also were gauntlets, or protective gloves, for the sword hand, along with scabbards, which left-handers wore on the right, right-handers on the left, so that, as the Italian master Angelo Viggiani (1575) explained, both could draw sword with the preferred hand. Some daggers also had a protective cross guard, which, like the guard for the sword, could be designed for either hand (Tarassuk, 1978, p. 41). Evidently, the only dispensation not granted to left-handers was the *name* for the dagger. Because right-handers held it in the left hand, it came to be called *la main gauche*. (Did left-handers, if only to themselves or with other left-handers, ever call it *la main droite*?)

What Fencing Masters and Others Said About the Left-Hander's Advantage

...The Kers were aye the deadliest faes [foes]/That e'er to Englishmen were known/

For they were all bred left handed men,/And fence against them there was none...

As I said, the left-hander's advantage in fencing has long been known. Today, perhaps the most familiar, or perhaps only known, historical examples are the Kers, or Kerrs, 16th century Scottish reivers, or raiders, in the continuing battle with the English over the disputed lands bordering their countries. The lines quoted earlier are from *The Raid of the Kers*, a ballad composed by Scottish poet James Hogg in 1830. A later stanza reads:

> When darkness wrapt the band around, the Kers harass'd their foemen sore,/
> Their left hand blows could not be borne; /Death spread behind, and dread before...

In 1900, another Scottish poet, Walter Laidlaw, paid them tribute in *The Reprisal*:

> The Castle, razed from tower to floor/Was built and garrisoned once more;/
> The Scots and French, led on by Kerr, Courageous and well-trained to war,...;/
> So well the Kerrs their left-hands ply/The dead and dying round them lie,/
> The castle gained, the battle won,/Revenge and slaughter are begun...

The castle "built and garrisoned once more" was Ferniehirst, seat of the Kerr clan, in Roxburgh County, and *The Reprisal* recalled how, after its siege and capture by the English in 1523, it was retaken by the Scots, with help from the French, in 1549. In the Scottish Borderland, the Kerrs were even said to have inspired left-handed sobriquets—*ker-handed, car-handed,* and *corry-handed* (Fraser, 1971, p. 51)—all derived from "cair" or "carr," for "left" (Jamieson, 2011; Vol. 1, p. 189), and, like those listed previously, all unpleasant in their secondary meanings; for example, to "ker or carry" signifies "awkward, devious, and in a moral sense is applied in the same way as *sinister* in English" (Wilson, 1872, p. 211).[6]

The Kerrs were not mentioned in the books I examined, not even those from Scotland and England. The fencing masters instead offered their own impressions of left-handed fencers or repeated what they said was generally known or believed. Possibly the first such account, however, did appear in the 16th century, contemporaneously with the Kerrs' exploits, but in Italy, not Scotland or England. The author was Acamillo Palladini, in his *Discorso sopra l'arte della scherma* [*Discourse on the art of fencing*], c.1560. I was unable

---

[6]An important detail about the story of the Kerrs' left-handedness, as told in James Hogg's poem, has been questioned. According to Anthony Kerr (1985, Chapter 4), a family descendent, only the patriarch Andrew Kerr was bred (i.e., born) left-handed and, upon discovering its advantage for fencing, taught his sons and armed men-servants to wield the sword with the left hand (in accord with custom, men-servants took the family name on joining the household). That would square with studies suggesting that left-handedness is not more common in persons with the surname Kerr or Carr (for review, see McManus, 2002, pp. 302–303).

to see this manual myself, but according to fencing master and historian William Gaugler (2014), Palladini observed that "many believe that a left-hander has an advantage over a right-hander" (p. 8).

Gaugler did not say whether Palladini named the believers. Whoever they were, more followed, among them many fencing masters themselves. Along with Domenico Angelo (1763), a partial list includes, in England, Joseph Swetnam (1617), John Godfrey (1747), J. Olivier (1771), Thomas Mathewson (1805), Joseph Roland (1809), and Richard Burton (1911); in Scotland, George Roland (1824); in France, Monsieur Valdin [Salomon Negri] (1729), Monsieur L'Abbat (1734), Guillaume Danet (1766), La Boëssière fils (1818), Gomard [A.J.J. Possellier] (1845), Cordelois (1862), and Walter Pollock, F.C. Grove, and Camille Prevost (1890); in Italy, Florio Blasco (1844) and Rosaroll Scorza and Pietro Grisetto (1871/1803); and in the United States, the French-trained Louis Rondelle (1892). All in their own ways expressed the same view. For example, Danet (1766) noted the left-hander's reputation for being dangerous (p. 219); Joseph Roland (1809) declared that the left-hander "will have the advantage of the right-handed" even with half the training (p. 162); Gomard [A.J.J. Possellier] (1845) called it a "grand advantage" (p. 284); Godfrey (1747) said, "I would rather contend with the right-handed Man with more Judgment, than [the left-hander] with less" (p. 17); Domenico Angelo (1763) described a right-hander greatly embarrassed [*fort embarassé*] fighting a left-hander (p. xxib); and Henry Angelo, in Volume 2 of his *Reminiscences* (1830, pp. 343–346), described a match in 1785 between two eminent swordsmen, the celebrated LeBrun, a left-hander, and Lapière, who had his own academy in Picadilly and reputed to be an "excellent master" and "superior antagonist." The result was an overwhelming victory for LeBrun and a defeat for Lapière so humiliating and distressing that, a few days later, he committed suicide.[7]

---

[7]Amberger (2011), who also recounts this story, added that Henry Angelo, an excellent fencer in his time, expressed his high regard for left-handers in a more personal way: that "after finding himself hard pressed by the lefty at his own club [the wording suggests that there was just one], he avoids a public match with the superior opponent, which could have damaged his reputation in case of a dramatic loss." Amberger did not name his source or identify the left-hander, and the story isn't mentioned, as far as I can tell, in Angelo's *Reminiscences*. Aylward (1953) intimates that the left-hander may have been none other than LeBrun: that Henry "sought every opportunity of measuring his skill against that of any master or amateur who presented himself" at his *salle*, for "he held it essential for a *maître d'armes* to keep in constant training, especially with strangers whose play was unknown to him." Among the visitors was LeBrun, who, according to Aylward (p. 149), was among the spectators in Rowlandson's drawing (Fig. 3.1) and who was a "most formidable opponent, particularly as he proved to have the advantage of being a left-handed fencer." Indeed, Henry went so far "as to hint that the Frenchman was one too many even for him!" (p. 150).

To this list of those believing in the left-hander's advantage, we can add Alexandre Dumas (père), whose many literary works celebrated the fencer's life. The favorite has always been *The Three Musketeers* [*Les Trois Mousquetaires*], first published in French in 1844 and later in English and other languages. In its best-known scene, the youth d'Artagnan, while chasing a thief, collides with the musketeer Athos, further injuring Athos' already wounded shoulder (his right, as we later learn) and offers him satisfaction in a duel. Athos agrees and announces:

> but I'll use my left hand, as is my habit in such circumstances. Don't think I'm doing you a kindness; I draw just as well with both hands; and there will even be a disadvantage for you: a left-handed man is very troublesome for people who are not forewarned [*un gaucher est très gênant pour les gens qui ne sont pas prévenus*]
> Dumas (2006/1844), Chapter 5, p. 52; translation by Richard Pevear.

That Athos, using his left, would indeed be "very troublesome" for the right-handed d'Artagnan,[8] we never learn because their duel was interrupted by the arrival of Cardinal Richelieu's guards. But how did Dumas know of the advantage? Dumas was a trained fencer and could have been repeating what was generally known or what he learned from personal experience. He also could have heard this from someone not yet mentioned, his own teacher Augustin Grisier, Fencing Master at L'École Royale Polytechnique, Paris. In his manual, *Les Armes et Le Duel* (1847), in a section called *Des Gauchers* [Left-handers], Grisier said the advantage had "always been known" (p. 262). Dumas wrote the manual's *Préface Anecdotique* and mentioned Grisier very respectfully in his memoirs and in two other swashbuckling novels, *The Count of Monte Cristo* and *The Corsican Brothers*.

Two Skeptics

So far, I have found just two persons skeptical of the common view about left-handed fencers. Only one was a fencing master: Vincentio Saviolo, who came to England from Padua in 1590 and was among the premier swordsmen of the Elizabethan age. His two-part work, *Vincentio Saviolo His Practice with the Rapier and Dagger*, published in 1595, consists of a dialogue between the author and his young student, Luke. In the last chapter of Book 1, "Entreating how a lefte handed man, shall plaie with

---

[8]We know, from context, that d'Artagnan was right-handed, even though he is never identified as such. He also is depicted as right-handed in Gustave Doré's monument to Alexandre Dumas, in the Place Malesherbes, Paris. On the back side, facing out, he is shown seated, his scabbard on his left hip and his sword resting near his right hand (Doré, 1880–1883).

one that is right handed," Luke reports knowing "many of opinion, that the left handed have a great advantage of the right," and yet:

> I see both doe their uttermost this morning, without any hurt of either partie, and in beholding both the one and the other diligently I could not discerne anie jot of advantage betweene them.

He therefore asks Saviolo whether left-handers had any advantage over right-handers, or right-handers over left-handers, and to teach him how to defend himself "from such a one, and how to offend him" (p. 1). Saviolo replies:

> Of this question, I have heard many times much reasoning, and many there are indeede which so think, but beleeve me, the left hand hath no advantage of the right hand, nor the right, of the lefte… (p. 1).

The other skeptic was neither a fencing master nor even a fencer. He was Alexander Dumas' long-time friend, Gustave Flaubert. Along with *Madame Bovary* and his many other literary works, there is *Le Dictionnaire des Idées Reçues*, compiled from Flaubert's notes taken from boyhood (he was born in 1821) and first published posthumously in 1913. Edward Fluck, who prepared the first English translation in 1954 under the title, *A Dictionary of Platitudes*, called it "a compendium of conversational clichés, blind beliefs, fashionable misconceptions, and fixed ideas" of the kind Flaubert found to be common among the French bourgeoisie (p. iii), the new middle class of merchants and capitalists he scorned. The *platitudes* included this one on *gauchers*: "*Terribles à l'escrime. Plus adroits que ceux qui se servent de la main droite*" ["redoubtable in fencing. More adroit than people who use the right hand"] (p. 84).

Because Flaubert did not date the entries, we cannot say whether *gauchers* was written before or after 1844, when Dumas published *The Three Musketeers*, but if after, could it have been inspired not just by what Flaubert heard people say but by what Athos told d'Artagnan? Dumas never saw the dictionary (like Flaubert, he died before it was published), but had he seen it and read the entry on left-handers, one could imagine him taking offense. After all, Flaubert regarded the claim about the left-hander's prowess as one of those conversational clichés repeated by persons lacking real knowledge, and here were Athos, Dumas' creation, and Grisier, Dumas' esteemed teacher, saying the same thing.[9]

---

[9]*The Three Musketeers* first appeared in serial form in the newspaper *Le Siècle*, which, given its circulation—52,000 at its peak in 1860 [*Le Siècle*, 2014]—could have been an important source of public opinion about left-handed fencers.

What Gave Left-Handers the Advantage?

For Grisier and other fencing masters with the conventional view, what did they think gave left-handers the edge, their nature or their nurture? Francis Galton made the phrase "Nature and Nurture" popular in 1874 as a way to frame debates about the roots of individual differences—he called it a "convenient jingle of words" (p. 12)—but the terms, singly or together, had been used before, by Shakespeare most famously.[10] The terms have also been used by some of the fencing masters. One was L'Abbat (1734), who said, "Most People imagine that a Left-handed Man has, by Nature, the Advantage of a Right-handed Man in Fencing" (p. 86). L'Abbat did not identify "Most People" (just as Luke did not identify "many of opinion" in his dialogue with Saviolo), but he probably did not mean other fencing masters, who, as we shall see, spurned that explanation, and if it was the general public, including the bourgeoisie, one wonders how they came to this view. Was it from repeating what others said, hearing about the Kerrs (before their celebration in verse), reading romantic stories earlier than Dumas', if there were such, or seeing left-handers in exhibitions or competition?[11] Or was L'Abbat referring to his students, not just right-handers looking perhaps for a way to excuse their defeats, but even left-handers on the possibility that winning made them feel *naturally* superior? Nor is it clear what "Most People" would have meant by "Nature," but if they were students, perhaps they meant qualities important for fencing: physical, such as speed, strength, and balance, or psychological, such as judgment, desire, and courage. Whoever they were and whatever they meant, L'Abbat himself favored Nurture: the advantage was mere habit owed to the left-hander's being a small minority and therefore "exercising oftener with Right-handed Men than a Right-handed Man with him" (p. 86; translation by A. Mahon).

According to Gaugler (1998, p. 8), Palladini reached the same conclusion nearly two centuries before L'Abbat. The "many believers," he said, "fool themselves," meaning that the advantage came only from more opportunities for practice. Joseph Roland expressed much the same sentiment

---

[10]In *The Tempest* (Act 4, Scene 1), Prospero described Caliban, the half-human son of the malevolent witch Sycorax, as "A devil, a born devil, on whose nature/Nurture can never stick."

[11]In France, the 1860s and 1870s saw significant growth of public interest in fencing; attendance at exhibitions rose dramatically, "with hundreds and occasionally thousands of spectators standing by to watch the feats of martial prowess." Known as "grand assaults," these exhibitions were important social events, "frequented by the brightest stars of both French and international society" (Anonymous, 2012, p. 3). If left-handers participated and performed as expected, it is surely conceivable that their success became known to the general public and not just to fencers and fencing masters.

75 years after. If, indeed, L'Abbat was referring to students when he said "Most People" believed in the Nature explanation, there was no doubt in Roland's case. Of the right-hander bested, presumably not once but repeatedly by a left-hander, he said:

> This circumstance appears to the young practitioner as very *extraordinary*, and he thence concludes that the left-handed fencer has *naturally* the superiority over him; whereas if he reflected properly he would find that a *left-handed* man has only the advantage by the *habit* of practising continually with right-handed men, and that, on the contrary, the right-handed man seldom or ever has met with a left-handed one before, which is the reason of his being so much puzzled on this occasion
> Roland (1809, pp. 162–163).

Other fencing masters wove variations on the theme. Saviolo (1595) assured Luke that "onelye use and knowledge giveth the better either to the right or the lefte…" (p. 3); Godfrey (1747) supposed that "as there are more right-handed, than left-handed, the latter must be more used to the former, than the former to the latter" (p. 16); Danet (1766) explained that if left-handers are a danger to right-handers, it is because right-handers "are not accustomed to drawing their swords against them" (p. 219); Olivier (1771) said that the reason was "as you are but seldom used to fence with them [left-handers]" (p. 187); George Roland (1824) was sure that "nature has given the left-handed man no advantages in fencing which the right-handed man does not also possess" (p. 126); Grisier (1847, pp. 261–262) and Cordelois (1862) attributed the advantage to, in Cordelois' words, "the relatively small number of left-handers" (p. 202); and Burton (1911) put it to "our being more familiar with right-handed men. Change the conditions, and the pair are absolutely equal in their chances of victory" (p. 13).

If the advantage came from more chances for the right kind of practice, then right- and left-handers should be alike in personal qualities important for success, like those named earlier. No one proposed a test, but Joseph Roland (1809) thought it was enough just to watch left-handers compete against each other: both will be "more embarrassed than the right [-hander] with the left [-hander]," and will "fence in the most ridiculous manner imaginable" (p. 163); and Rondelle (1892) remarked, when they fence together, "they seldom exhibit grace or finish" (p. 189), or as Cyril Burt (1937) might have said, "they fumble and bungle."

Advice for Right-Handers

The whole art of fencing consists in just two things, to hit and not to be hit.
The Fencing Master in Molière's *Le Bourgeois Gentilhomme*, 1670, Act 2, Scene 3.

If it was just practice, the solution for right-handers was straightforward, and again starting perhaps with Palladini, everyone had the same advice when facing left-handers: in the words of Molière's Fencing Master, if one is "to hit and not to be hit," get more practice against them. That way, George Roland (1824) promised that "any difficulties... arising from the [left-handed] positions will be easily overcome..." (p. 126).

To increase such opportunities, Roland (1824) also recommended "occasionally getting lessons from your master with his left hand" (p. 126). So did others. Burton (1911) said, "The *maître d'armes* may always annul the incognito of the left-handed man by representing him at times in lessons to his pupils" (p. 14). Domenico Angelo (1763), along with insisting that his pupils practice "various strokes left-handed," would "give some lessons left handed" (p. xxiv). La Boëssière fils (1818) called it "indispensable" (p. 245). Henry Angelo (1830) did not mention doing the same, but, thinking it would be "beneficial" for his students to "accustom themselves to practice against a left-handed fencer," he told the left-handed Monsieur Le Bron that "he would be welcome to us all" (p. 344) (This was before Le Bron's contest with Lapiere, the outcome of which must have made Angelo even more confident of the wisdom of his invitation.).

Roland's (1824) "only useful advice" for right-handers was "frequent practice" against left-handers (p. 125), and Saviolo (1595) merely said to do everything in reverse, or, as Hope (1692) put it, to act "contrary to what ye are to observe in playing against a Right-Handed Man" (Preface, p. 2). Others were more specific: oppose the left-hander's point thrust with a parry to the outside and riposte to the chest or face (Palladini, c.1560; cited in Gaugler, 1998, p. 14); and engage the left-hander "always on the outside of the arm, that you may perform small strokes or glizades along his blade, to thrust under the arm" (Olivier, 1771, pp. 188–189).

Along with recommending practice against left-handers, with the master himself as occasional model, some advised right-handers to practice with their own left hand. That way, L'Abbat (1734) explained, they will not be "so much surprised when [meeting] a Left-Handed Man, as they would otherwise be" (p. 87); and Domenico Angelo (1763), while acknowledging that the exercise would be difficult, promised that "with good will and hard work," the skill achieved will be "advantageous for oneself and [do] honor to one's teacher" (p. xxiv). Hope (1707, p. 191), although not referring specifically to encounters against left-handers, promised that by using the left hand:

> a Man may become more dexterous, at both Opposing and Parieing his Adversary's Sword with it...indeed, it is too good and useful an assistance for a Man's Defence, to be wholly laid aside or neglected.

Angelo's rationale for left-hand practice was clear; for the others, less so. L'Abbat perhaps meant it would help one think like a left-hander so as to have a better plan of attack and defense when facing a left-hander, whereas Hope perhaps meant that *during* the match, whether facing a right- or left-hander, one could switch to the left, surprising one's opponent by attacking from either side. It was something that Herger, the swordsman of Norse myths, did with deadly effect:

> Then, Herger threw his own sword from one hand to the other, for these Northmen can fight as well with either hand, and equally strong. And quickly Herger turned and cut off Ragnar's head from behind with a single blow (quoted in Crichton, 1977, pp. 130–131).

If switching during the match was what Hope had in mind, the only master I found who was clear on this point was Edward Blackwell (1734), except that he saw it not as a tactic but as a way to manage fatigue: "When your Right Hand is tired in the Engagement, you may flip your sword into your Left Hand"(p. 87).

Of all the masters, Saviolo (1595) was perhaps best able to model left-hand use because, according to his contemporary John Florio, he handled the sword equally well with either hand. In *Second Frutes*, Florio's (1591) guide to self-improvement, not just in fencing but in etiquette, public speaking, and learning new languages, Saviolo (V.S.) is portrayed in a conversation between two gentlemen, Geordano (G) and Edward (E) (Chapter 7, pp. 117–119):

> G:...of whom doo you learne to plaie at your weapon?
> E: Of master V.S.
> G. Who, that Italian that lookes like Mars himselfe.
> E. The verie same
> ...
> G. I have heard him reported to be a notable talle man.
> E. Hee will hit any man, bee it with a thrust or floccada, with an imbrocada or a charging blow, with a right or reverse blowe, be it with the edge, with the back, or with the flat, even as it liketh him.
> G. Is he left or right handed?
> E. Both, all is one to him.

When Saviolo (1595) reassured Luke that "onelye use and knowledge giveth the better either to the right or the lefte," he evidently was speaking from experience.

Advice for Left-Handers

Unlike Florio, most writers on education and self-improvement, whether in writing, etiquette, or public speaking, presented the rules as though left-handers barely existed, as in Putnam's (1856) unqualified statement, quoted earlier, that "principal gestures are to be made with the right arm." They only occasionally explained why, as when Hill (1754) called left-hand gestures "strangely distasteful." By contrast, fencing masters not only recognized left-handers and let them fence with the left, they told them how. But unlike their often detailed instructions for right-handers, their instructions for left-handers were perfunctory: just do everything in reverse. For example, "if the Scholar is left-handed, his left Hand is to be conducted with the same Instructions as the right" (Valdin, 1729, p. 17); and two left-handers facing each other "should fence as would two right-handers" (Scorza & Grisetti, 1871, p. 95). Saviolo (1595) was the exception. After assuring Luke that neither hand had any natural advantage, Luke asked, "if you would teach a [left-handed scholar], how would you begin?", and Saviolo answered in detail, although, as in other manuals, his drawings illustrating positions and movements showed only right-handers.

If only Saviolo gave detailed instructions and no one provided left-hand drawings, perhaps the fencing masters thought left-handers had enough advantage already. But neither did they advise them to practice against other left-handers so that when facing them, they would *not*, as Roland (1809) remarked, fence in "the most ridiculous manner imaginable." Gomard [A.J.J. Possellier] (1845), however, did note that left-handers also would profit if the fencing master used his left hand "because their trouble is even greater [than it is for right-handers] when they encounter a left-hander" (p. 284). He presumably meant that left-handers had even fewer opportunities than right-handers for the right kind of practice, meaning against other left-handers.

Did Fencing Masters Follow Their Own Advice?

Did fencing masters follow their own advice and serve as left-handed models? Some did, including Palladini (c.1560), Domenico Angelo (1763), Danet (1766), and La Boëssière fils (1818), but most did not. As Danet (1766) remarked, "if left-handers are a danger to right-handers," it is not just because right-handers have little or no experience fencing against them, it is "because most masters do not from time to time use their left hand in giving lessons" (p. 219). Likewise, La Boëssière fils (1818) complained that "The old masters were not sufficiently concerned" to do so (p. 244). Of the "old masters," Palladini and Saviolo were the apparent exceptions.

A "Serious Disadvantage" for the Left-Hander

While recognizing the left-hander's advantage, several masters observed that in one crucial respect, it was not only nullified but reversed. As Roland (1824, p. 126) explained:

> In actual combat the left-handed person labours under a serious disadvantage, as many wounds of the lungs alone have been known to do well, which, if carried to an equal depth on the left side, would immediately have produced fatal consequences by wounding the heart.

He presumably meant that when wounded by an opponent of opposite handedness, a right-hander more likely would be struck on the right side, injuring the lung, usually a nonmortal injury, whereas a left-hander would be struck on the left, so that a wound of equal depth could pierce the heart directly or the left ventricle behind the lung. Still, no one advised left-handers to fence with the right hand. Perhaps they assumed that any increased risk of using the left was outweighed by the lesser chance of being grievously injured in the first place.

Roland's statement came before similar observations by the Scottish essayist Thomas Carlyle (1871; cited in Froude, 1885) and the English physician Philip H. Pye-Smith (1871). Neither, however, evidently saw any compensating benefit for the left-hander; they instead incorporated this element into their "heart-shield" theories to explain the origins and ascendancy of right-handedness. In Carlyle's version, choice of the right hand "probably arose in fighting; most important to protect your heart and its adjacencies, and to carry the shield in [the left] hand" (quoted in Froude, 1885, pp. 348–349).

Pye-Smith's (1871, p. 145) version differed only in reflecting the new ideas of the Darwinian era:

> If a hundred of our ambidextrous ancestors made the step in civilization of inventing a shield, we may suppose that half would carry it on the right arm and fight with the left, the other half on the left and fight with the right. The latter would certainly, in the long run, escape mortal wounds better than the former, and thus a race of men who fought with the right hand would gradually be developed by a process of natural selection.[12]

Did Fencing Masters Welcome Left-Handers or Merely Accept Them, and Were Left-Handers Themselves Drawn to the Sport?

In baseball, the abundance of left-handers shows their attraction and value to the sport. In early times, were left-handers similarly drawn to fencing so that, as in baseball, they outnumbered left-handers in the general population, and did fencing masters not only accept but welcome them for the success they might bring to their academies? If so, there are no signs in the books and manuals I examined. To the contrary, other than noting, explicitly or implicitly, that left-handers were a minority in the population, the only ones mentioning or alluding to their representation among *fencers* implied, in one instance, that it was "relatively small"

---

[12]The theory did not fare well. One critic declared that the heart is displaced so little to the left that "it must be denied, in the name of anatomy, that there is more than a very slight difference in the danger of wounds between the two sides" (Dwight, 1891, p. 475). Others pointed out that right-handedness was dominant in cultures not using swords and shields. Neither advocates nor critics, however, cited medical evidence.

(Cordelois, 1862, p. 202); in another, under 10% (the right-hander "scarcely meets one left-hander in 10 adversaries"; Gomard [A.J.J. Possellier] (1845), p. 284); in another, under 5% ("a [right-handed] man may play with 40 men, and not meete with too [two] left-handed men, except it be a great chance"; Swetnam, 1617, p. 166); and in still another, even less than that ("the right-handed man seldom or ever has met with a left-handed one before"; Roland, 1809, pp. 162–163). These statements, all based on personal impression, at most suggest no difference or even an *under*representation of left-handers. In contrast, there is one piece of physical evidence suggesting that left-handed fencers *were* overrepresented just as they are today. It comes from Leonid Tarassuk (1978). In the 1970s, Tarassuk was a research associate in the Department of Arms and Armor at the New York Metropolitan Museum of Art and former Curator of European and American Arms at the Hermitage in St. Petersburg. In his account of di Grassi's (1570) instructions for use of the dagger, which I cited previously, although Tarassuk noted that daggers with handguards designed for left-handers were "considerably fewer than those preserved for right-handers," the proportions he found (mainly from specimens in both museums) were higher than those from the fencing masters quoted above—"about one to three," or 33% (p. 44).

Something else must be considered about these or any estimates. Inasmuch as use of the right hand was seen as the mark of a "Gentleman," it follows that right-hand customs were taught and enforced especially among the wealthier and better educated. As previously noted, training normally was only for writing, using utensils, shaking hands, and the like, and not for acts that, as Broca (1865, p. 382) noted, were "spontaneously performed." Ogle (1871), however, remarked that even "untaught actions" are "sometimes gradually modified" by the child's efforts to "imitate its playfellows and avoid their ridicule," that "this feeling of shame... is of course much stronger in the well-nurtured than in the uneducated," and that this explained why "left-handedness is apparently much less common in the upper and middle classes than in the lower." In support, he added, "One can hardly look at a village cricket match without seeing one or more left-handed players, while among gentlemen such is quite exceptional" (p. 291). (If so, one wonders which matches Lundie was watching in 1896 when, as quoted earlier, he noted the "trouble" a left-handed batsman "causes to his opponents.") Likewise, the British anthropologist Gordon Harrower (1928) observed that among "uneducated" Chinese laborers, left-hand use is "as common as the right," whereas "among the more educated," the "majority" use the right (p. 138). Ogle's and Harrower's statements and estimates are vague; still, if "untaught actions" that are "sometimes gradually modified" included the hand used not just for cricket but for fencing, it conceivably could have lowered the number of left-handed fencers in "Gentlemen's" academies.

Did Accepting Left-Handed Fencers Mean Accepting Left-Handedness?

I said there is no reason to suppose that fencing masters endorsed right-hand customs any less strictly than other teachers. Still, since they accepted left-handers as students, however many there were, could they have been more open to left-handedness generally, even for writing, eating, and other public acts? If they were, Godfrey (1747) surely was not. His contempt for the condition was palpable: "I dare say no Body would chuse to be left-handed," and he called left-handers an "undesired Race." He did not elaborate, but it prompts the question whether he personally found left-handers to be "trouble" in competition. In any case, it is hard to imagine him accepting, much less welcoming, left-handers as students. That may be why his manual was among the few *not* to include special instructions for them, although that would not explain the lack of the same for right-handers. Even if he shielded his students from members of the "undesired Race," they still might have to face them elsewhere.

Did Fencing Masters Think Left-Handers Were "Odd," "Peculiar," or "Crazy"?

Finally, unlike the descriptions of Babe Ruth and certain other left-handed athletes, the manuals I examined never called left-handed fencers "odd," "peculiar," or "crazy" or implied that others saw them this way. But could Godfrey (1747) have thought so, and could that have sharpened his animus against left-handers generally?

LEFT-HANDEDNESS AND FENCING: THE VIEW TODAY

These are just a few examples of what fencing masters said in the past. They say much the same today but now can point to empirical evidence, so we can suppose that Athos would indeed have been trouble for d'Artagnan and that the bourgeousie, *pace* Flaubert, were correct about left-hander's prowess. And like their predecessors, fencing masters today credit the advantage to left-handers' smaller numbers (e.g., Crosnier, 1965; Manley, 1979), advise left-hand practice for right-handers (e.g., Czajkowski, 2005; Terrone, 1959), and note left-handers' difficulties when facing each other. As Manley (1979) remarked, "About the worst panic scene in fencing occurs when two novice left-handers meet in competition" (p. 125).

The Frequency-Dependency Effect

That the advantage comes from left-handers' smaller numbers is what ecologists and evolutionary biologists refer to as a "frequency-dependency" effect (Ayala & Campbell, 1974). It seems to be the consensus explanation among laterality researchers (e.g., Brooks et al., 2004; Grouios et al., 2000), just as it was and remains for fencing masters. It also finds support in studies that take the kind of sport into account. Raymond et al. (1996) compared the numbers of left-handers in two kinds: *interactive*, as in fencing and the other sports listed earlier, including tennis, boxing, and, for baseball, in the contest between batter and pitcher, where the action of one directly affects the action of the other; and *non-interactive*, such as in swimming, gymnastics, and skiing. If the advantage is frequency-dependent, left-handers should be overrepresented only in the former, which is what Raymond et al. (1996) found as did Grouios et al. (2000) and Wood and Aggleton (1989). The explanation also implies that as left-handers ascend the ranks in competition, they will be increasingly likely to face each other, so the advantage of left-handedness per se should diminish and the outcome will depend increasingly on nonhandedness-related differences in ability.

Other Possibilities: Differences in Reaction Time, Motor Control, Attention, and Speed of Interhemispheric Transfer of Information

Along with the frequency-dependency effect, some researchers have asked whether the advantage reflects real differences in ability, especially of the kinds important in *close* interactive sports like fencing. Of course, at the individual level, ability counts (along with quality of training, amount of deliberate practice, and motivation, among other factors), and some athletes are more richly endowed than others. The question is whether left-handers as a group are better endowed than right-handers.

Several possibilities can be contemplated. Speed of arm and hand movement are critical in fencing, so if left-handers can thrust and parry faster, the benefits would be clear. Speed differences favoring left-handers are found in peg-moving and finger-tapping tasks (Annett & Manning, 1989; Nalçaci, Kalaycioğlu, Çiçek, & Genç, 2001) but so far, not in fencing (e.g., Ketlinski & Pickens, 1973; Singer, 1968).

Another potentially important difference is in comparability of speed as well as strength and skill *between* the limbs. On strength and skill tests, as well as on hand preference questionnaires, laterality quotients are consistently lower for left-handers. For example, whereas right-handers' strength of grip is 10–30% greater on the right, differences for left-handers are smaller, sometimes even absent (Clerke & Clarke, 2001). They also are smaller on peg-moving and tapping tasks (Bryden & Roy, 2005; Kilshaw & Annett, 1983) and on tasks requiring the coordination of reaching movements as measured by movement curvature, initial direction error, accuracy, and precision (Przybyla, Good, & Sainburg, 2012). In all these tasks, the hands are tested individually, but could the results also mean better overall performance when both hands are used simultaneously and, if so, for any sports in particular? The most direct advantage, or so it would seem, would be for sports requiring use of both hands such as boxing and wrestling or baseball and cricket (and tennis for a two-handed backhand). In fencing, though, the advantage presumably would have been only in times before those reviewed here, when heavier two-handed weapons were favored, like the Norseman Herger's battle-axe. For the lighter weapons of the fencing era, there are other possibilities, including blocking or grabbing an opponent's weapon (as shown by the fencer on the right in the bottom panel of Fig. 3.2), parrying incoming thrusts with a dagger or other off-hand weapon, and *switching* hands, although here again it would depend on the historical period. For those reviewed here, as already noted, blocking and grabbing were often permitted, and the dagger, until falling from favor, served as an off-hand weapon. Today, daggers are not used in competition, and using the other hand defensively is prohibited. Hand-switching is allowed but only between, not during, matches, unless the referee gives special permission because of an injury to the hand (Fencing Rules, 2012).[13]

Could left-handers also react faster to an opponent's moves? Support for this possibility comes from a study of world-class épée fencers and beginners; although the former were not faster lunging in response to a light going on, when a fencing-like starting procedure was used, they not only were faster, but their performance was correlated with their success in competition (Harmenberg, Ceci, Barvestad, Hjerpe, & Nystrom, 1991). Handedness was not considered, so it remains to be seen whether left-handers were faster than right-handers.

In fencing, *spatial* attention is important as well. The right hemisphere normally controls attention across the entire extrapersonal space, whereas the left primarily controls attention in the right hemispace (Mesulam, 1999). Bisiacchi, Ripoll, Stein, Simonet, and Azémar (1985) proposed that because fencers are trained to respond quickly and accurately, then in situations calling for spatial attention and cued recall, left-handers will have the advantage insofar as the right hemisphere also controls the left hand. To find out, they gave a cued reaction-time test to 6 right-handed and 6 left-handed fencers and to 12 athletes in other sports. The targets were lights placed 8 or 24 degrees to either side of midline fixation, and the cues for each trial indicated target side and number of degrees. On half the trials, subjects responded by pressing a button with the right hand, on the other half with the left. Although fencers overall were not faster,

---

[13]Recall that the musketeer Athos was able to switch to his left following injury (to his right shoulder, not his hand). So could Edoardo Mangiarotti, who, on being struck on his left index finger in the semifinals at the 1951 Olympics, changed to his right hand, which he could still use with great skill, and won his last two semifinal matches and the silver medal in the finals (Cohen, 2002, p. 382).

they were more accurate, with left-handers best of all: the authors saw this as "a good [speed-accuracy] trade-off" (p. 511). Ten of the 12 fencers, regardless of handedness, also were more accurate with the left. Should the right-handers among these 10 consider switching to the left?

Fencers also must respond quickly and accurately to attacks from either side, which means anticipating opponents' moves, including lateral shifts in position. Hagemann (2009) found a handedness effect in tennis: left-handers were better at predicting the stroke direction of opposite-handed opponents. Since tennis is a "close-interactive" sport—even at the net, the players are usually at least 10 feet apart—the effect should be even stronger for fencing, a "close" sport, where opponents are only arms' (and swords') length apart. That comparison remains to be made.

Hagemann called this advantage a "perceptual frequency" effect after Faurie and Raymond (2005), implying that, like the frequency-dependent effect itself, it comes from left-handers' more frequent opportunities to practice against right-handers than right-handers have against them. But could there also be real differences in attention, possibly due to a weaker directional attentional bias in left-handers (Buckingham, Main, & Carey, 2011), and at the neural level due to faster interhemispheric transfer of primary-level sensory and motor information (e.g., Cherbuin & Brinkman, 2006)?

Individual Differences

Fencing masters in the past evidently assumed that all left-handers were cut from the same cloth, never supposing that the advantage might be greater for some than for others, and if they saw differences in advantage, they presumably would have attributed them to further differences among left-handers in opportunities for practice against right-handers. We now know that left-handers are phenotypically far more heterogeneous than right-handers (for reviews, see Harris, 1992; Peters, 1996). Their smaller group-laterality quotients, noted previously, therefore reflect larger individual differences, with proportionately fewer left-than right-handers in the strongly-, or consistently-handed, subgroups in the tails of the distribution, and with more in the weakly-, or inconsistently-handed, subgroups between. On self-report hand-use inventories, many more left- than right-handers therefore not only report weaker biases, more report preferring the *other* hand. In cricket, already mentioned is Charles Wordsworth, who bowled left but batted right. In baseball, there is the great Ty Cobb, who did the reverse—threw right but batted left—and had the all-time batting average at 0.367. (Ruth was consistent, throwing left and batting left.) Similarly, on tests of grip strength, when the nonpreferred hand is stronger, it is more often in left-handers. If certain motor and attentional factors do give left-handers an advantage in fencing and other close-interactive sports, it may be only in certain left-handers.

Type of Weapon, Fencing Distance, and Type of Movement

Whether or not the advantage for left-handed fencers is natural, its appearance could depend on the weapon used. In Azémar and Stein's (1994) survey of elite fencers, the advantage was greatest for foil competition, less for épée, and least for sabre (Table 3 in Raymond et al., 1996). Raymond et al. (1996) propose that the differences reflect different rules and tactics for each weapon: for the sabre, opponents stand farther apart than for épée or foil, despite the sabre's shorter length, because, by convention, the hand and arm can be targets only in sabre competition (p. 1631). Alternatively, as Boulinguez, Velay, and Nougier (2001) suggest, the advantage has to do with the spatial constraints of the movement, with left-handers favored for movements requiring mostly sagittal and proactive control (foil and épée) and with right-handers favored for movements requiring mostly lateral and retroactive control (sabre), although this is not completely consistent with the pattern in Table 1 in Azémar (2003).

For Left-Handers, Will the Advantage Continue?

In fencing, the left-hander has long held the edge, but will it continue? As Loffing, Hagemann, and Strauss (2012) noted, if there are no natural differences at work and since professional athletes' training regimens continuously improve, the advantage could diminish. If, however, it is natural, then, as Holtzen (2000) proposed, left-handers might be expected to profit *more* than right-handers from long, intense training so that the advantage would *increase*. Holzen's example was tennis. To put the question to test, Loffing et al. (2012) analyzed world rankings for left- and right-handed tennis players from 1968 to 2011. They found that the advantage not only did *not* increase, it significantly weakened so that left-handers no longer had a high probability of being highly ranked. Among amateurs, however, the advantage held. The authors therefore concluded that natural differences were not at work. As already noted, tennis is a "far-interactive" sport, with lower spatiotemporal constraints on performance. What would be the cumulative effects of intense training on fencing, a close-interactive sport, with higher spatiotemporal constraints? Would the left-hander's advantage be harder or easier to counteract? We shall have to wait and see.

The Hand Shake

I leave to the end of my review a note on a fencing custom that comes at the end of a match: the hand shake. Although not mentioned in the manuals I examined, it too would have been essential in the "breeding of a Gentleman." What makes it notable is that, judging from current practices, right-handers shake with the *left*, not the right. That way, they do not have to shift the sword from right hand to left, or remove the now sweat-moistened glove from the right (the left normally being ungloved) (Fencing.net, 2014). But in that case, what is the protocol for fencers of opposite handedness? Who shifts the sword and removes the glove to accommodate the opponent? If it is the left-hander, then so much for the warning about the stranger who "greets thy hand with proffered left," and how odd, fittingly so, that the customary right-hand shake would occur only when both combatants are *left*-handed.

CONCLUSION

In conclusion, fencing masters were correct: left-handers *are* trouble for right-handers, and the consensus, past and present, is that it comes from "Nurture," not "Nature." If, however, some left-handers are more naturally enabled for *close* interactive sports like fencing, and if at least those left-handers continue to excel as training regimens improve, it would mean that the few fencing masters who laid the advantage to "Nature" were also correct. The lesson will resonate with every behavioral scientist: To understand individual differences in fencing as in virtually all talents, proclivities, and skills, the reasons must be sought in the mix of both. As the Elizabethan schoolmaster Richard Mulcaster (1582, p. 35) said in his treatise on the "right writing of our English tung," "Nature makes the boy toward, nurture sees him forward." Or as the biologist Anna Fausto-Sterling (2005, p. 1510) observed, "we are always 100 percent" of each. And as always, the devil is in the details. It's up to us to draw them out.

Acknowledgments

I first described fencing masters' views about left-handers in an article in *Laterality* (Harris, 2010). This essay draws on that work, with permission from the publisher, Taylor and Francis. I completed research for that article in 2007, and my principal sources, as already noted, came from the Charles and Ruth Schmitter Fencing Collection at Michigan State University. Since then, along with important additions to the collection, other historic manuals too valuable to lend have been digitized and made available on the Internet, letting me expand my survey beyond what was initially available. For my original article as well as for the current essay, along with published reports of studies of laterality in fencing and other sports, I have profited from Internet postings from sports writers, scholars, and practitioners.

Along with my thanks to the late Professor Charles Schmitter for his remarkable gift of books and manuals to the Michigan State University Library, and to the other collectors and authors noted above, I am grateful to Peter Berg, the Library's Head of Special Collections and the members of his staff, past and present, who were always generous in their assistance; to Alessandra Passarotti and Anne Meyering for advice on Italian and French translation, respectively; to William Lee Martin for telling me about Herger, the Norse swordsman; to Chris McManus, coeditor of *Laterality*, and an anonymous reviewer for comments and suggestions about the original version of this essay; and to Norbert Hagemann and Florian Loffing for comments and suggestions about the current version. As I said in my acknowledgments to my original article, my only regret was not starting this project while Charles Schmitter was still alive because, apart from the general advice he would have offered, he was a left-handed fencer whose experiences and reflections I would have been eager to hear about, both from the perspective of the student he had been and the Maestro di Scherma that he became. Luckily, Alessandra Passarotti, a fencer in her student days at the University of Padova, is left-handed (what are the odds!) and gave helpful accounts of her own experiences. With all this good advice, I should have gotten the story right. For any failures large or small, the fault is mine.

References

Amberger, J. C. (2011). *Henry Angelo: Strategic planning in running a salle. The secret history of the sword: Fencing classics from the secret archives of fencing and dueling.* Retrieved July 26, 2014, from http://fencingclassics.wordpress.com/2011/09/21/.

Angelo, D. (1763). *The school of fencing.* London: R. & J. Dodsley, Pall-Mall (2nd ed. In French and English, 1765; English translation by Henry C. W. Angelo).

Angelo, D. (1787). *The school of fencing. With a general explanation of the principal attitudes and positions peculiar to the art.* London: R. & J. Dodsley, Pall-Mall. Reduced and translated from the original French version (1763) by Henry C.W. Angelo.

Angelo, H. (1830). *Reminiscences of Henry Angelo, with memoirs of his late father and friends, including numerous original anecdotes and curious traits of the most celebrated characters that have flourished during the last eighty years* (Vol. 2). London: Henry Colburn and Richard Bentley. https://archive.org/details/reminiscenceshe00angegoog.

Annett, M., & Manning, M. (1989). The disadvantages of dexterity for intelligence. *British Journal of Psychology, 80,* 213–226.

Anonymous. (1875). Left-handed people. May 8. *All The Year Round,* 136–140.

Anonymous. (1915). Left-hander Ruth puzzles Yankees. *The New York Times.* June 3. Retrieved May 25, 2015, from http://query.nytimes.com/mem/archive-free/pdf.

Anonymous. (2012). *The grand assault. Notes on its history. Association for historical fencing.* 7 pp. Retrieved, May 29, 2015, from http://ahfi.org/wp-content/upload/GA-article.pdf.

Anonymous. (2014). *Parrying dagger (2014).* Retrieved August 9, 2014, from: http://en.wikipedia.org/wiki/Parrying_dagger.

Antonen, M. (2005). When it comes to pitching, left-handers get extra benefits. *USA Today,* June 6, 2005. Retrieved July 20, 2014, from: http://usatoday30.usatoday.com/sports/baseball/draft/2005-06-06-pitching_x.htm.

Ayala, F. J., & Campbell, C. A. (1974). Frequency-dependent selection. *Annual Review of Ecology and Systematics, 5,* 115–138.

Aylward, J. D. (1953). *The house of Angelo: A dynasty of scientific swordsmen.* London: The Bathworth Press.

Azémar, G. (2003). *L'homme asymmétrique: Gauchers et droitiers face à face.* Paris: CNRS éditions.

Azémar, G., Ripoll, H., Simonet, P., & Stein, J.-F. (1983). Etude neuropsychologique du comportement des gauchers en escrime. *Cinesiologie, 22,* 7–18.

Azémar, G., & Stein, J.-F. (1994). Surrepréséntation des gauchers, en fonction de l'arme, dans l'élite mondiale de l'escrime. In Paper presented at the Congrès International de la Société Française du Sport, Poitiers, September.

Baker, J., & Schorer, J. (2013). The southpaw advantage? – Lateral preference in mixed martial arts. *PLoS One, 8*(11), 1–3 e79793.

Bisiacchi, P. S., Ripoll, H., Stein, J. F., Simonet, P., & Azémar, G. (1985). Left-handedness in fencers: an attentional advantage? *Perceptual and Motor Skills, 61,* 507–513.

Blackwell, E. (1734). *A compleat system of fencing: or, the art of defence, in the use of the smallsword.* Williamsburg, VA: Printed by William Parks.

Blasco, F. (1844). *La scienza della scherma.* Catania, Italy.

Boulinguez, P., Velay, J.-L., & Nougier, V. (2001). Manual asymmetries in reaching movement control. II. Study of left-handers. *Cortex, 37,* 123–138.

Broca, P. (1865). Sur le siège de la faculté du langage articulé. *Bulletins de la Société d'Anthropologie de Paris, 6*, 377–393.

Brooks, R., Bussière, L. F., Jennions, M. D., & Hunt, J. (2004). Sinister strategies succeed at the cricket World Cup. *Proceedings of the Royal Society London, 271*(Suppl. 3), S64–S66.

Bryden, P. J., & Roy, E. A. (2005). A new method of administering the Grooved Pegboard Test: performance as a function of handedness and sex. *Brain and Cognition, 58*, 258–268.

Buckingham, G., Main, J. C., & Carey, D. P. (2011). Asymmetries in motor attention during a cued bimanual reaching task: left and right handers compared. *Cortex, 47*(4), 432–440.

Burt, C. (1937). *The backward child*. New York: Appleton-Century.

Burton, R. (1911). *The sentiment of the sword: A country-house dialogue (Part VII)*. London: Horace Cox. Reprinted from *Journal of Non-Lethal Combat*, March, 2000. Retrieved April 13, 2015, from http://ejmas.com/jnc/jncart_burtonsentimentsword07_0300.htm.

Caesar. (2009). *Left-handed batsmen*. Posted December 28, 2009 on BigCricket Forum. Retrieved September 5, 2014, from http://www.bigcricket.com/community/threads/left-handed-batsmen.46524/.

Carlyle, T. (1871). *The Right Hand*. Entry from Carlyle's Journal, June 15; quoted in Froude, J. A. (1885). *Thomas Carlyle: A history of his life in London, 1834–1881 Vol. II* (4th ed.) (pp. 407–408). London: Longmans, Green.

Castle, E. (1885). *Schools and masters of fence, from the middle ages to the eighteenth century*. London: G. Bell and Sons.

Charles and Ruth Schmitter Fencing Collection, Michigan State University Library, East Lansing, Michigan. http://wwwlib.msu/spc/collections/fencing2/

Cherbuin, N., & Brinkman, C. (2006). Hemispheric interactions are different in left-handed individuals. *Neuropsychology, 20*(6), 700–707.

Clement. (1587–1966). *The petie schole with an English orthographie*. Gainesville, Florida: Scholars' Facsimiles & Reprints. Facsimile reproduction with an introduction by R.D. Pepper.

Clerke, A., & Clarke, J. (2001). A literature review of the effect of handedness on isometric grip strength differences of the left and right hands. *American Journal of Occupational Therapy, 55*, 206–211.

Cohen, R. (2002). *By the sword: A history of gladiators, musketeers, samurai, swashbucklers, and olympic champions*. New York: Random House.

Cordelois. (1862). *Leçons d'armes. Du duel et de l'assaut. Edition illustrée*. Paris: Chez l'auteur.

Crichton, M. (1977). *Eaters of the dead (the manuscript of Ibn Fadlan, relating his experiences with the Northmen in A.D. 922)*. New York: Bantam Books.

Crosnier, R. (1965). *Fencing with the sabre; instruction and technique*. London: Faber and Faber Ltd.

Czajkowski, Z. (2005). *Domenico Angelo – Great fencing master of the XVIII century, champion of fencing as a sport*. Retrieved May 15, 2006, from http://www.fencing.ca/coaching/domenico_angelo_cza_eng.pdf.

Danet, G. (1766). *L'art des armes, ou la maniere la plus certaine de se servir utilement de l'épée,...* Paris: Chez Herissant, Fils, Libraire, rue S. Jacques.

Doré, G. (1880–1883). *Monument to Alexandre Dumas*. Paris: Place Malesherbes. Retrieved October 19, 2014, from http://www.artandarchitecture.org.uk/images/conway/e58bf710.html?ixsid=pn6Aja0QeXV.

Dumas, A. (2006). *The three musketeers. Translated with an introduction by Richard Pevear*. New York: Viking (Original title, *Les trois mousquetaires*, first published 1844).

Dwight, T. (1891). Right and left handedness. *Journal of Psychological Medicine, 4*, 535–542.

Edwards, S., & Beaton, A. B. (1996). Howzat?! Why is there an over-representation of left-handed bowlers in professional cricket in the UK? *Laterality: Asymmetries of Body, Brain and Cognition, 1*, 45–50.

Faurie, C., & Raymond, M. (2005). Handedness, homicide and negative frequency-dependent selection. *Proceedings of the Royal Society of London B, 272*, 25–28.

Fausto-Sterling, A. (2005). The bare bones of sex: Part 1. *Signs, 30,* 1491–1527.

Fencing. (2014). Retrieved October 20, 2014, from http://en.m.wikipedia.org/wiki/Fencing.

Fencing Rules. (2002). Retrieved November 8, 2012, from http://olympics.sporting99.com/london-2012/sports/fencing-rules.html.

Fencing.net. (2014). *Why do fencers shake with their left hand?* Retrieved August 27, 2014, from http://www.fencing.net/forums/thread25966.html.

Fiore, J. (1983). En garde: coach Schmitter's grand gift. *The University Library (Newsletter of the Michigan State University Libraries), 15,* 1–2.

Flaubert, G. (1913). *A dictionary of platitudes. Being a compendium of conversational cliches, blind beliefs, fashionable misconceptions, and fixed ideas.* Paris: L. Conard. Translation with preface and notes by Edward J. Fluck of *Le dictionnaire des idées reçues.* Emmaus, Pennsylvania, and London, England. Classic Firsts, 1954.

Florio, J. (1591–1953). *Second frutes. London.* Gainesville, Florida: Scholars' Facsimiles & Reprints. Printed for Thomas Woodcock. Facsimile reproduction, with an introduction by R.C. Simonini, Jr.

Fraser, G. M. (1971). *The Steel Bonnets: The story of the Anglo-Scottish border reivers.* London: Barrie & Jenkins Ltd.

Froude, J. A. (1885). *Thomas Carlyle: A history of his life in London, 1834–1881 Vol. II* (4th ed.). London: Longmans, Green.

Galton, F. (1874). *English men of science: Their nature and nurture.* London: Macmillan and Co.

Gaugler, W. M. (1998). *The history of fencing. Foundations of modern European swordplay.* Bangor, Maine: Laureate Press. Foreward by Malcolm Fare.

Gaugler, W. M. (2014). *The discourse of Acamillo Palladini.* Retrieved July 17, 2014, from http://www.classicalfencing.com/articles/Palladini.php (Originally published in *The Sword*).

Georgian Index. (2014). *Henry Angelo's fencing school.* Retrieved July 26, 2014, from http://www.rakehell.com/article.php?id=165&Title=Henry-Angelos-Fencing-School.

Gilbert, A. N., & Wysocki, C. J. (1992). Hand preference and age in the United States. *Neuropsychologia, 30,* 601–608.

GitHub. (2014). Retrieved August 17, 2014, from http://github.com/dsbmac/SABR101X%20History%20Lindsey%2011.txt

Godfrey, J. (1747). *A treatise upon the useful science of defence, connecting the small and back-sword, and shewing the affinity between them.* London: T. Gardner.

Goldstein, S. R., & Young, C. A. (1996). "Evolutionary" stable strategy of handedness in major league baseball. *Journal of Comparative Psychology, 110,* 164–169.

Gomard [A.J.J. Possellier]. (1845). *La théorie de l'escrime enseignée par une méthode simple basée sur l'observation de la nature….* Paris: Librarie Militaire de J. Dumaine.

Grassi, G. de (1570). *Raggione di adoprar sicuramente l'arme.* Venice.

Grisier, A. E. (1847). *Les armes et le duel.* Paris: Chez Garniers Frères, Libraires. Préface anecdotique by Alexandre Dumas.

Grondin, S., Guiard, Y., Ivry, R. B., & Koren, S. (1999). Manual laterality and hitting performance in major league baseball. *Journal of Experimental Psychology: Human Perception & Performance, 25,* 747–754.

Grouios, G., Tsorbatzoudis, H., Alexandris, K., & Barkoukis, V. (2000). Do left-handed competitors have an innate superiority in sports? *Perceptual and Motor Skills, 90,* 1273–1282.

Gursoy, R. (2009). Effects of left- or right-hand preference on the success of boxers in Turkey. *British Journal of Sports Medicine, 43,* 142–144.

Hagemann, N. (2009). The advantage of being left-handed in interactive sports. *Attention, Perception, & Psychophysics, 71*(7), 1641–1648.

Harmenberg, J., Ceci, R., Barvestad, P., Hjerpe, K., & Nystrom, J. (1991). Comparison of different tests of fencing performance. *International Journal of Sports Medicine, 12,* 573–576.

Harris, L.J. (1992). Left-handedness. In I. Rapin & S.J. Segalowitz (Eds.), *Handbook of neuropsychology: child neuropsychology,* vol. 6, section 10, Part 1 (pp. 145–208) (Series editors: F. Boller & J. Grafman). Amsterdam: Elsevier Science Publishers B.V.

Harris, L. J. (2003). What to do about your child's handedness: advice from five eighteenth-century authors, and some questions for today. *Laterality: Asymmetries of Body, Brain and Cognition, 8*(22), 99–120.

Harris, L. J. (2010). In fencing, what gives left-handers the edge? Views from the present and the distant past. *Laterality: Asymmetries of Body, Brain and Cognition, 15*(1–2), 15–55.

Harrower, G. (1928). A note on right-handedness. *Man, 28*, 137–139.

Hécaen, H. (1984). *Les gauchers: Étude neuropsychologique.* Paris: Presses Universitaires de France.

Hill, J. (1754). *On the management and education of children.* London: Printed for R. Baldwin. Microfilm: Charlottesville, Virginia: Micrographics II, 1986. Part 1 of microfilm reel/ Eighteenth century sources for the study of English literature and culture; reel no. 598.

Hogg, J. (1830). The raid of the Kers. *Blackwood's Magazine* (Edinburgh), 28 (168), July-December. Retrieved July 10, 2014, from *Blackwood's Magazine* https://books.google.de/ books?id=y7MCAAAAIAAJ; or http://www.clanker.co.uk/songs%20%26%20stories/ the%20raid-2.html

Holtzen, D. W. (2000). Handedness and professional tennis. *International Journal of Neuroscience, 105*, 101–119.

Hope, W. (1692). *The compleat fencing-master; in which is fully described the whole guards, parades and lessons, belonging to the small sword…* (2nd ed.). London: Printed for D. Newman.

Hope, W. (1707). *A new, short, and easy method of fencing: or the art of the broad and small sword rectified and compendiz'd.* Edinburgh: James Watson. Reprinted in M. Rector (Ed.), *Highland swordsmanship: Techniques of the scottish swordmasters* (pp. 89–195). Union City, California: Chivalry Bookshelf. 2001.

Huston, W. (1950). *The asphalt jungle.* Screenplay by B. Maddow from the 1949 novel by W.R. Burnett. Distributed by Metro-Goldyn-Mayer.

Jackson, J. H. (1880). On aphasia with left hemiplegia. *The Lancet (April 24)*, 637–638.

James, B. (1988). *The Bill James historical baseball abstract.* New York: Villard Books.

Jamieson, J. (2011). *Scottish dictionary and supplement in four volumes. A-Kut* (Vol. 1). Reproduction. BiblioBazaar. Retrieved May 25, 2015, from https://books.google.com/books/ about/Scottish_Dictionary_and_Supplement.html?id=Dp9AygAACAAJ&hl=en.

Kerr, A. J. C. (1985). *Ferniehurst castle: Scotland's frontier stronghold.* Roxburgh, Scotland: A. Kerr.

Ketlinski, R., & Pickens, L. (1973). Characteristics of male fencers in the 28th annual NCAA fencing championships. *Research Quarterly, 44*, 434–439.

Kilshaw, D., & Annett, M. (1983). Right- and left-hand skill 1: effects of age, sex, and hand preference showing superior skill in left-handers. *British Journal of Psychology, 74*, 253–268.

L'Abbat, M. (1734). *The art of fencing, or, the use of the small sword.* Dublin: James Hoey, Printer. Trans. from the French by Andrew Mahon.

La Boëssière fils. (1818). *Traité de l'art des armes: À l'usage des professeurs et des amateurs.* Paris: De l'imprimiere de Didot, l'aîné.

Laidlaw, W. (1900). *The siege & the reprisal.* Retrieved on July 20, 2014, from *Home Origins Ferniehirst Songs & Stories,* http://www.clankerr.co.uk/reprisal.html (first published in 1900 in *Prose and Poetry,* Jedburgh, Scotland: T.S. Smail).

Le Siècle (2014). Retrieved July 17, 2014, from http://en.wikipedia.org/wiki/Le_Si%C%A8cle.

Lehman, H. C., & Webb, F. E. (1951). Left-handedness among major league baseball players. *Motor Skills Research Exchange, 3*, 5–10.

Locke, J. (1693–1989). *Some thoughts concerning education. Edited with introduction, notes, and critical apparatus by John and Jean S. Yolton.* Oxford, England: Clarendon Press.

Loffing, F., & Hagemann, N. (2015). Pushing through evolution? Incidence and fight records of left-oriented fighters in professional boxing history. *Laterality: Asymmetries of Body, Brain and Cognition, 20*(3), 270–286.

Loffing, F., Hagemann, N., & Strauss, B. (2012). Left-handedness in professional and amateur tennis. *PLoS One, 7*, e49325.

Lundie, R. A. (1896). Left-handedness. *Chambers's Journal of Popular Literature, Science and Arts, 13,* 9–12.

Manley, A. (1979). *Complete fencing.* Garden City, NY: Doubleday & Co.

Martin, D. (2012). Edoardo Mangiarotti, Fencer, dies at 93; won six Gold medals in Olympic Games. *The New York Times.* May 25, p. B7.

Mathewson, T. (1805). *Fencing familiarized; or, a new treatise on the art of the scotch broad sword: Shewing the superiority of that weapon, when opposed to an enemy, armed with a spear, pike, or gun and bayonet.* London: printed by W. Cowdroy.

McManus, I. C. (2002). *Right hand, left hand. The origins of asymmetry in brains, bodies, atoms and cultures.* Cambridge, Mass: Harvard University Press.

McManus, I. C. (2009). The history and geography of human handednesss. In I. C. E. Sommer, & R. S. Kahn (Eds.), *Language lateralization and psychosis* (pp. 37–57). Cambridge, England: Cambridge University Press.

Mesulam, M.-M. (1999). Spatial attention and neglect: parietal, frontal and cingulate contributions to the mental representation and attentional targeting of salient extrapersonal events. *Philosophical Transactions of the Royal Society B/Biological Sciences, 354*(4), 1325–1346.

Molière. (1670). *Le bourgeois gentilhomme.* Retrieved August 10, 2014, from http://www.gutenberg.org/ebooks/2992.

Mulcaster, R. C. (1582). *The first part of the elementaris, which intreateth of right writing of our english tung.* London.

Nalçaci, E., Kalaycioğlu, C., Çiçek, M., & Genç, Y. (2001). The relationship between handedness and fine motor performance. *Cortex, 37,* 493–500.

Neft, D. S., & Cohen, R. M. (1988). *The sports encyclopedia: Baseball* (8th ed.). New York: St. Martin's Press.

Ogle, W. (1871). On dextral pre-eminence. *Medical-Chirurgical Transactions (Transactions of the Royal Medical and Chirurgical Society of London), 54,* 279–301.

Olivier, J. (1771). *Fencing familiarized: Or, a new treatise on the art of sword play.* London: Printed for John Bell, near Exeter Change in the Strand, and C. Etherington, at York.

Palladini, A. (undated, c.1560). *Discorso sopra l'arte della scherma* (Publisher unnamed).

Peters, M. (1996). Hand preference and performance in left-handers. In D. Elliott, & R. Roy (Eds.), *Manual asymmetries in motor performance* (pp. 123–142). Boca Raton: Florida: CRF Press.

Peters, M. (1997). Commentary left and right in classical Greece and Italy. *Laterality: Asymmetries of Body, Brain and Cognition, 2*(1), 3–6.

Plutarch. (1533). *The education or Bringinge up of Children/Translated Oute of Plutarche. Translation by Thomas Elyot.* London: Thomas Berthelet. University Microfilms No. 20057.

Pollock, W. H., Grove, F. C., & Prevost, C. (1890). *Fencing.* London: Longmans, Green, and Co (bound with *Boxing,* by E.B. Michell, and *Wrestling,* by W. Armstrong).

Przybyla, A., Good, D. C., & Sainburg, R. L. (2012). Dynamic dominance varies with handedness: reduced interlimb asymmetries in left-handers. *Experimental Brain Research, 216,* 419–431.

Putnam, W. (1856). *The science and art of elocution and oratory.* New York and Auburn: Miller, Orton & Mulligan.

Pye-Smith, P. H. (1871). Left-handedness. *Guy's Hospital Reports (3rd Series), 16,* 141–146.

Raymond, M., Pontier, D., Dufour, A.-B., & Moller, A. P. (1996). Frequency-dependent maintenance of left handedness in humans. *Proceedings of the Royal Society, London B, 263,* 1627–1633.

Robinson, G. (2012). *The left-handed advantage in cricket.* Retrieved June 2, 2015, from http://theroar.comau/2012/05/15/the-left-handed-advantage.

Roland, J. (1809). *The amateur of fencing, or a treatise, on the art of sword-defence theoretically and experimentally explained, upon new principles, designed chiefly for persons who have only acquired a superificial knowledge of the subject.* London: Printed by the author.

Roland, G. (1824). *A treatise on the theory and practice of the art of fencing.* London: William Sams, and Edinburgh: Archibald Constable and Co.

Rondelle, L. (1892). *Foil and sabre; a grammar of fencing in detailed lessons for professor and pupil.* Boston: Estes and Lauriat.

Rowlandson, T. (1787). Angelo's fencing academy. In *Georgian Index (2006)* Retrieved November 10, 2006, from http://www.georgianindex.net/Sport/Angelo/Henry_Angelo.html.

Saviolo, V. (1595). *Vincentio Saviolo his practice: In two bookes. The first entreating of the use of the rapier and dagger. The second, of honor and honorable quarrels.* London: John Wolfe. Retrieved April 24, 2015, from http:www.umass.edu/renaissance/lord/pdfs/Saviolo_1595.pdf http://www.cs.unc.edu/%7Ehudson/saviolo/firstbook.html1.

Scorza, R., & Grisetti, P. (1871). *La scienza della scherma/espostia dai due amici Rosaroll Scorza e Pietro Grisetti e Pietro Grisetti.* Nocera Inferiore: Tippgrafoa Agrocola G. Orlando. First published, 1803.

Selzer, C. A. (1933). *Lateral dominance and visual fusion.* Cambridge, Mass: Harvard University Press. Harvard Monographs in Education, No. 12: Studies in educational psychology and educational measurement.

Shakespeare, W. (undated). The tempest. In *The works of William Shakespeare gathered into one volume* (pp. 1135–1159). New York: The Shakespeare Head Press Edition. Oxford University Press.

Shaughnessy, D. (1989). Baseball '89: the invaluable lefty. *The Boston Globe, 52,* 55–56 March 31.

Singer, R. N. (1968). Speed and accuracy of movement as related to fencing success. *Research Quarterly, 39,* 1080–1083.

Smith, W. H. (1903). Concerning a certain minority. *School and Home Education, 22*(7), 328–330.

Southpaw. (2011). *Oxford English dictionary* (3rd ed.). Online. Retrieved June 6, 2015, from. http://www.oed.com/viewdictionaryentry/Entry/67623.

Southpaw. (2014). *The American Heritage dictionary of the English language* (5th ed.). New York: Houghton Mifflin Harcourt.

Stewart, D. (2014). *What percentage of MLB pitchers are left-handed?.* Retrieved August 17, 2014, from http://www.quora.com/What-percentage-of-MLB-pitchers-are-left-handed?

Swetnam, J. (1617). *The schoole of the noble and worthy science of defence. (Part 2).* A facsimile copy transcribed by Steve Hick and scanned by Stuart Huntley, May 2000, from the original provided by Patri Pugliese. Retrieved April 20, 2015, from: http://swetnam.org/SwetnamSchoolofDefence.pdf.

Tarassuk, L. (1978). Some notes on parrying daggers and poniards. *Metropolitan Museum Journal, 12,* 33–53.

Terrone, L. F. (1959). *Right and left hand fencing. With a biographical preface by L.M. Fleisher.* New York: Dodd, Mead, & Company.

Uhrbrock, R. S. (1970). Laterality of champion athletes. *Journal of Motor Behavior, 2,* 285–291.

Valdin, M. [Salomon Negri] (1729). *The art of fencing, as practiced by Monsieur Valdin.* London: Printed for J. Parker in Pall-Mall.

Viggiani, A. (1575). *The defense of Angelo Viggiani.* Venice: Giorgo Angelieri, printer. English translation by William Jherek Swanger, 2002. Retrieved April 20, 2015, from http://www.books.google.de/books?id=t2zBibZPOUcC.

Walsh, J. (2007). *The advantage of batting left-handed.* Posted November 15 in The *Hardball* Times. Retrieved April 1, 2015, from http://www.hardballtimes.com/the-advantage-of-batting-left-handed/.

Webster's new international dictionary of the English language, Second Edition, unabridged (1937). Springfield, Mass.: G. & C. Merriam Company.

Wilson, D. (1872). Righthandedness. *The Canadian Journal of Science, literature, and history. New Series, 75,* 199–231.

A. LATERALITY – AN IMPORTANT AND OFTEN DISREGARDED TOPIC

Wolf, T. (November 2001). Inside two Georgian schools of arms. *Journal of Manly Arts*. Retrieved June 19, 2015, from http://jmanly.ejmas.com/articles/2001/jmanlyart_wolf_1101.htm.

Wolf, T. (February 2002). Singlestick fencing: 1787–1923. *Journal of Manly Arts*. Retrieved June 19, 2015, from http://ejmas.com/jmanly/articles/2002/jmanlyart_wolf_0202.htm.

Wood, C. J., & Aggleton, J. P. (1989). Handedness in 'fast ball' sports: do left-handers have an innate advantage? *British Journal of Psychology, 80*, 227–240.

Wordsworth, C. (1891). *Annals of my early life, 1806-1846: With occasional compositions in Latin and English verse*. London: New York: Longmans, Green, and Co.

Ziyagil, M. A., Gursoy, R., Dane, Ş., & Yuksel, R. (2010). Left-handed wrestlers are more successful. *Perceptual and Motor Skills, 111*, 65–70.

4

Measurement of Laterality and Its Relevance for Sports

Till Utesch, Stijn Valentijn Mentzel, Bernd Strauss

University of Münster, Münster, Germany

Dirk Büsch

University of Health and Sport, Technique and Art, Berlin, Germany

The aim of laterality assessments is to find out the laterality characteristics of an individual, for example, handedness, footedness, eyedness, earedness, or preferences such as the rotation preference. A reliable and valid assessment of laterality is important, not only for research purposes but also for sport, clinical, and intervention reasons (e.g., to improve top performance sports).

Laterality is a multidimensional construct (Corballis, 2010), which includes development as an active process affected by both environmental and genetic factors (Musálek, 2015). A wide range of assessment methods to measure an individual's laterality as well as different understandings of the phenomenon in terms of definition and theoretical construct are continuously altered and developed. The one who endeavors to fully understand laterality and to make reasonable efforts to adequately measure laterality might encounter an onerous challenge.

This obstacle becomes apparent when examining existing assessment tools, which underlie various definitions and assumptions of the latent variable laterality (discussed in this chapter), which incorporate sometimes different and sometimes similar manifest (observable) variables such as items in a questionnaire. In addition, different definitions are partially caused by the prior-made theoretical assumptions. Hence, thresholds between left, right, or ambivalent are drawn at different thresholds, also depending on the number and form of items.

Firstly, *laterality as latent type* can be understood solely as a *discrete phenomenon* differentiating between groups (categories), meaning that individuals are simply categorized into left, right, ambidexterity, or more differentiated hybrid categories, depending on the assessment used and underlying theoretical assumptions. Within this definition the average proportion of left-handed individuals usually ranges around 10–12% (see Chapter 2: Origins, Development and Persistence of Laterality in Humans in this book), which has been shown to be remarkably consistent across cultures (Marchant, McGrew, & Eibl–Eibesfeldt, 1995). However, laterality might be influenced by specific individual characteristics such as age, gender, and season of birth (e.g., Tran et al., 2014; Tran, Stieger, & Voracek, 2014a).

Secondly, *laterality as latent trait* can be specified as a *continuous phenomenon*, from consistent right-sided in continuous degrees of laterality to consistent left-sided, and can be seen as a bipolar dimension. This definition results in the typically displayed J-curve of laterality, in which relative manual proficiency is typically normally distributed with a shift toward superior performance of the right side (Annett, 1972).

Alternatively, *laterality* can be defined as both a *discrete* latent type and as a *continuous* variable (respecting dimension or latent trait) within one type. This means, for example, that someone can be categorized qualitatively as a left-hander, but within this category, individuals differ quantitatively in terms of how well they can perform with their left hand (e.g., Büsch, Hagemann, & Bender, 2010).

It is a fundamental and enduring rationale in general theory development to decide between categorical and dimensional models of a latent variable. A lack of clarity occurs not only between the different concepts of laterality; within one definition the concept can be ambiguous. Laterality is not yet a taxonomic concept. While some authors indicate ambidexterity already in the presence of one deviating item of an assessment, others claim that subjects need to show no side preference for all items (Coren, 1993; Overbeck, 1989), causing arbitrary thresholds of laterality. Therefore it is not surprising that reported percentages of left-sided people range from 1% to 30% (Hécaen & Ajuriaguerra, 1964; Overbeck, 1989).

AN ASSESSMENT-ORIENTED PERSPECTIVE

In the beginning, laterality research focused exclusively on the asymmetry of the upper limbs due to the prominent appearance in many everyday tasks (Musálek, 2015; see also Chapter 2: Origins, Development and Persistence of Laterality in Humans in this book). However, laterality is not only expressed by handedness. For a wide field of different sports, further aspects of laterality play major roles (e.g., footedness in soccer, rotation preference in gymnastics, etc.; Loffing, Sölter, & Hagemann, 2014).

In the current literature, three types of assessment tools (the so-called manifest variables or observations to measure the underlying latent variables, as discussed earlier) are predominantly used (see Table 4.1 for an overview of laterality tests; see Schachter, 2000):

1. Performance tasks
2. Preference tasks
3. Self-report questionnaires

In general, performance tasks are developed to evaluate the outcome and quality of tasks executed with both the left and right side. Preference tasks are designed to elicit motor responses as an indication of laterality. Finally, self-report questionnaires inspect preferences in different motor activities based on individual's responses.

Altogether, the different approaches underlie certain understandings and consequently address various concepts of laterality, although few underlie verified latent structures (for an overview, Musálek, 2014). Within the performance approach, performance differences between opposing motor extremities indicate laterality, whereas within the preference approach, laterality is concluded solely from an individual's level of preference executing certain tasks. Self-report preference questionnaires define laterality based on specific individual self-indications of side preference.

For all three approaches the variable measured has mostly a quantitative, continuous character, and therefore follows the "idea" of a single dimension, although, seen from a methodological standpoint, it remains on a manifest level. Besides, for example, time or error in performance tasks, the degree of laterality (LQ; laterality quotient; to our knowledge first mentioned by Humphrey, 1951; see Musálek, 2014) is often measured in laterality assessments. The LQ is formalized by Eq. [4.1] where L is defined by the number of tasks/items performed or preferred with the left side, and the number of tasks/items performed or preferred with the right side defines R. The result is the degree of laterality in a percentage, which has a continuous interval from consistent right (100% right) to consistent left (100% left). Alternatively the laterality score (LS) is used as a measure of laterality (e.g., Bryden, 1977; White & Ashton, 1976). The LS is also calculated on a manifest level simply cumulating left-sided responses coded negatively and right-sided responses coded positively.

$$LQ = 100 * \frac{(R-L)}{(R+L)}$$

[4.1]

The phenomenon of laterality has been investigated in numerous ways and in various age groups. Unfortunately, due to the diversity of approaches, neither "best practice" examples for assessing an individual's laterality, nor a fixed term for the concept of laterality, are available.

TABLE 4.1 Exemplary Overview of Different Laterality Tests

Assessment Type	Name	Author(s) and Year	Assessment of	# Items	Validity/Reliability
Performance tests	Harris Scale/Harris Tests of Lateral Dominance	Harris (1947)	Hand, eye, and foot	11	$R = 0.83-0.89$
	Hand-Dominanz-Test (HDT)	Steingrüber and Lienert (1971)	Hand	6	$R = 0.64$, $R_{Author} = 0.77$
	WatHand Cabinet Test (WHQ)	Bryden et al. (2007)	Hand	1	TBD
	Foot tapping	Peters and Durding (1979)	Foot	1	TBD
	Dot task	Tapley and Bryden (1985)	Hand	4	TBD
	Purdue pegboard task	Tiffin and Asher (1948)	Hand	1	$R = 0.60-0.91$, Validity shown across 14 studies
	Manual aiming task	Roy and Elliott (1986)	Hand	36-12	TBD
Preference tests	Variety of footedness tasks to determine location and nature of impairment regarding motor dominance	Markoulakis, Scharoun, Bryden, and Fletcher (2012)	Foot	4	TBD
	Hand preference test for 4–6 year olds	Kastner-Koller et al. (2007)	Hand	14	$R = 0.97$
	Lateral preferences test for children	Groden (1969)	Hand, foot, eye, ear	16	TBD
	Handedness and footedness in infancy	Berger, Friedman, and Polis (2011)	Hand and Foot	2	TBD
	Foot preference in sprinting	Ziyagil (2011)	Foot	1	TBD

Self-report questionnaires

Edinburgh Handedness Inventory	Oldfield (1971)	Hand	10	$R = 0.8$
Fazio Laterality Inventory (FLI)	Fazio et al. (2013)	Hand	12-10	12 items; $R = 0.92$ 10 items; $R = 0.94$
Annett Handedness Questionnaire	Annett (1970)	Hand	12	$R = 0.8$
The Sherman-Kulhavy Laterality Assessment Inventory	Sherman, Kulhavy, and Bretzing (1976)	Hand, arms, legs, feet	45	$R = 0.98$
Lateral Preference Inventory	Coren (1993)	Hand, foot, eye, ear	16	TBD
Waterloo Footedness Questionnaire-Revised	Elias, Bryden, and Bulman-Fleming (1998)	Foot	13	TBD
Waterloo Handedness Questionnaire-Revised	Elias et al. (1998)	Hand	38	TBD
The Flinders Handedness Survey (FLANDERS)	Nicholls, Thomas, Loetscher, and Grimshaw (2013)	Hand	10	TBD
Foot preference test	Chapman, Chapman, and Allen (1987)	Foot	11	$R = 0.89$
Hand Dominance Questionnaire	Chapman and Chapman (1987)	Hand	13	$R = 0.96$-0.97
Paraense Lateral Preference Inventory	Martin and Machado (2005)	Hand, foot	13 (10 Hand, 3 Foot)	TBD
18-item Laterality Inventory	Saudino and McManus (1998)	Hand, foot, eye, ear	18	TBD

Performance Approach

Within the performance approach, motor performance tests are used to assess performance and sometimes the quality of performance. Performance tasks include, for example, foot tapping or grip strength (e.g., Kraemer, Canavan, Brannigan, & Hijikata, 1983; Peters & Surfing, 1978; Triggs, Calvanio, Levine, Heaton, & Heilman, 2000). These tests are designed to induce actions from which the degree of laterality can be deduced. Most performance-orientated assessments focus on the upper limbs (e.g., Bryden, Roy, & Spence, 2007; Kraemer et al., 1983) and compare the results of both left and right motor extremities to indicate the level of laterality on an interval scale. Within the performance task approach, laterality is mostly regarded as a quantitative, continuous variable.

Performance tasks can be categorized into two groups: firstly in tests assessing neuromuscular activity in terms of speed or strength and secondly in tests focusing on fine motor performance, for example, accuracy (Rigal, 1992). Typical neuromuscular activity tests are stability in static targeting, grip strength, or different types of tapping, for example, dot-filling without a constrained area (Peters & Surfing, 1978). Fine motor tasks include tests with area constraints (Tapley & Bryden, 1985), tests where specifically shaped objects have to be put in holes (e.g., the well-known pegboard test, Tiffin & Asher, 1948), and many others. Measurements often include counting errors made, time needed, or a combination of both (Borod, Caron, & Koff, 1984).

Performance tasks underlie the presumption that the preferred side is naturally also the stronger and more skilled side. The proponents of the performance approach argue that performance is automatically linked to preference (Corey, Hurley, & Foundas, 2001; Peters, 1998), although some studies state that this relationship might be weak (Porac & Coren, 1981) and both approaches should be used in parallel (Doyen & Carlier, 2002). Since performance is considered multidimensional (Elliott & Roy, 1996), performance tasks can experience the problem of short-term transfer. Hence, using performance tasks entails the difficulty of determining why and which of the performance dimensions are most important for the identification of laterality (Elliott & Roy, 1996). Performance tasks accompany the problem that in everyday life, left-sided people experience many motor tasks designed for the mainly right-sided population, such as opening a twist-capped bottle (Provins, 1997). Büsch and Hagemann (2013) showed that these daily experiences moderate the results of related performance tasks in their study using a computer mouse.

Preference Tasks

Preference tasks are motor activities aimed at inducing direct spontaneous actions to given instructions. The main difference with performance tasks is that only the preferred side is recorded and not the actual performance. Within this approach, individuals are supposed to implicitly choose their preferred side to successfully complete the given task, which generally results in a dichotomous variable left or right. Some examples of preference tasks are kicking a ball, hopping on one foot, and drawing imaginary letters (Groden, 1969; Ziyagil, 2011). Most known preference tasks use multiple items in order to determine lower and upper limb preference and also to enhance test reliability.

Motor preference tasks indicate a tendency of an individual's laterality but do not reveal the degree of lateralization in particular settings such as sport. The most prominent items aiming at the lower limbs are kicking a ball, hopping on one leg, or moving an object (Bryden, 2000; Ziyagil, 2011), while items like writing and drawing are part of most general preference assessments for upper limbs (Musálek, 2014). In general, preference tasks concentrate mainly on the upper limbs (e.g., Kastner-Koller, Deimann, & Bruckner, 2007) but also include a few items assessing lower limb preferences as well as ocular dominance (e.g., Humphrey, 1951; see Musálek, 2014). Alternative procedures, such as video-based assessments, have been developed to assess children (e.g., Tirosh, Stein, Harel, & Scher, 1999) but are quite time-consuming. Overall, many preference tasks neglect to determine any diagnostic tool structure and lack diagnostic quality. This seems mainly due to the fact that these tests are mostly based on logical validity instead of analyzing factorial structures or generic reliability of constructs to create meaningful assessments (Musálek, 2014).

Self-Report Questionnaires

A self-report preference questionnaire is the least time-consuming approach to assess an individual's laterality. Questionnaires are designed to determine preference in different motor activities for which individuals only decide whether they prefer to use their left or right side. The scores consist of different scales depending on the questionnaire used. Some questionnaires use dichotomous scales, where individuals only have to decide between left and right (Eyre & Schmeeckle, 1933), and some use scales with an option that a given task is performed with both sides, the left side, or the right side (van Strien, 2003). Others provide a five-point scoring system, where the degree of lateral preference can be expressed (Bryden, Mandal, & Ida, 2000). In most cases, an individual's laterality is indicated by a continuous variable formalized by Eq. [4.1], while in some questionnaires an individual's laterality is indicated by the algebraic sign of the sum of all items with the answers operationalized as positive (+1) for the right limb, negative (−1) for the left limb, and neutral (0) for both limbs. That means one is classified as left- or right-sided simply based on the side with which one performs relatively more actions, while ambidexterity in some cases is already argued in presence of one item deviating from the consistent side. Some researchers propose the option to differentiate laterality into both, qualitative types and a quantitative degree of laterality within one qualitative type (see Fig. 4.1; Büsch et al., 2010). Regrettably, different researchers use different items to indicate an individual's laterality and make apparent random decisions regarding the scaling of the questionnaire, and consequently, subgroups of different lateral preferences are built inconsistently (Annett, 2002; Dragovic & Hammond, 2007; Musálek, 2014). Nevertheless, self-report preference questionnaires are regarded as the most reliable and valid type of assessment of an individual's laterality (Bryden et al., 2000). This is, in part, attributed to the fact that questionnaires as an assessment tool incorporate the largest amount of items.

The most common questionnaire is the Edinburgh Handedness Inventory (EHI; Oldfield, 1971; discussed in the next section). An adaptation of this questionnaire was recently developed by Fazio, Dunham, Griswold, and Denney (2013), named the Fazio Laterality Inventory (FLI). Other examples are the Lateral Preference Inventory (LPI; Coren, 1993),

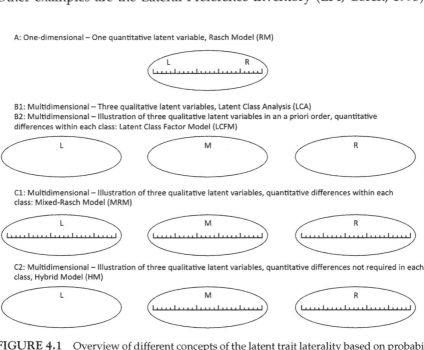

FIGURE 4.1 Overview of different concepts of the latent trait laterality based on probabilistic models. Laterality can be regarded as a one-dimensional quantitative continuous variable (A), as a qualitative variable (B1 and B2), or as a combination of both qualitative and quantitative characteristics of the latent variable (C1 and C2). L, left-sided; M, mixed-sided; and R, right-sided. *Adapted from Büsch, D., Hagemann, N., & Bender, N. (2010). The dimensionality of the Edinburgh Handedness Inventory: an analysis with models of the item response theory. Laterality: Asymmetries of Body, Brain and Cognition, 15(6), 616.*

Annett Hand Preference Questionnaire (AHPQ; Annett, 1967), and the Waterloo Handedness Questionnaire (WHQ; Bryden, 1977).

Only a few questionnaires that include multiple dimensions of laterality have been developed. One popular example is the LPI, which consists of 16 items and is based on handedness, footedness, eyedness, and earedness (each subscale is four items). It has been validated with behavioral data and shows 92% concordance (Büsch, Hagemann, & Bender, 2009; Coren, 1993; Coren, Porac, & Duncan, 1979).

EDINBURGH HANDEDNESS INVENTORY

The most frequently used tool to assess laterality is the Edinburgh Handedness Inventory questionnaire (EHI; Oldfield, 1971) with a total number of 16,156 citations in July 2015 (scopus.com).

The questionnaire was developed as a fast and simple method for assessing handedness as a one-dimensional latent variable on a quantitative scale (see A in Fig. 4.1). At that time, laterality was determined either using eye dominance (Parson, 1924) or by using performance tasks. The issue Oldfield had with these methods was that they were time-consuming, could be influenced by differences in experience of the tasks, and could be influenced by gender, age, and cultural differences. Originally the assessment consisted of 20 items with set instructions, which were analyzed for gender, cultural and socioeconomic factors, and interrelationships between the different items. The definitive version of the EHI included 10 items listed in Table 4.2. The items are to be rated as being executed solely with one hand (++), predominantly with one hand (+), or as indifferent (+for both hands). The degree of laterality (*LQ*) is measured by Eq. [4.1]. The EHI was designed as a self-report preference questionnaire and has been shown to have an acceptable to good test–retest reliability of about 0.80 (McMeekan & Lishman, 1975) as well as high internal consistency (Williams, 1991).

However, research has also shown that the original instructions for the test are often misinterpreted and consequently are not executed properly (Fazio, Coenen, & Denney, 2012; Fazio et al., 2013). This limitation seems to hold irrespective of participants' education or handedness. Furthermore, Fazio and colleagues suggest the usage of a 0–4 and Büsch et al. (2010) suggest the usage of a 0–2 or 0–3 Likert scale, improving reliability and validity. Not only misinterpretations regarding the instructions have occurred, but also greater issues regarding the concept of laterality itself have been discussed on the basis of the EHI from a test theoretical perspective over the years (see next section).

continued

EDINBURGH HANDEDNESS INVENTORY *(cont'd)*

TABLE 4.2   The Edinburgh Handedness Inventory and Instructions

Instructions: *Please indicate your preferences in the use of hands in the following activities by putting one + in the appropriate column. Where the preference is so strong that you would never try to use the other hand unless absolutely forced to, <u>put two ++</u>. If in any case you are really indifferent put + in both columns*
    Some of the activities require both hands. In these cases the part of the task, or object, for which hand preference is wanted is indicated in brackets.
    Please try to answer all the questions and only leave a blank if you have no experience at all of the object or task.

Comment: Based on the results of Fazio et al. (2012) the scale should be used as a 0–4 Likert scale. Büsch et al. (2010) suggest the usage of a 0–2 or 0–3 Likert scale to improve reliability and validity.

	Left	Right
1. Writing		
2. Drawing		
3. Throwing		
4. Scissors		
5. Toothbrush		
6. Knife (without fork)		
7. Spoon		
8. Broom (upper hand) (should be excluded according to e.g., Büsch et al., 2010; Dragovic, 2004b; Milenkovic & Dragovic, 2013; Williams, 1986)		
9. Striking match		
10. Opening box (lid) (should be excluded according to e.g., Büsch et al., 2010; Dragovic, 2004b; Milenkovic & Dragovic, 2013; Williams, 1986)		
i. Which foot do you prefer to kick with?		
ii. Which eye do you use when using only one?		
L.Q. Leave the spaces blank DECILE		

Taken and modified from Oldfield, R. C. (1971). The assessment and analysis of handedness: the Edinburgh inventory. Neuropsychologia, 9(1), 97–113.

LATERALITY AS LATENT STRUCTURE FROM A TEST THEORETICAL PERSPECTIVE

The EHI has been examined in numerous studies and from different test theoretical perspectives. Even though the EHI is an assessment solely aimed at handedness, the wide range of approaches to determine its latent structure demonstrates the methodological and test theoretical entanglements in appropriately assessing laterality. Therefore this paragraph will mainly focus on the EHI and handedness as an important aspect of laterality.

Self-report preference questionnaires such as the EHI consist of itemsets representing different motor tasks. The argument that only one item can be sufficient to indicate one's lateral preference leads to problems regarding reliability and sensitivity/specificity of the measure. The fundamental rationale underlying this approach has been that all items are homogeneous and indicate one latent variable. The items are then summed up or transformed to a general score of laterality. The most common interpretation method of the EHI is the LQ formalized by Eq. [4.1] or alternatively the LS (e.g., Ransil & Schachter, 1994; Schachter, Ransil, & Geschwind, 1987). Both options understand laterality as a continuous and not discrete variable ranging from consistent left-sided via continuous degrees of ambilaterality to consistent right-sided as a quantitative continuum. Hence, in this approach laterality is regarded as a one-dimensional trait (see Fig. 4.1A). Following this understanding of laterality, the first studies examining the quality criteria of self-report preference questionnaires used item-centered approaches and conducted traditional factorial analysis procedures (e.g., Richardson, 1978). Most studies conducting factorial analysis found that one-factor solutions representing laterality explained the majority of variance (e.g., Bryden, 1977; White & Ashton, 1976; Williams, 1986). As an example, Williams (1986) found one factor ($N = 161$) with 8 out of 10 items (see Table 4.2) showing acceptable factor loadings ($0.75 \leq \lambda \leq 0.89$). Only the items "using a broom" (0.60) and "opening a box" (0.56) showed insufficient loadings, which led to an eight-item short form of the EHI. Similar findings were reported by Dragovic (2004b), who conducted a confirmatory factor analysis to the EHI and also found insufficient factor loadings for the items "using a broom" and "opening a box". A seven-item short form was created because drawing was seen as overlapping with writing. The results were confirmed by another study by Milenkovic and Dragovic (2013). Recently, Veale (2014) examined the EHI with 1514 participants finding a poor fit to a one-factor model using confirmatory factorial analysis. The author concluded a four-item short form of the EHI where all items formed a scale, which represents both a continuous and ordinal variable. Fazio et al. (2013) developed an alternative questionnaire, named the Fazio Laterality Inventory (FLI).

The FLI demonstrated single-factor dissociation into two factors: fine motor/ballistic movements and expressive/instrumental movements. This was in contrast to the EHI, for which they found only a single factor loading (Fazio & Cantor, 2015). The insufficient model fits reported in the majority of studies did not lead to questioning the assumed latent structure of laterality as a one-dimensional quantitative variable. However, the omission of nonfitting items led to short forms of self-report preference questionnaires.

Conducting factorial analysis can entail methodological issues regarding the analysis of dimensionality: firstly, the number of items examined in relation to the response formats and secondly the dependency with respect to the sample composition. Especially sample size and composition must be based on a sensible consideration in the context of laterality research, due to the skewed distribution regardless of the theoretical understanding of laterality (Coren, 1993). Few studies utilizing classical test methods tried to refine laterality research by conducting person-centered cluster analyses to questionnaire data to further examine the concept of laterality. A three-dimensional construct was found consisting of left-handers, inconsistent left-handers, and right-handers: see Fig. 4.1(B1) (Gilbert & Wysocki, 1992; Peters & Murphy, 1992). This structure distinguishes between qualitative (discontinuous), unordered categories of laterality without considering quantitative differences within one type.

Ida, Mandal, and Bryden (2000) stated that the examination of the dimensionality of handedness is not feasible within the framework of classical test theory-conducting methods such as factor analysis or cluster analysis. Additionally, if an assessment uses a sum score build out of several items with ordinal-scaled response categories, classical models are not adequate to validate the linearity between the sum score and the latent variable (for a deeper discussion in the field of handedness, see Richardson, 1976).

An alternative approach is the examination of laterality from a trait-orientated perspective. Models of item response theory (IRT; also probabilistic test theory) can be valuable for theory examination and development (e.g., Strauss, Büsch, & Tenenbaum, 2007, 2012). They are capable of linking practical issues such as validating sum scores as interpretation measures or investigating different concepts of laterality within specific test theoretical assumptions. IRT models are used in a variety of different fields such as medicine, biology, economics, psychology, or motor development to measure abilities, attitudes, or other latent variables (see for an overview of IRT models in sport science Safrit & Wood, 1989; Strauss et al., 2007, 2012; Wood & Zhu, 2006). They define a probabilistic relationship between dichotomous or polytomous item responses and the assumed latent variable (e.g., laterality) (Alagumalai, Curtis, & Hungi, 2005), where the latter can be a type (latent class models), a trait (latent trait models), or a mixture of both (mixture distribution models). One of the main advantages of IRT Models is the invariance of parameters, which means that within a measured latent trait model, conform data are indicator distribution free and sample distribution free. Additionally, certain IRT models can be used to validate sum scores, which most laterality assessments are based on. This approach provides models that address certain measurement issues in laterality and can help to acquire a deeper understanding of laterality. As illustrated in Fig. 4.1, laterality can be regarded as a one-dimensional quantitative variable (A), a qualitative variable (B), or a combination of both qualitative and quantitative characteristics of the latent variable (C). IRT provides models, which can analyze laterality precisely in respect to these different structures. They are adequate to analyze homogeneity on both a person level and an item level in the context of construct validity examination. To address these issues, IRT models have found their way to laterality research, yet only in a modicum of studies.

Two major families of probabilistic models have been developed over the years: latent trait models and latent class models.

Firstly, latent trait models, addressing laterality regarded as (A) in Fig. 4.1, assume the latent variable to be on a continuous, quantitative scale. The basic latent trait model is the one-parameter Rasch model for manifest dichotomous data (Rasch, 1960). A large number of extension models have been developed to address a wide variety of measurement issues, for example, the Partial Credit Model (PCM, Masters, 1982) or the mixed-Rasch model (MRM, Rost, 1990). This model assumes that the probability of a certain response is based not only on a person's ability but also on the item difficulty. In a valid model, both are measured on the same scale and a person's value represents a sufficient statistic of a person's ability. Secondly, latent class models (or types), addressing laterality regarded as (B) in Fig. 4.1, assume the latent variables to be categorical and without a specific order (Strauss et al., 2012). Within one class, all persons show homogeneity regarding their pattern characteristics, whereas between classes persons are considered nonhomogeneous. This means that only the item difficulty varies between latent classes resulting in qualitative differences. Thirdly, according to latent class factor models, addressing laterality regarded as (B2) in Fig. 4.1, laterality can be regarded as qualitative latent classes. The latent classes resulting from the analysis are a priori aligned in a numerical order. Fourthly, mixture distribution models (MDM; see e.g., von Davier & Carstensen, 2007), addressing laterality regarded as (C1) in Fig. 4.1, such as the MRM (Rost, 1990), were developed combining the characteristics of latent trait and latent class models to test multidimensionality. A one-class solution would be congruent with the ordinary Rasch model indicating unidimensionality. In the MRM an individual's characteristics depend on both a nonhomogeneous qualitative latent variable and a homogeneous quantitative latent trait within a single class (for an overview see von Davier & Carstensen, 2007; Rost, 2004). Beyond, hybrid models, addressing laterality regarded as (C2) in Fig. 4.1, do not require quantitative differences in every class (Rost, 2004).

Only a few studies are known that have applied probabilistic models to laterality data, and then mostly to self-report preference questionnaires due to the given data characteristics. Dragovic (2004a) was one of the first to apply IRT models to laterality data. He examined the dimensionality of the EHI using latent class analysis (LCA), assuming handedness to be only a qualitative latent variable (see B1 in Fig. 4.1). A three-dimensional structure was found consisting of 74% right-handers, 16% mixed-handers, and 10% left-handers. In contrast to prior findings using classical methods (Dragovic, 2004b), the items "opening a box" and "using a broom" showed the highest explanatory power (Dragovic, 2004a). Dragovic and Hammond (2007) also conducted the LCA to the AHPQ and could confirm three-dimensionality. They found a slightly differing distribution of 66% right-handers, 24.2% mixed-handers, and 9.8% left-handers. Büsch et al. (2010) applied the mixed-Rasch model to the EHI to test the construct validity in terms of homogeneity. This model implies handedness to be a qualitative latent variable with quantitative differences within each class (see A/C1 in Fig. 4.1). A two-class solution of the latent trait was found, resulting in 91% right-handers and 9% left-handers, which can be discriminated quantitatively within each class. They did not find evidence for either handedness as a one-dimensional latent variable (as most factorial analyses seem to reveal) or for the existence of a so-called mixed-handers group. Furthermore, the authors demonstrated the usefulness of the mixed-Rasch model in detecting nonfitting items and recommend excluding the items "using a broom" and "opening a box" from the questionnaire.

Further IRT models have been applied to other assessment tools than the EHI. For example, Merni, Di Michele, and Soffritti (2014) applied the latent class factor model to a preference task assessment, in which an operator recorded the used hand for each item on a dichotomous scale. This model implies handedness to be a priori-ordered qualitative latent variable (see B2 in Fig. 4.1). Further, the authors compared the results obtained from a latent class factor model with results from a LCA (see B1 in Fig. 4.1). A total of 2236 young sportspeople completed the assessment consisting of 10 everyday activities: writing, throwing, hammering, brushing one's teeth, combing one's hair, crumpling up paper, lifting a glass, blowing one's nose, cutting with a knife, and stirring with a spoon. The authors reported the best model fit was found for four latent classes in the latent class factor model containing 75.94% consistent right-handers (1), 15.13% also consistent right-handers (2), 4.30% mixed-handers (3), and 4.63% left-handers (4). Based on detailed analyses, the authors conclude that the first two classes should be accumulated because very high probabilities for the right hand in both classes indicate no practical relevance of dividing right-handers into two classes even though the statistics indicate a four-class solution. In addition, they reported a two-class solution for the LCA with 90.84% right-handers and 9.16% left-handers. The authors conclude that the usage of mixed-Rasch models could be the most promising method due to the joint understanding of handedness or even laterality, consisting of both a qualitative latent variable and a continuous latent trait (Merni et al., 2014). Consistent with the results from handedness, Tran, Stieger, and Voracek (2014b) question laterality as being one-dimensional. The authors investigated the latent variable underlying handedness (10-item EHI), footedness, eyedness, and earedness (three scales of the LPI) using structural equation modeling and LCA in 15,175 participants and suggest a three-dimensional approach to laterality.

The studies applying probabilistic models to handedness assessments provide promising results. Until now, predominantly for handedness (as a major component of laterality) it has been shown that the assumption of laterality as a one-dimensional latent trait, for example interpreting a single score on a quantitative continuum as the *LQ*, should not be used in the future. In conclusion, the mentioned studies showed that laterality should no longer be regarded as a one-dimensional trait and, from a methodological-statistical point of view, the relevance of mixed-handers can be questioned (e.g., Büsch et al., 2010; Dragovic, 2004b; Dragovic & Hammond, 2007; Merni et al., 2014). Although this paragraph focused on the EHI, it can be assumed and discussed to what extent the results can be transferred to further laterality aspects than handedness. More existing assessment tools, also including performance tests, should be put in a test theoretical focus to gain deeper insight into the latent structure of laterality. Using probabilistic models, laterality assessments can be enhanced on the one hand by validating used interpretation methods as sum scores by detecting nonfitting items. On the other hand, probabilistic models can valuably contribute to enhance the structural understanding of laterality.

CONCLUSION

Comparing the above-mentioned concepts, no consistent assumptions concerning the structure of laterality have currently been made. This is not only due to the heterogeneous approaches, but also due to the changing definition of laterality (Musálek, 2015). Although this chapter mainly focuses on handedness, many aspects can be transferred to other dimensions of laterality. Without a given context, it cannot be decided which approach is most suitable, but it can be stated that there is not a single best way to indicate an individual's laterality, not even handedness (Bishop, Ross, Daniels, & Bright, 1996). For instance, studies comparing performance tests to other types of assessments, such as preference tests or self-report preference questionnaires, did not find additional information given by the more time-consuming performance tests (van Strien, 2003). Performance tests might even be biased in many motor tasks due to everyday experiences (Büsch & Hagemann, 2013; Provins, 1997). For these reasons, performance tests are often not favored as a singular diagnosis tool in practice. Nevertheless, it can be valuable to observe the quality of performances to gain additional objective information about one's laterality in comparison to subjective assessments via self-reports (Elliott & Roy, 1996). In general, conducting self-report preference questionnaires shows the highest reliability and validity compared to their popular alternative assessment counterparts and requires the least amount of time (Bryden et al., 2000). Yet, diagnosing an individual's laterality solely on self-report preference questionnaires can cause problems. Some researchers question preference tasks to be reliable predictors of laterality (Annett, 1970). In preference or performance tasks an individual responds in a relatively spontaneous manner and cannot influence the results in a subjective way due to a given number of options (Brown, Roy, Rohr, & Bryden, 2006; Bryden et al., 2000). Particularly in specific sport settings a questionnaire might not be the gold standard. The development of sport-specific test instruments is required in order to ensure reliable and valid estimations of an individual's laterality, because reliability can often only be achieved by a combination of tests (Loffing et al., 2014; Overbeck, 1989). Nevertheless, not only the amount of approaches (upper limb, lower limb, eyedness, earedness, turning preference) assessing laterality, but also the different theoretical assumptions of the concept of laterality due to the character of the measured variables, can exert influence.

Especially in specific sport settings a lack of valid assessments can be observed. It is important to assess the intrinsic importance of laterality depending on situation and purpose. Hence, alternative sport-specific test instruments can provide additional valuable information and deeper insight in an individual's laterality compared to their conventional counterparts. This means assessing laterality, especially functional laterality, has to be considered in respect to the given research question, especially in sports. For instance, for a wide field of sports, turning preference (e.g., gymnastics, motorsports, winter sports) or dominant eye (e.g., archery) can play major roles (see Arnold-Schulz-Gahmen, Siefer, & Ehrenstein, 2006; Overbeck, 1989). The assessment of these preferences of laterality is mostly limited to the performance of sport-specific skills, for instance jumping 360 degrees in gymnastics (Olislagers, 1983), performing a pirouette in figure skating (Stein, 1959), or performing a breaststroke turn in swimming (Fetz & Werner, 1981). In summary the results of sport-specific laterality assessment can indicate specific laterality distributions, which might be incongruent in comparison to, for example, handedness (Loffing et al., 2014). Studies evaluating quality criteria of assessments aiming on sport-specific phenomena of laterality remain almost completely absent to date. Furthermore, investigating laterality in sports comprises some specific challenges. The development of laterality is in many situations not solely determined based on experience. It can for instance be influenced by critical events such as serious injuries (Kuhn, 1987). Moreover, in complex sport settings such as mastering and enhancing specific movements or sequences, initial side preferences can lead to disadvantages in beneficial end-state movement positions. Also everyday training processes can play an important role, when specific instructions due to coaching style or coach preferences lead to individual learning trajectories or fundamental relearn processes among athletes.

One major issue regarding the three described test forms is that these focus predominantly on adults. Thus assessment tools need to be validated for specific populations and varying age groups (Obrzut, Dalby, Boliek, & Cannon, 1992; Tran et al., 2014, 2014a). The lack of research on younger children is sometimes attributed to the tasks requiring both hands when performed by children potentially having trouble to appropriately identify the test's intention. For example, in the item writing (EHI), the nondominant hand is still used to fixate the paper. Moreover, specific items are composed of skills where the process of execution is not yet automatic. Also some complex tasks place high demands on coordination, which is not as well developed in children (Musálek, 2014) and therefore could possibly assess intelligence and learning effects more than actual laterality. The same could be stated for populations with physical or mental impairment, such as patients with Parkinson's Disease (Berardelli, Rothwell, Thompson, & Hallet, 2001). Another issue with assessing specific populations is that laterality assessment requires large sample sizes to obtain findings with acceptable statistical power (Coren, 1993) and a clear and concise definition of laterality (Dragovic & Hammond, 2007).

Three different scale types of laterality have been introduced (Fig. 4.1). The given differences can be quite important not only from a test theoretical point of view, but also because they reflect the heterogeneity of the different concepts of laterality. Merni et al. (2014) state that, from a practical view, an assumed difference between qualitative and quantitative latent variables is not important. They argue that measuring a continuous latent variable was always discrete, and therefore it is possible to approximate the distribution of the continuous latent variable by a discrete distribution (Heinen, 1996). From a meta-perspective, these differences in the latent variable are the most important aspect in terms of concept, model evaluation, and development, since laterality assessment can only be valid to the degree of which the underlying concept itself is valid. There are some promising studies using probabilistic models to gain deeper insight into this concept. Until today, it has been most commonly stated that laterality is a one-dimensional trait, which is shown by the interpretation of laterality as a summed-up score or a certain LQ in the majority of assessments. Using the probabilistic approach, several studies have shown that laterality should not be seen as a one-dimensional trait. The field of laterality provides numerous unanswered questions, since only a few steps have been made in applying probabilistic models to preference data or self-report preference questionnaires. For instance, no study was found conducting probabilistic models to performance data.

In summary, the use of inappropriate interpretation methods to indicate laterality can lead to major misinterpretations (see the detailed analysis of the EHI). In the future, modeling laterality as a latent trait using probabilistic models seems the most promising way to further develop a structural understanding of laterality. Especially practical applications can benefit from a solid theoretical foundation.

References

Alagumalai, S., Curtis, D. D., & Hungi, N. (2005). *Applied Rasch measurement: A book of exemplars*. Dordrecht: Springer.

Annett, M. (1967). The binomial distribution of right, mixed and left handedness. *Quarterly Journal of Experimental Psychology*, 19(4), 327–333.

Annett, M. (1970). A classification of hand preference by association analysis. *British Journal of Psychology*, 61(3), 303–321.

Annett, M. (1972). The distribution of manual asymmetry. *British Journal of Psychology*, 63(3), 343–358.

Annett, M. (2002). *Handedness and brain asymmetry: The right shift theory*. Hove: Psychology Press.

Arnold-Schulz-Gahmen, B. E., Siefer, A., & Ehrenstein, W. H. (2006). Sensomotorische Seitenbevorzugung und sportliche Spezialisierung [Senso-motor laterality preference and sport specialisation]. In B. Halberschmidt, & B. Strauß (Eds.), *Elf Freunde sollt ihr sein!? 38. Jahrestagung der Arbeitsgemeinschaft für Sportpsychologie (asp) gemeinsam mit dem Bundesinstitut für Sportwissenschaft vom 25–27.05.2006 in Münster [Proceedings]* (p. 24). Hamburg: Czwalina.

Berardelli, A., Rothwell, J. C., Thompson, P. D., & Hallet, M. (2001). Pathophysiology of bradykinesia in Parkinson's disease. *Brain*, 124(11), 2131–2146.

Berger, S. E., Friedman, R., & Polis, M. C. (2011). The role of locomotor posture and experience on handedness and footedness in infancy. *Infant Behavior and Development*, 34(3), 472–480.

Bishop, D. V. M., Ross, V. A., Daniels, M. S., & Bright, P. (1996). The measurement of hand preference: a validation study comparing three groups of right-handers. *British Journal of Psychology*, 87, 269–285.

Borod, J. C., Caron, H. S., & Koff, E. (1984). Left–handers and right–handers compared on performance and preference measures of lateral dominance. *British Journal of Psychology*, 75(2), 177–186.

Brown, S., Roy, E., Rohr, L., & Bryden, P. (2006). Using hand performance measures to predict handedness. *Laterality: Asymmetries of Body, Brain and Cognition*, 11(1), 1–14.

Bryden, M. P. (1977). Measuring handedness with questionnaires. *Neuropsychologia*, 15(4), 617–624.

Bryden, P. J. (2000). Lateral preference, skilled behaviour and task complexity: hand and foot. In M. K. Mandal, M. B. Bulman-Fleming, & G. Tiwari (Eds.), *Side bias: A neuropsychological perspective* (pp. 225–248). Dordrecht: Springer.

Bryden, M. P., Mandal, M. K., & Ida, Y. (2000). Factor structure of hand preference question-naires. In M. B. Bulman-Fleming, M. K. Mandal, & G. Tiwari (Eds.), *Side bias: Neuropsychological perspective* (pp. 175–190). Dordrecht: Springer.

Bryden, P. J., Roy, E. A., & Spence, J. (2007). An observational method of assessing handedness in children and adults. *Developmental Neuropsychology, 32*(3), 825–846.

Büsch, D., & Hagemann, N. (2013). Leistungsasymmetrien von Linkshändern in Abhängigkeit manueller Erfahrungen [Performance asymmetry of left-handers depending on manual experiences]. *Zeitschrift für Sportpsychologie, 20*(2), 65–71.

Büsch, D., Hagemann, N., & Bender, N. (2009). Das Lateral Preference Inventory: Itemhomogenität der deutschen Version [The Lateral Preference Inventory: item homogeneity of the German version]. *Zeitschrift für Sportpsychologie, 16*(1), 17–28.

Büsch, D., Hagemann, N., & Bender, N. (2010). The dimensionality of the Edinburgh Handedness Inventory: an analysis with models of the item response theory. *Laterality: Asymmetries of Body, Brain and Cognition, 15*(6), 610–628.

Chapman, L. J., & Chapman, J. P. (1987). The measurement of handedness. *Brain and Cognition, 6*(2), 175–183.

Chapman, J. P., Chapman, L. J., & Allen, J. J. (1987). The measurement of foot preference. *Neuropsychologia, 25*(3), 579–584.

Corballis, M. C. (2010). Handedness and cerebral asymmetry: an evolutionary perspective. In K. Hugdahl, & R. Westerhausen (Eds.), *The two halves of the brain: Information processing in the cerebral hemispheres* (1st ed.) (pp. 65–88). Cambridge: MIT Press.

Coren, S. (1993). Failure to find statistical significance in left-handedness and pathology studies: a forgotten consideration. *Bulletin of the Psychonomic Society, 31*(5), 443–446.

Coren, S., Porac, C., & Duncan, P. (1979). A behaviorally validated self-report inventory to assess four types of lateral preference. *Journal of Clinical and Experimental Neuropsychology, 1*(1), 55–64.

Corey, D. M., Hurley, M. M., & Foundas, A. L. (2001). Right and left handedness defined: a multivariate approach using hand preference and hand performance measures. *Cognitive and Behavioral Neurology, 14*(3), 144–152.

von Davier, M., & Carstensen, C. H. (2007). *Multivariate and mixture distribution Rasch models: Extensions and applications.* Berlin: Springer.

Doyen, A. L., & Carlier, M. (2002). Measuring handedness: a validation study of Bishop's reaching card test. *Laterality: Asymmetries of Body, Brain and Cognition, 7*(2), 115–130.

Dragovic, M. (2004a). Categorization and validation of handedness using latent class analysis. *Acta Neuropsychiatrica, 16*(4), 212–218.

Dragovic, M. (2004b). Towards an improved measure of the Edinburgh Handedness Inventory: a one-factor congeneric measurement model using confirmatory factor analysis. *Laterality: Asymmetries of Body, Brain and Cognition, 9*(4), 411–419.

Dragovic, M., & Hammond, G. (2007). A classification of handedness using the Annett hand preference questionnaire. *British Journal of Psychology, 98*(3), 375–387.

Elias, L. J., Bryden, M. P., & Bulman-Fleming, M. B. (1998). Footedness is a better predictor than is handedness of emotional lateralization. *Neuropsychologia, 36*(1), 37–43.

Elliott, D., & Roy, E. A. (1996). *Manual asymmetries in motor performance.* Boca Raton: CRC Press.

Eyre, M. B., & Schmeeckle, M. M. (1933). A study of handedness, eyedness, and footedness. *Child Development, 4*(1), 73–78.

Fazio, R. L., & Cantor, J. M. (2015). Factor structure of the Edinburgh Handedness Inventory versus the Fazio Laterality Inventory in a population with established atypical handedness. *Applied Neuropsychology: Adult, 22*(2), 156–160.

Fazio, R., Coenen, C., & Denney, R. L. (2012). The original instructions for the Edinburgh Handedness Inventory are misunderstood by a majority of participants. *Laterality: Asymmetries of Body, Brain and Cognition, 17*(1), 70–77.

Fazio, R., Dunham, K. J., Griswold, S., & Denney, R. L. (2013). An improved measure of handedness: the Fazio Laterality Inventory. *Applied Neuropsychology: Adult, 20*(3), 197–202.

Fetz, F., & Werner, I. (1981). Trainingsbedingte Ausprägung der Wendigkeit [Training-induced characteristics of maneuverability]. *Leibesübungen[Leibserziehung], 20*, 132–133.

Gilbert, A. N., & Wysocki, C. J. (1992). Hand preference and age in the United States. *Neuropsychologia, 30*(7), 601–608.

Groden, G. (1969). Lateral preferences in normal children. *Perceptual and Motor Skills, 28*(1), 213–214.

Harris, A. J. (1947). *Harris tests of lateral dominance: Manual of directions for administration and interpretation.* New York: Psychological Corporation.

Hécaen, H., & Ajuriaguerra, J. (1964). *Left-handedness: Manual superiority and cerebral dominance.* New York: Grune & Stratton.

Heinen, T. (1996). *Latent class and discrete latent trait models: Similarities and differences.* Thousand Oaks: Sage Publication Inc.

Humphrey, M. (1951). *Handedness and cerebral dominance* (B.Sc. thesis). Oxford University.

Ida, Y., Mandal, M. K., & Bryden, M. P. (2000). Factor structures of hand preference questionnaires: are "skilled" and "unskilled" factors artifacts? In M. K. Mandal, M. B. Bulman-Fleming, & G. Tiwari (Eds.), *Side bias: Neuropsychological perspective* (pp. 175–190). Dordrecht: Springer.

Kastner-Koller, U., Deimann, P., & Bruckner, J. (2007). Assessing handedness in pre-schoolers: construction and initial validation of a hand preference test for 4–6-year-olds. *Psychology Science, 49*(3), 239–254.

Kraemer, D., Canavan, P., Brannigan, G. G., & Hijikata, S. (1983). The torque test as a measure of lateral dominance. *The Journal of Genetic Psychology, 143*(2), 251–258.

Kuhn, W. (1987). *Zum Phänomen des kontralateralen Transfers [The phenomenon of contralateral transfer].* Cologne: BPS.

Loffing, F., Sölter, F., & Hagemann, N. (2014). Left preference for sport tasks does not necessarily indicate left-handedness: sport-specific lateral preferences, relationship with handedness and implications for laterality research in behavioural sciences. *PLoS One, 9*, e105800.

Marchant, L. F., McGrew, W. C., & Eibl–Eibesfeldt, I. (1995). Is human handedness universal? Ethological analyses from three traditional cultures. *Ethology, 101*(3), 239–258.

Markoulakis, R., Scharoun, S. M., Bryden, P. J., & Fletcher, P. C. (2012). An examination of handedness and footedness in children with high functioning autism and Asperger syndrome. *Journal of Autism and Developmental Disorders, 42*(10), 2192–2201.

Martin, W. L. B., & Machado, A. H. (2005). Deriving estimates of contralateral footedness from prevalence rates in samples of Brazilian and non-Brazilian right-and left-handers. *Laterality: Asymmetries of Body, Brain and Cognition, 10*(4), 353–368.

Masters, G. N. (1982). A Rasch model for partial credit scoring. *Psychometrika, 47*(2), 149–174.

McMeekan, E. R. L., & Lishman, W. A. (1975). Retest reliabilities and interrelationship of the Annett hand preference questionnaire and the Edinburgh Handedness Inventory. *British Journal of Psychology, 66*(1), 53–59.

Merni, F., Di Michele, R., & Soffritti, G. (2014). Assessment of handedness using latent class factor analysis. *Laterality: Asymmetries of Body, Brain and Cognition, 19*(4), 405–423.

Milenkovic, S., & Dragovic, M. (2013). Modification of the Edinburgh Handedness Inventory: a replication study. *Laterality: Asymmetries of Body, Brain and Cognition, 18*(3), 340–348.

Musálek, M. (2014). *Development of test batteries for diagnostics of motor laterality manifestation: Link between cerebellar dominance and hand performance.* Prague: Karolinum Press.

Musálek, M. (2015). Skilled performance tests and their use in diagnosing handedness and footedness at children of lower school age 8–10. *Frontiers in Psychology, 5*, 1513.

Nicholls, M. E., Thomas, N. A., Loetscher, T., & Grimshaw, G. M. (2013). The Flinders Handedness survey (FLANDERS): a brief measure of skilled hand preference. *Cortex, 49*(10), 2914–2926.

A. LATERALITY – AN IMPORTANT AND OFTEN DISREGARDED TOPIC

Obrzut, J. E., Dalby, P. R., Boliek, C. A., & Cannon, G. E. (1992). Factorial structure of the Waterloo Handedness Questionnaire for control and learning-disabled adults. *Journal of Clinical and Experimental Neuropsychology, 14*(6), 935–950.

Oldfield, R. C. (1971). The assessment and analysis of handedness: the Edinburgh inventory. *Neuropsychologia, 9*(1), 97–113.

Olislagers, P. (1983). Die Längsrotationen des Körpers beim Turnen [The axial rotation of the body in gymnastics]. In H. Rieder, K. Bös, H. Mechling, & K. Reischle (Eds.), *Motorik und Bewegungsforschung. Ein Beitrag zum Lernen im Sport* (pp. 209–215). Schorndorf: Hofmann.

Overbeck, H. (1989). *Seitigkeitsphänomene und Seitigkeitstypologie im Sport [Laterality phenomena and laterality typology in sports]*. Schorndorf: Hofmann.

Parson, B. S. (1924). *Left-handednesss*. New York: Macmillan Co.

Peters, M. (1998). Description and validation of a flexible and broadly usable handedness questionnaire. *Laterality: Asymmetries of Body, Brain and Cognition, 3*(1), 77–96.

Peters, M., & Durding, B. (1979). Left-handers and right-handers compared on a motor task. *Journal of Motor Behavior, 11*(2), 103–111.

Peters, M., & Murphy, K. (1992). Cluster analysis reveals at least three, and possibly five distinct handedness groups. *Neuropsychologia, 30*(4), 373–380.

Peters, M., & Surfing, B. (1978). Handedness measure by finger tapping: a continuous variable. *Canadian Journal of Psychology, 32*(4), 257–261.

Porac, C., & Coren, S. (1981). *Lateral preferences and human behaviour*. New York: Springer.

Provins, K. (1997). The specificity of motor skill and manual asymmetry: a review of the evidence and its implications. *Journal of Motor Behavior, 29*(2), 183–192.

Ransil, B. J., & Schachter, S. C. (1994). Test-retest reliability of the Edinburgh Handedness Inventory and Global Handedness preference measurements, and their correlation. *Perceptual and Motor Skills, 79*(3), 1355–1372.

Rasch, G. (1960). *Probabilistic models for some intelligence and achievement tests*. Copenhagen: Danish Institute for Educational Research.

Richardson, J. S. (1976). Handedness of crossover connections in beta sheets. *Proceedings of the National Academy of Sciences, 73*(8), 2619–2623.

Richardson, J. T. (1978). A factor analysis of self-reported handedness. *Neuropsychologia, 16*(6), 747–748.

Rigal, R. A. (1992). Which handedness: preference or performance? *Perceptual and Motor Skills, 75*(3), 851–866.

Rost, J. (1990). Rasch models in latent classes: an integration of two approaches to item analysis. *Applied Psychological Measurement, 14*(3), 271–282.

Rost, J. (2004). *Lehrbuch Testtheorie – Testkonstruktion [Textbook of test theory – Test construction]*. Bern: Huber.

Roy, E. A., & Elliott, D. (1986). Manual asymmetries in visually directed aiming. *Canadian Journal of PsychologyRevue canadienne de psychologie, 40*(2), 109–121.

Safrit, M. J., & Wood, T. M. (1989). *Measurement concepts in physical education and exercise science*. Champaign, IL: Human Kinetics.

Saudino, K., & McManus, I. C. (1998). Handedness, footedness, eyedness and earedness in the Colorado Adoption Project. *British Journal of Developmental Psychology, 16*(2), 167–174.

Schachter, S. C. (2000). The quantification and definition of handedness: implications for handedness research. In M. K. Mandal, M. B. Bulman-Fleming, & G. Tiwari (Eds.), *Side bias: A neuropsychological perspective* (pp. 155–174). Dordrecht: Kluwer.

Schachter, S. C., Ransil, B. J., & Geschwind, N. (1987). Associations of handedness with hair color and learning disabilities. *Neuropsychologia, 25*(1), 269–276.

Sherman, J. L., Kulhavy, R. W., & Bretzing, B. H. (1976). The Sherman-Kulhavy Laterality Assessment Inventory: some validation data. *Perceptual and Motor Skills, 42*(3c), 1314.

Stein, F. (1959). Der "natürliche Drehsinn" [The "natural sense of rotation"]. *Sportarzt, 10*(4), 84–85.

Steingrüber, H. J., & Lienert, G. A. (1971). *Hand-dominanz-test: HDT* [*Hand-dominance-test: HDT*]. Göttingen: Hogrefe.

Strauss, B., Büsch, D., & Tenenbaum, G. (2007). New perspectives on measurement and testing in sport psychology. In G. Tenenbaum, & R. C. Eklund (Eds.), *Handbook of sport psychology* (3rd ed.) (pp. 735–756). Hoboken: John Wiley & Sons, Inc.

Strauss, B., Büsch, D., & Tenenbaum, G. (2012). Rasch modeling in sports. In G. Tenenbaum, R. C. Eklund, & A. Kamata (Eds.), *Handbook of measurement in sports* (pp. 75–80). New York: Human Kinetics.

van Strien, J. W. (2003). *The Dutch handedness questionnaire*. Rotterdam: Faculty of Social Sciences (FSS), Erasmus University Rotterdam.

Tapley, S. M., & Bryden, M. P. (1985). A group test for the assessment of performance between the hands. *Neuropsychologia, 23*(2), 215–221.

Tiffin, J., & Asher, E. J. (1948). The purdue pegboard: norms and studies of reliability and validity. *Journal of Applied Psychology, 32*(3), 234–247.

Tirosh, E., Stein, M., Harel, J., & Scher, A. (1999). Hand preference as related to development and behavior in infancy. *Perceptual and Motor Skills, 89*(2), 371–380.

Tran, U. S., Koller, I., Nader, I. W., Pietschnig, J., Schild, A. H., Stieger, S., … Voracek, M. (2014). Lateral preferences for hand clasping and arm folding are associated with handedness in two large-sample latent variable analyses. *Laterality: Asymmetries of Body, Brain and Cognition, 19*(5), 602–614.

Tran, U. S., Stieger, S., & Voracek, M. (2014a). Latent variable analysis indicates that seasonal anisotropy accounts for the higher prevalence of left-handedness in men. *Cortex, 57*, 188–197.

Tran, U. S., Stieger, S., & Voracek, M. (2014b). Evidence for general right-, mixed-, and left-sidedness in self-reported handedness, footedness, eyedness, and earedness, and a primacy of footedness in a large-sample latent variable analysis. *Neuropsychologia, 62*, 220–232.

Triggs, W. J., Calvanio, R., Levine, M., Heaton, R. K., & Heilman, K. M. (2000). Predicting hand preference with performance on motor tasks. *Cortex, 36*(5), 679–689.

Veale, J. F. (2014). Edinburgh handedness inventory–short form: a revised version based on confirmatory factor analysis. *Laterality: Asymmetries of Body, Brain and Cognition, 19*(2), 164–177.

White, K., & Ashton, R. (1976). Handedness assessment inventory. *Neuropsychologia, 14*(2), 261–264.

Williams, M. S. (1986). Factor analysis of the Edinburgh Handedness Inventory. *Cortex, 22*, 325–326.

Williams, S. M. (1991). Handedness inventories: Edinburgh versus Annett. *Neuropsychology, 5*(1), 43–48.

Wood, T. M., & Zhu, W. (Eds.). (2006). *Measurement theory and practice in kinesiology*. Champaign, IL: Human Kinetics.

Ziyagil, M. A. (2011). Handedness and footedness: relations to differences in sprinting speed and multiple sprint performance in prepubertal boys. *Perceptual and Motor Skills, 112*(2), 440–450.

Laterality and Its Role in Talent Identification and Athlete Development

Jörg Schorer, Judith Tirp, Christina Steingröver
University of Oldenburg, Oldenburg, Germany

Joseph Baker
York University, Toronto, ON, Canada

In medieval times, palm reading was often used to predict a person's future. At this time (and today for those keen to spend their money on quackery and shams), palm readers used length and disturbances in "life lines" and "heart lines" to make predictions about the future. While palm reading has been long disputed and obviously has little relevance to predicting future sport performances, other characteristics that on the surface might seem equally questionable could help those interested in understanding talent in some sports. Over the last decade in team handball, for example, form, size, and strength of the hand have been investigated as potential predictors of success (Visnapuu & Jürimäe, 2007). The main assumption of this line of research is that size and strength have a direct influence on performance in shooting, catching, and/or dribbling, although this evidence is far from conclusive (Pabst, Büsch, Wilhelm, & Schorer, 2010). Another flourishing area of research considers the ratio between the length of the index and ring fingers (Bennett, Manning, Cook, & Kilduff, 2010; Hönekopp & Schuster, 2010). In talented young handball players, Baker et al. (2013) showed that athletes' digit ratio was smaller than in the normal population, which suggests a greater exposure to testosterone during important phases on prenatal development.

While these findings in "palmistry" are fascinating, this chapter focuses on another "hand-related" variable, specifically how laterality (most commonly associated with "handedness" but including other lateral preferences as well) might influence the identification and selection of talented or promising athletes during the early stages of their career. For better or worse, talent selection is an important and very difficult process on the road to sporting excellence, and an athlete's laterality has rarely been considered in athlete development research. The discussion that follows examines the potential relevance of laterality for talent identification and development.

TALENT IDENTIFICATION AND SELECTION

Before considering whether talent can be identified, it is first important to consider the evidence regarding whether talent actually exists. This might seem counterintuitive, but several researchers have concluded that the notion of talent, that is, an identifiable potential for later success in a domain (Baker, Cobley, & Schorer, 2012), is not viable. For instance, in their article *Innate talent: Reality or myth?*, Howe, Davidson, and Sloboda (1998) concluded that talent was a myth and was not supported by a strong body of evidence. This debate can be framed within larger discussions of nature versus nurture, which has been hotly argued for at least the last century. Although there is still passionate discussion of this debate among the lay public (cf. Epstein, 2013; Gladwell, 2008), most researchers generally agree that environment and genetics interact to hinder or promote athlete success (Baker & Davids, 2007).

There are several complex models of talent; for example, Joch (2000) defined talent using two main components. The first, *static talent*, includes dispositions, motivation, social environment, and current results, while the second, *dynamic talent*, includes the athlete's active development, the availability of structured training, and the pedagogical care taken by an advisor on life development. Similarly, Gagné's Differentiated Model of Giftedness and Talent (2004) makes a distinction between natural abilities (i.e., giftedness) and those qualities that reflect learning and environmental adaptations (i.e., talent). Interestingly, all talent models are based on two assumptions: the first is that talent is identifiable, and the second is that adult performance can be predicted by earlier performance. While these assumptions are hard to prove, they form the basis for research on talent identification and selections.

APPROACHES TO RESEARCHING TALENT

Talent research has generally used two main approaches, as illustrated in Fig. 5.1: the ability approach and the expertise approach (cf. Hohmann, 2009). The *ability approach* focuses on identifying specific sets of stable

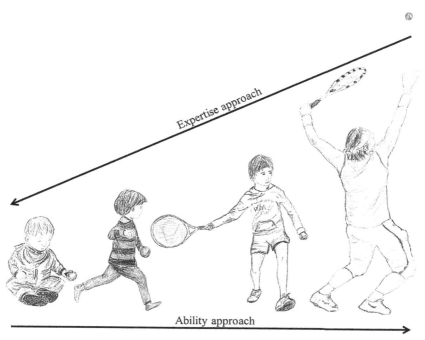

FIGURE 5.1 Graphical description of ability and expertise approach.

abilities in athletes that may give insight into their later performances. Early identification is thought to be necessary by the sporting federations because they have a limited resource pool (e.g., money, coaches) to develop athletes. The abilities examined as part of this approach are generally based on factors drawn from developmental and educational psychology (e.g., motor intelligence or motor abilities).

The *expertise approach* generally uses retrospective methods to look back on the development of top athletes to determine what factors differentiate experts from lesser skilled groups (e.g., novices, nonexperts, or near-experts; Ericsson, 2007; Ericsson & Williams, 2007). Early findings from this approach focused on the role of engagement in "deliberate practice" as the primary explanation for who achieves elite level performance (Ericsson, Krampe, & Tesch-Römer, 1993). Initial work suggested over 10,000h of deliberate practice is required for tasks like chess (Gobet & Charness, 2006; Simon & Chase, 1973) or football and field hockey (Helsen, Starkes, & Hodges, 1998), while other research indicates sporting tasks have varying requirements (Baker, Côté, & Deakin, 2005; Hodges & Starkes, 1996; Starkes, Deakin, Allard, Hodges, & Hayes, 1996).

Arguably, both of these approaches have their benefits, and a combined model for talent selection might best represent the "state of the science".

However, research in this area is surprisingly sparse and, as a result, our understanding of talent prediction is limited (cf. Schorer & Elferink-Gemser, 2013). In the upcoming sections, we summarize what is known about the influence of laterality on this process and speculate regarding areas where laterality could significantly hinder or facilitate talent identification and development.

INFLUENCE OF LATERALITY ON TALENT DEVELOPMENT

Laterality and Genes

To understand the possible relationships between laterality and talent development, it is necessary to consider the influence of different genetic, biological, and environmental factors on laterality. Annett (1985) conducted one of the first studies concerning lateral development, establishing the *right-shift theory*. This theory explained the formation of asymmetries not through the direct influence of varying genes, but through an indirect influence, specifically the presence and absence of cerebral asymmetries which are induced by genes. The basis of this theory is a dominant allele (RS+) (right shift) that is responsible for the development of speech in the left hemisphere, which leads to a higher probability of being right-handed. The presence of a recessive allele (rs-) did not lead to this systematical drift, neither for speech nor for handedness. Referring to the Punnett square and the assumption that all alleles are uniformly distributed, Annett was able to charge the proportion of handedness. The result of the model is almost equal with the actual distribution. This theory influenced Geschwind and Galaburda (1985a, 1985b, 1985c) in their research. They refined Annett's model and assumed a cerebral asymmetry as a normal condition which could be suspended to symmetry by a *left shift factor*. Additionally, this factor might permit an asymmetry which prefers the right hemisphere. In conclusion the basis of this theory is a principal dominance of the left hemisphere. Geschwind and Galaburda (1985b) postulated that the *left shift factor* is influenced by genetic and nongenetic factors. Geschwind and Galaburda (1985b) discussed environmental influences on the development of handedness as well. They stated that cerebral asymmetries, which influence handedness, were characterized by the prenatal proportion of testosterone. The authors evolved a model which considered the greater involvement of the right hemisphere on the dominant hand in men with a higher proportion of prenatal testosterone. This theory was supported by different studies which found a higher amount of left-handers in men (Oldfield, 1971;

Raymond, Pontier, Dufour, & Møller, 1996). Considering handedness and its association with talent development, it is unavoidable to take account of the brain development and structure.

The Role of Laterality in Talent Identification and Development

Talent identification and development in sports invariably involves navigating a series of selection steps. To our knowledge, the only study that has examined the influence of laterality on the probability of being selected during a talent camp is from Baker et al. (2013). In their study, data from German handball national selection camps were analyzed. On the basis of 474 athletes from regional selections, they found a significant overrepresentation of left-handers compared to the normal population in the male subsample, but no effect in young female players. While the results for the males were as expected (cf. Grouios, 2004; Grouios, Tsorbatzoudis, Alexandris, & Barkoukis, 2000; Holtzen, 2000; Raymond et al., 1996), the findings for the females were intriguing. To explain these counterintuitive results, they hypothesized that since the female sample was the younger of a two-year group, the older part of this sample might have been "rich" in left-handers and therefore fewer left-handers were needed (cf. Baker et al., 2013, p. 7).

The authors emphasized that this conclusion required verification, and for this book chapter, we investigated this topic in more depth, analyzing data from three talent selection camps. As can be seen in Table 5.1, the effect was replicated in two other national selection camp years, undermining the hypothesis suggested by Baker et al. (2013). Another potential explanation might be the number of players in female and male youth handball. As Baker, Schorer, Cobley, Bräutigam, & Büsch (2009); Schorer, Cobley, Büsch, Bräutigam, & Baker (2009) noted earlier, in Germany there are far fewer players in female youth handball than in male youth handball, which might

TABLE 5.1 Handedness of German Handball Talents Differentiated by Several Selection Camps and Sexes

Year	Sexes	Left	Right	Chi²-inferentials
2009	Females	30	206	$\chi^2(1, n = 236) = 1.93, p = 0.16$
	Males	37	202	$\chi^2(1, n = 239) = 7.98, p < 0.01$
2010	Females	31	208	$\chi^2(1, n = 239) = 2.34, p = 0.13$
	Males	53	181	$\chi^2(1, n = 234) = 41.60, p < 0.01$
2011	Females	18	216	$\chi^2(1, n = 234) = 1.38, p = 0.24$
	Males	51	185	$\chi^2(1, n = 236) = 35.34, p < 0.01$

affect the strength of the left-hander effect in this sport. Obviously, this explanation requires further exploration, but the paucity of research looking at the potential role of being left-handed in talent selections is surprising given the consistency of the advantage for left-handers in many sports in adulthood (e.g., Grouios, 2004; Raymond et al., 1996).

We also know little about the role of laterality throughout talent development. Sterkowicz, Lech, and Blecharz (2010) investigated throwing direction and lateral dominance of 13- to 14-year-old judoka during an international tournament. From a thrower's perspective, four different throwing directions can be distinguished: front right, front left, rear right, and rear left. Results revealed a significant relationship between handedness and throwing direction. Left-handers chose front left and rear left as their most frequently used throwing option while right-handers primarily chose front right as a throwing direction. Similar results were revealed for footedness as an independent variable: judoka competing with a dominant right foot mostly direct their throws to front right while athletes with a dominant left foot throw primarily to the front left and rear left. Throws directed to the rear right were rarely conducted. The study shows that handedness and footedness correlate with the choice of throwing direction. Additionally, Sterkowicz et al. (2010) demonstrated that athletes in the under 15 age-cohort with a dominant technique on their left body side had significantly better chances of winning medals at the tournament compared to their right-sided counterparts. Left-sided judoka advantages are multifaceted and related to athletes' techniques, strategies, and situational factors. Using the opposite stance, they face their opponents with their left body side and use the grip called *Kenka-yotsu* instead of *Ai-yotsu*. For many right-sided judoka, this is an unusual situation because they compete more frequently against right-sided judoka using the *Ai-yotsu*. Due to the differing initial position, left-sides judokas' actions are harder to predict, and therefore their attacks are more effective. In addition, the less familiar situation might implicate further elements of uncertainty for a right-sided opponent such as unpredictability and the lack of situational control. For the athlete fighting with a dominant left body side, the same situation might have a reversed effect; for example, the left-sided judoka is used to the *Kenka-yotsu*, and this could positively affect his or her self-confidence (Sterkowicz et al., 2010).

Does Left-Handedness Prevent Young Talents From Being Affected by the Relative Age Effect?

Among the variables affecting the development of expert performance in sport are primary (direct) and secondary (indirect) factors (Baker & Horton, 2004). While primary factors are obvious, including training, genes, and psychological qualities, secondary factors are less obvious.

Consider, for example, relative age effects, which appear in many sport systems due to the use of arbitrary cut off dates to determine age cohorts and create homogenous groups. Although well meant, children born shortly after the cut off date are up to 1 year older than later-born children in their respective age group (Musch & Grondin, 2001). Relative age effects in sports are a worldwide phenomenon, existing in many competitive sports (see Cobley, Baker, Wattie, & McKenna, 2009).

One sport where both relative age (Baxter-Jones, Helms, Baines-Preece, & Preece, 1995; Dudink, 1994) and laterality effects (Loffing, Hagemann, & Strauss, 2009, 2010) have been noted is tennis. Loffing, Schorer, and Cobley (2010) examined whether handedness mediated relative age effects in this sport. Birth date and players' handedness were collected for all left- and right-handed professional tennis players ranked among the top 500 at the final Association of Tennis Professionals (ATP) tables of 2000–2006. Not surprisingly, results revealed a clear relative age effect for the total sample including left- and right-handers. Interestingly, when the data were analyzed by laterality, significantly skewed birthdate distributions were revealed only for right-handers with no relative age effects for left-handed tennis players. Loffing, Schorer, et al. (2010) suggested that left-handed players were less affected by relative age effects than their right-handed counterparts. While right-handed players might use maturity-related advantages to defeat their opponents at early stages of their career, left-handed players seem to benefit from performance advantages associated with *negative frequency-dependent effects* (Hagemann, 2009; Raymond et al., 1996; see also Faurie, Uomini, & Raymond, in this book).[1] Possibly, relatively younger tennis players can counterbalance possible disadvantages caused by differences in biological age when they are left-handed. For example, owing to left-handed players' relative rarity compared to right-handers (Schorer, Loffing, Hagemann, & Baker, 2012), athletes have difficulties predicting left-handers' action outcomes and adapting to left-handers' playing style (cf. Loffing, Schorer, Hagemann, & Baker, 2012). This, in turn, might give left-handed players a performance advantage.

Since relative age effects remain an unsolved problem in many sports where cut off dates are used and selection processes take place, the fact that left-handers overcome possible disadvantages is an important issue. Identifying further moderators of the relative age effect and understanding the underlying mechanisms is essential for sporting success as well as talent detection and successful individual development.

[1] Alternatively, from a "biological" perspective, proponents of the *innate superiority hypothesis* argue that left-handers benefit, among others, from more efficient neuropsychological processes associated with right hemisphere specialization (e.g., Geschwind & Galaburda, 1985a, 1985b, 1985c, 1987; Gursoy, 2009; Holtzen, 2000). For more detailed discussion of hypotheses and related findings, we would like to direct our readers to Loffing and Hagemann (in this book).

In a related study, Schorer et al. (2009) considered laterality and playing positions as possible moderators of relative age effects in handball. On some positions (especially wing and backcourt players), performance may benefit from both physical attributes such as height and strength and from laterality, that is, the preferred hand used in throwing. The fact that up to 28% of the players in a handball team are left-handed (compared to only 10–13% in the normal population; Raymond et al., 1996) suggests that being left-handed provides some advantage in this sport. Schorer et al. (2009) demonstrated that the size of relative age effects (RAEs) interacts with playing positions affected by laterality, with positions that are advantageous to left-handers demonstrating weaker relative age effects. However, the need for left-handers on certain handball playing positions may be one mechanism that protects players from relative age effects and therefore from one of the most prevalent selection bias in talent development systems.

Collectively, studies indicate that laterality is one of numerous factors influencing an athlete's development (e.g., Loffing, Schorer, et al., 2010). Left-handers seem to benefit primarily from the fact that they represent a minority in the normal population, and that this specific characteristic causes problems for their opponents in several interactive sports (*negative frequency-dependent effect hypothesis*; Faurie & Raymond, 2005, 2013; Raymond et al., 1996). More research, however, is needed to determine the particular role laterality plays in the complex process of talent identification and development.

EXPERTISE RESEARCH AND LATERALITY: REAL EXPERTS ARE RARE IN THEIR OCCURRENCE

When considering expert performances, often researchers look for similarities between athletes. Experts in varying disciplines share left- including Lionel Messi and Diego Maradona (soccer), Muhammad Ali (boxing), Wayne Gretzky (ice hockey), John McEnroe and Monica Seles (tennis), Toni Kukoc (basketball), and Ted Williams (baseball). Beyond such anecdotal evidence of exceptional left-handed athletes, however, it is important to ask, with the potential role of laterality for talent identification and development in mind, whether there is solid empirical evidence to suggest that left-handers are more likely to be successful than right-handers?

Overrepresentation of Functional Left Dominance in Various Fields of Sporting Activity

As noted earlier, the incidence of left-handers relative to right-handers in the general population is about 10–13% (Europe, North America). Although this proportion can range between 3.3% and 26.9% across different cultures

(Faurie, Schiefenhovel, Le Bomin, Billiard, & Raymond, 2005; Raymond et al., 1996), the proportion of left-handers in the normal population overall is obviously lower compared to right handers. An overrepresentation of left-handers has been shown in sporting disciplines such as tennis (Holtzen, 2000), baseball (Grondin, Guiard, Ivry, & Koren, 1999), or boxing (Gursoy, 2009). This effect does not seem to be limited to handedness. For example, Grouios, Kollias, Koidou, and Podrei (2002) considered the representation of footedness (defined using the Waterloo Footedness Questionnaire-Revised) between professional soccer players and nonsporting university students as a marker of laterality. Results showed an overrepresentation of mixed-footed and left-footed soccer players compared to normal population estimates. Similarly, Grouios, Kollias, Tsorbatzoudis, and Alexandris (2002) considered the relationship between the representations of footedness with different expertise levels in soccer, showing that left-footedness is overrepresented in professional and semiprofessional soccer players compared to amateur soccer players and nonsporting students.

These exemplar findings of left-dominant athletes' overrepresentation in various sporting domains lead to the question of whether these athletes may have benefits compared with their right-dominant counterparts in different sporting disciplines. Gobet and Campitelli (2007) investigated whether handedness was related to skill and expertise among skill levels of Argentinian chess players (3 grandmasters, 10 international masters, 13 FIDE Masters, 39 international players untitled, 39 noninternational players, and 87 nonchess athletes). Their study collected skill level (ranking place, birth date, chess rating, started age, etc.), training (hours per week, tournament games, studying, and practicing with others), and handedness as assessed by both self-definition and the Edinburgh Handedness Inventory (EHI; Oldfield, 1971). With regard to self-defined handedness, an overrepresentation of nonright-handed (i.e., left-handed or ambidextrous) chess players (17.9%) compared to a normal population control sample (10.2%) was found. Further analysis of degree of handedness, as obtained from the EHI, revealed lower mean scores for the chess players compared to the control group. Within chess sample comparisons did not indicate any relationship between handedness and chess skill. Additionally, the authors investigated whether there is a critical period (i.e., starting age) in the development of chess expertise. Results indicated that chess players who became experts later joined a chess club at the age of 12 or earlier. Two exceptions were one international and one FIDE master who joined a club at the age of 15, who, interestingly, were either self-defined left-handed or ambidextrous.

Performance Advantages of Left-Dominant Athletes

Holtzen (2000) investigated whether left-handed professional tennis players have advantages compared to their right-handed counterparts.

In addition to considering whether left-handers were more likely to become a professional tennis player, Holtzen (2000) examined whether left-handed tennis players were more successful in competition than right-handed athletes. The latter issue was investigated using different success factors including world number one ranking, world top ten ranking, different single Championships, and finalists at Grand Slam competitions. For male athletes, data from 1981, 1986, 1987, and 1999 were analyzed. Similarly, data for female tennis players from 1981, 1986, and 1999 were used. Although there was *no significant overrepresentation* of left-handers compared to the general population, there was an overrepresentation of left-handers among the success variables in both genders. In all factors the frequency of left-handers was much higher than in the general population. In a separate analysis, Holtzen (2000) considered the frequency of all left-handed tour members from 1999. The results showed an overrepresentation of left-handed male athletes for the ranking range 1–250 but not for female athletes. He noted that left-handed tennis players have a significant advantage in professional tennis compared to their right-handed counterparts (but see Loffing, Hagemann, & Strauss, 2012).

Puterman, Schorer, and Baker (2010) focused on laterality differences in elite ice hockey players. They investigated laterality occurrence in different hockey leagues (study 1: 2006–2007), strategic advantages between laterality and performance (study 2: 1917–2006), and the specific strategic advantage of laterality in penalty shots (study 3: 2005–2007). In study 1, for example, they considered data from three different hockey leagues: Ontario Hockey League (semiprofessional), American Hockey League (professional league), and National Hockey League (highest professional hockey league in America). The shot side of the field players and the catch side of the goalkeepers were examined based on the hypothesis that higher expertise levels would show different laterality occurrences. Data from 2187 male ice hockey players showed that the proportion of left-shooting players increased slightly with expertise level (OHL 59%, AL 60%, NHL 64%). There were positional differences, however. The proportion of right shooters in the right wing position decreased with expertise level (OHL 85%, AHL 82%, NHL 71%). Similarly, there was a significant increase in left-catching goalkeepers with competition level (OHL 66%, AHL 86%, NHL 90%).

Carey et al. (2001) analyzed the footedness of players participating at the 1998 FIFA World Cup. The authors tested the assumption that, in professional soccer, most players are mixed-footed. To this end, they analyzed performances of 236 players from 16 teams by recording how players used their left and right feet for passing, shooting, stopping, etc. Accordingly, 79% of players were classified as right-footed and about 21% of players were left-footed, indicating no overrepresentation of left-footed players relative to normal population estimates (see also Carey et al., 2009). Consideration of success rates of left- and right-footed players revealed no significant relationship.

Performance Advantages of Left-Dominant Athletes in Combat Sports

Combat sports have regularly considered the strategic and tactical value of left- versus right-orientations, and researchers have performed several investigations of these effects. Gursoy (2009), for example, considered success rates of 14 right-handed and 8 left-handed semiprofessional or amateur boxers from a Turkish boxing club. Boxers' handedness was assessed by the EHI (Oldfield, 1971). The author found that left-handed athletes lost significantly fewer fights compared to their right-handed counterparts, and he attributed this finding to left-handers' superior spatiomotor skills. As one limitation, however, Gursoy (2009) did not consider the boxers' combat stance, and it is unclear from this work whether findings may not alternatively be explained by a performance advantage of relatively rarer left-oriented fighters as suggested by the negative frequency-dependent effect hypothesis (cf. Raymond et al., 1996).

In a related study, Tirp, Baker, Weigelt, and Schorer (2014) considered the association between laterality and success at different competition levels in judo. To this end, they identified left and right combat stance preference of 840 male judoka in three different competition levels (Olympic Games $n = 204$, German National Championships $n = 203$, and German University Championships $n = 433$). Competition level data were obtained from five Olympic Games (1996–2012), six German Championships (2005–2011) and five German University Championships (2008–2012). The authors used lateral preference data from athletes ranked 7th or worse at the 2011 German University Championships as the baseline for normative combat stance distribution, because for participating at the University Championships, no qualification is needed (i.e., every student within a judo program is allowed to participate at this tournament without preceding selection). Compared to the baseline distribution a significant overrepresentation of the ranked judoka (all tournaments, ranked 1st–5th) was found. Between-tournament comparisons revealed that the proportion of left-fighters was highest in the Olympic Games, while the German Championships showed a lower percentage of left-fighters compared to the German University Championships.

Similarly, Baker and Schorer (2013) investigated lateral preferences of mixed martial arts (MMA) fighters. They analyzed data from 1468 MMA fighters and considered the association of combat stance and winning percentage by categorizing the athletes in groups with nearly the same number of fights. The results showed significant differences in the number of fights with left-sided fighters (i.e., "southpaws") having more fights, but there was no statistical relationship between combat stance and winning percentage.

It is conspicuous that the left-dominant athletes' advantage seems to be more dominant in interactive sports. Grouios et al. (2000) tried to categorize the advantage of left-handers in varying disciplines. First, they divided sporting disciplines into two groups: interactive (i.e., handball, judo, boxing) and noninteractive (i.e., swimming, gymnastics) sports. They also divided the interactive disciplines into direct disciplines (i.e., judo, boxing, fencing) and indirect disciplines (i.e., basketball, tennis). They investigated the occurrence of left-handers in athletes from these disciplines and nonsporting athletes with a *12-item handedness inventory* from Briggs and Nebes (1975). The results showed only an overrepresentation in interactive sporting disciplines and none in the other disciplines or nonsporting athletes.

SOME ADVANTAGES COME AND GO: AN EVOLUTIONARY PERSPECTIVE ON LATERALITY

The use of frequency-dependent approaches, such as those outlined above, has received much attention in explaining laterality advantages. In addition, the term *frequency-dependent selection* is used in evolutionary biology to explain the variation between organisms in the genotypes and phenotypes they display in a given environment (Ayala & Campbell, 1974). In many complex biological systems, the viability (or success) of a given trait is related to the frequency of the trait within a population. For instance, in many systems, advantages are provided to organisms that possess traits that are relatively rare, which may provide them with selection advantages. In biology, negative frequency-dependent selection refers to increasing "fitness" of a phenotype when a trait is rare, while positive frequency-dependent selection refers to increased fitness when a trait is common.

In their paper on the stability of left-handedness in humans over time, Raymond et al. (1996) suggested that the increased frequency of left-handers in many sporting domains was not due to lateralization itself, but rather it was due to the evolutionary mechanisms driving the "value" of left-handed (or left-oriented) performers in specific competitive domains. The basic premise of modern evolutionary theory is that traits found to be advantageous in a domain will be more valued (and more likely to be selected) over traits that are less advantageous traits. The authors used this notion to explain the overrepresentation of left-handers in combat sports such as boxing and fencing. More specifically, they argued that because right-handed (or right-oriented) competitors were so common, combatants grew accustomed to predicting their attacks, but the relatively scarcity of left-handers made them harder to predict and therefore at an advantage in this competitive domain.

These concepts are relevant to our understanding of the role of laterality in talent identification and development because it is important to recognize that proportions of left-versus right-oriented competitors change over time. Loffing, Hagemann, et al. (2012) showed that the proportion of left-handed players has fluctuated over the history of tennis with current distributions at the elite level, suggesting no advantage for left-dominant competitors. Historical examinations of sport performance such as these reinforce the notion that these types of complex systems undergo significant change over time (e.g., Chatterjee & Yilmaz, 1999; Yilmaz & Chatterjee, 2000). Several researchers (e.g., Taylor & Jonker, 1978) have used models from the field of Game Theory to explain these changes. For instance, studies have examined the notion of an "evolutionarily stable strategy" that reflects a population's ability to develop and adjust over time until optimal conflict strategies are found and equilibrium is attained (e.g., Goldstein & Young, 1996).

Several studies have examined changes in the laterality distributions between pitchers and batters in baseball (e.g., Chatterjee & Yilmaz, 1999; Clotfelter, 2008; Goldstein & Young, 1996). In Goldstein and Young's (1996) analysis of the evolution of laterality interactions between pitchers and batters in Major League Baseball from 1876 to 1985, the authors noted stability on the basis of observed frequency-dependent population patterns. Their analysis noted an interaction between handedness of batters and pitchers such that the proportion of left-handedness in baseball reflected the interaction of different handedness strategies across the history of the league (however, see Clotfelter, 2008). Similar interactions between batter and bowler have been found in cricket (Brooks, Bussière, Jennions, & Hunt, 2004).

This evolutionary relationship is not limited to handedness. Puterman et al. (2010) examined changes in lateral distributions over the history of ice hockey, a sport where shooting and catching side (in skating players and goalkeepers, respectively) are not exclusively determined by handedness. In a series of studies, they showed that the proportion of left-shooting players increased over the 90-year history of the National Hockey League (NHL); however, right-sided orientations (i.e., shooting from the right side) were associated with scoring more goals over time while left-side orientations were associated with scoring more assists. In goalkeepers, right-sided catching orientations were associated with a better save percentage than left-sided orientations across the history of the league.

Understanding how the "ebb and flow" of laterality distributions change over time in response to changes in the competition environment is important for predicting future constraints on athlete development. For instance, until recently it would have been advantageous to be left-handed in tennis, but that advantage seems to have disappeared. In addition, Schorer et al. (2012) have shown that a video intervention can improve anticipation against lefties and increased use of this type of training will likely decrease the perceptual advantage of left-handers in interactive sports.

This research highlights the importance of conceptualizing performance differences within a system's unique constraints as they change over time. Gould (1996) found that Major League Baseball performance over time should be conceptualized using evolutionary theory because it showed consistent improvement within a relatively controlled system, as evidenced by a decreasing deviation in batting performance and winning percentage, as well as increased fielding averages. Understanding these types of changes is important: as noted by Chatterjee and Yilmaz (1999), without accounting for baseball's evolutionary performance, one could easily make the erroneous assumption that a 0.420 batting average in 1911 is better than a 0.390 average in 2000. Collectively, these studies highlight the utility of applying evolutionary theory to understanding sport performance.

TWO CASES AS EXAMPLES FOR PRACTICAL IMPLICATIONS

Finally, we provide two examples regarding how laterality has been considered in the real world of talent development. As we have pointed out above, talent selection and development is difficult because one tries to predict the future. In the two following subsections, we present two cases who took into account the role of laterality for later success: Rafael Nadal and the German Judo federation.

Left-Hander, Right-Hander, or Both in Tennis? The Case of Rafael Nadal

As discussed above, laterality has repeatedly been regarded as an influential factor for an athlete's talent development (Schorer et al., 2009; Sterkowitz et al., 2010). In some sports, being left-handed may be disadvantageous, because the regulations do not consider left-handers' needs and requirements. For example, in polo the racket must be held in the right hand. Similarly, young athletes in shooting sports might have to face the condition that local sport clubs can only afford equipment designed for right-handers.

In contrast to some isolated disadvantages, research highlights that being left-handed may enhance the probability of success in sports such as tennis (del Corral & Prieto-Rodríguez, 2010). A recent number one tennis player is Rafael Nadal, who challenges his opponents with strong and precise left-handed forehand strokes. A unique characteristic about this famous left-handed player is that he is actually right-handed. He acquired tennis-specific left-handedness as a young athlete and therefore benefits from the strategic advantage of being left-handed. Before his coach and uncle made him change at age nine or ten to a one-handed forehand, Nadal used to play a two-handed forehand and backhand. Nadal's case nicely demonstrates the interaction of primary and secondary influences throughout the development of sport expertise. Obviously, his unique combination of physical and mental faculties enabled Nadal to meet the high requirements of elite tennis. Born into a family passionate about sport and whose members had collected some experience at high levels of sport performance, Nadal grew up in a supportive and fostering environment. Though he was actually predisposed to be right-handed, his coach focused on training Nadal's left arm until it became his dominant arm, characteristic of his style to play. Nadal's story highlights the complex interaction of biological and psychosocial factors underpinning ultimate performance (Baker & Horton, 2004).

The Case of German Judo

Earlier in the chapter, we discussed the Tirp et al. (2014) study of laterality in elite judo athletes. In this study, the proportion of left-standers was highest among athletes who participated in the Olympic Games and lowest among judoka in the German Championships, with left-stander proportion at German University Championships in between. This finding was counterintuitive since the German Championships were hypothesized to have a greater proportion of left-oriented athletes because they are more competitive than the German University Championships. The authors suggested that a possible explanation might be the training structure for talent development in the German judo system (i.e., = Rahmentrainingskonzeption). The German judo federation has a training structure that focuses on combat stance very early in the career of the athletes. The first exposure to training and competition occurs at the U12 level, where athletes are trained by coaches from their club and their region. However, from the U14 level and higher (i.e., up to the senior level) the German judo federation works via national education programs that focus relatively early on the orientation of the combat stance. Athletes in these programs regularly train and develop strategies against both right- and left-oriented opponents (*Ai-yotsu*: the opponent has the same combat stance orientation and *Kenka-Yotsu*: the opponent has the other combat stance orientation). The complexity of this technical-tactical component of training increases as athletes progress through the age groups. Due to this unique training structure, the relatively early education in both combat stance orientations may decrease the strategic advantage of left-oriented fighters in the case of judo, an effect that seems particularly manifested in the German national Championships (i.e., since the majority of German judoka followed the same training approach).

These two case studies highlight the potential role of coaching and instruction for either accentuating or minimizing the left-orientation advantage in interactive sports. It would be interesting to have other sporting disciplines encourage the education of strategies against both orientations (right/left handedness, right/left footedness, etc.) within their early talent development programs. This approach may do much to minimize or remove the left-side advantage. This chapter has highlighted the various ways that left-orientations in sport affect talent identification and athlete development. In particular, the relative scarcity of left-orientations seems to drive this advantage and lead to greater likelihoods of being selected as talent, superior performance in competitive settings, and higher levels of attainment at the elite or professional levels.

References

Annett, M. (1985). *Left, right, hand and brain: The right shift theory*. Hillsdale, NJ: Erlbaum.

Ayala, F. J., & Campbell, C. A. (1974). Frequency dependent selection. *Annual Review of Ecological Systems, 5*, 115–138.

Baker, J., Cobley, S., & Schorer, J. (Eds.). (2012). *Talent identification and development in sport: International perspectives*. New York: Routledge.

Baker, J., Côté, J., & Deakin, J. (2005). Expertise in ultra-endurance triathletes early sport involvement, training structure, and the theory of deliberate practice. *Journal of Applied Sport Psychology, 17*(1), 64–78.

Baker, J., & Davids, K. (2007). Nature, nurture and sport performance–Introduction. *International Journal of Sport Psychology, 38*(1), 1–3.

Baker, J., & Horton, S. (2004). A review of primary and secondary influences on sport expertise. *High Ability Studies, 15*, 211–228.

Baker, J., Kungl, A. M., Pabst, J., Strauss, B., Büsch, D., & Schorer, J. (2013). Your fate is in your hands? Handedness, digit ratio (2D:4D), and selection to a national talent development system. *Laterality: Asymmetries of Body, Brain and Cognition, 18*(6), 710–718.

Baker, J., & Schorer, J. (2013). The southpaw advantage?–lateral preference in mixed martial arts. *PLoS One, 8*(11), e79793.

Baker, J., Schorer, J., Cobley, S., Bräutigam, H., & Büsch, D. (2009). Gender, depth of competition and relative age effects in team sports. *Asian Journal of Sport & Exercise Science, 6*, 7–13.

Baxter-Jones, A., Helms, P., Baines-Preece, J., & Preece, M. (1995). Growth and development of male gymnasts, swimmers, soccer and tennis players: a longitudinal study. *Annals of Human Biology, 22*, 381–394.

Bennett, M., Manning, J. T., Cook, C. J., & Kilduff, L. P. (2010). Digit ratio (2D:4D) and performance in elite rugby players. *Journal of Sports Sciences, 28*(13), 1415–1421. .

Briggs, G. G., & Nebes, R. D. (1975). Patterns of hand preference in a student population. *Cortex, 11*(3), 230–238.

Brooks, R., Bussière, L. F., Jennions, M. D., & Hunt, J. (2004). Sinister strategies succeed at the cricket World Cup. *Proceedings of the Royal Society B: Biological Sciences, 271*(Suppl. 3), S64–S66.

Carey, D. P., Smith, D. T., Martin, D., Smith, G., Sktivet, J., Rutland, A., & Shepherd, J. W. (2009). The bi-pedal ape: plasticity and asymmetry in footedness. *Cortex, 45*(5), 650–661. .

Carey, D. P., Smith, G., Smith, D. T., Shepherd, J. W., Skriver, J., Ord, L., & Rutland, A. (2001). Footedness in world soccer: an analysis of France '98. *Journal of Sports Sciences, 19*(11), 855–864.

Chatterjee, S., & Yilmaz, M. R. (1999). The NBA as an evolving multivariate system. *The American Statistician, 53*(3), 257–262.

Clotfelter, E. D. (2008). Frequency-dependent performance and handedness in professional baseball players (*Homo sapiens*). *Journal of Comparative Psychology, 122*, 68–72.

Cobley, S., Baker, J., Wattie, N., & McKenna, J. M. (2009). Annual age-grouping and athlete development: a meta-analytical review of relative age effects in sport. *Sports Medicine, 39*(3), 235–256.

del Corral, J., & Prieto-Rodríguez, J. (2010). Are differences in ranks good predictors for Grand Slam tennis matches? *International Journal of Forecasting, 26*(3), 551–563.

Dudink. (1994). Birthdate and sporting success. *Nature, 368*, 592.

Epstein, D. (2013). *The sports gene: Inside the science of extraordinary athletic performance*. Westminster, UK: Penguin Books.

Ericsson, K. A. (2007). Toward a science of expert and exceptional performance in sport: a reply to the commentaries. *International Journal of Sport Psychology, 38*, 109–123.

Ericsson, K. A., Krampe, R. T., & Tesch-Römer, C. (1993). The role of deliberate practice in the acquisition of expert performance. *Psychological Review, 100*, 363–406.

Ericsson, K. A., & Williams, A. M. (2007). Capturing naturally occurring superior performance in the laboratory: translational research on expert performance. *Journal of Experimental Psychology: Applied, 13*(3), 115–123.

Faurie, C., & Raymond, M. (2005). Handedness, homicide and negative frequency-dependent selection. *Proceedings of the Royal Society B: Biological Sciences, 272*, 25–28.

Faurie, C., & Raymond, M. (2013). The fighting hypothesis as an evolutionary explanation for the handedness polymorphism in humans: where are we? *Annals of the New York Academy of Sciences, 1288*, 110–113.

Faurie, C., Schiefenhovel, W., Le Bomin, S., Billiard, S., & Raymond, M. (2005). Variation in the frequency of left-handedness in traditional societies. *Current Anthropology, 46*(1), 142–147.

Gagné, F. (2004). Transforming gifts into talents: the DMGT as a developmental theory. *High Ability Studies, 15*(2), 119–147.

Geschwind, N., & Galaburda, A. M. (1985). Cerebral lateralization. Biological mechanisms, associations, and pathology: I. A hypothesis and a program for research. *Archives of Neurology, 42*(5), 428–459.

Geschwind, N., & Galaburda, A. M. (1985). Cerebral lateralization. Biological mechanisms, associations, and pathology: II. A hypothesis and a program for research. *Archives of Neurology, 42*(6), 521–552.

Geschwind, N., & Galaburda, A. M. (1985). Cerebral lateralization. Biological mechanisms, associations, and pathology: III. A hypothesis and a program for research. *Archives of Neurology, 42*(7), 634–654.

Geschwind, N., & Galaburda, A. M. (1987). *Cerebral lateralization*. Cambridge, MA: MIT Press.

Gladwell. (2008). *Outliers*. New York, USA: Little, Brown and Company.

Gobet, F., & Campitelli, G. (2007). The role of domain-specific practice, handedness, and starting age in chess. *Developmental Psychology, 43*(1), 159–172.

Gobet, F., & Charness, N. (2006). Expertise in chess. In K. A. Ericsson, N. Chaness, P. J. Feltovich, & R. R. Hoffmann (Eds.), *The Cambridge handbook of expertise and expert performance* (pp. 523–538). New York: Cambridge University Press.

Goldstein, S. R., & Young, C. A. (1996). "Evolutionary" stable strategy of handedness in major league baseball. *Journal of Comparative Psychology, 110*(2), 164–169.

Gould, S. J. (1996). *Full house: The spread of excellence from Plato to Darwin*. New York: Three Rivers.

Grondin, S., Guiard, Y., Ivry, R. B., & Koren, S. (1999). Manual laterality and hitting perfor-mance in major league baseball. *Journal of Experimental Psychology: Human Perception & Performance*, 25(3), 747–754.

Grouios, G. (2004). Motoric dominance and sporting excellence: training versus heredity. *Perceptual and Motor Skills*, 98(1), 53–66.

Grouios, G., Kollias, N., Koidou, I., & Poderi, A. (2002). Excess of mixed-footedness among professional soccer players. *Perceptual and Motor Skills*, 94(2), 695–699.

Grouios, G., Kollias, N., Tsorbatzoudis, H., & Alexandris, K. (2002). Over-representation of mixed-footedness among professional and semi-professional soccer players: an innate superiority or a strategic advantage? *Journal of Human Movement Studies*, 42(1), 19–29.

Grouios, G., Tsorbatzoudis, H., Alexandris, K., & Barkoukis, V. (2000). Do left-handed com-petitors have an innate superiority in sports? *Perceptual and Motor Skills*, 90(3), 1273–1282.

Gursoy, R. (2009). Effects of left- or right-hand preference on the success of boxers in Turkey. *British Journal of Sports Medicine*, 43(2), 142–144.

Hagemann, N. (2009). The advantage of being left-handed in interactive sports. *Attention, Perception, & Psychophysics*, 71(7), 1641–1648.

Helsen, W. F., Starkes, J. L., & Hodges, N. J. (1998). Team sports and the theory of deliberate practice. *Journal of Sport and Exercise Psychology*, 20(1), 12–34.

Hodges, N. J., & Starkes, J. (1996). Wrestling with the nature of expertise: a sport specific test of Ericsson, Krampe and Tesch-Römer's (1993) theory of "deliberate practice". *Interna-tional Journal of Sport Psychology*, 27(4), 400–424.

Hohmann, A. (2009). *Entwicklung sportlicher Talente an sportbetonten Schulen [Development of sporting talents at sport-accentuated schools.]*. Petersberg: Michael Imhof.

Holtzen, D. W. (2000). Handedness and professional tennis. *International Journal of Neurosci-ence*, 105(1–4), 101–119.

Hönekopp, J., & Schuster, M. (2010). A meta-analysis on 2D:4D and athletic prowess: sub-stantial relationships but neither hand out-predicts the other. *Personality and Individual Differences*, 48(1), 4–10.

Howe, M. J. A., Davidson, J. W., & Sloboda, J. A. (1998). Innate talents: reality or myth? *Behav-ioral and Brain Sciences*, 21(3), 399–442.

Joch, W. (2000). *Das sportliche Talent [The sporting talent.]* (4th ed.). Aachen: Meyer & Meyer Verlag.

Loffing, F., Hagemann, N., & Strauss, B. (2009). The serve in professional men's tennis: effects of players' handedness. *International Journal of Performance Analysis in Sport*, 9, 255–274.

Loffing, F., Hagemann, N., & Strauss, B. (2010). Automated processes in tennis: do left-handed players benefit from the tactical preferences of their opponents? *Journal of Sports Sciences*, 28(4), 435–443.

Loffing, F., Hagemann, N., & Strauss, B. (2012). Left-handedness in professional and amateur tennis. *PLoS One*, 7(11), e49325.

Loffing, F., Schorer, J., & Cobley, S. (2010). Relative age effects are a developmental problem in tennis: but not necessarily when you're left-handed!. *High Abilities Studies*, 21, 19–25.

Loffing, F., Schorer, J., Hagemann, N., & Baker, J. (2012). On the advantage of being left-handed in volleyball: further evidence of the specificity of skilled visual perception. *Attention, Perception, & Psychophysics*, 74, 446–453.

Musch, J., & Grondin, S. (2001). Unequal competition as an impediment to personal develop-ment: a review of the relative age effect in sport. *Developmental Review*, 21(2), 147–167.

Oldfield, R. C. (1971). The assessment and analysis of handedness: the Edinburgh inventory. *Neuropsychologia*, 9, 97–113.

Pabst, J., Büsch, D., Wilhelm, A., & Schorer, J. (2010). Haben es gute Handballer (selbst) in der Hand? [Do good players in team-handball have it in their own grip?]. *Leipziger Sportwissenschaftliche Beiträge*, 51(2), 140–154.

Puterman, J., Schorer, J., & Baker, J. (2010). Laterality differences in elite ice hockey: an inves-tigation of shooting and catching orientations. *Journal of Sports Sciences*, 28, 1581–1593.

Raymond, M., Pontier, D., Dufour, A. B., & Møller, A. P. (1996). Frequency-dependent maintenance of left handedness in humans. *Proceedings of the Royal Society of London Series B: Biological Sciences*, 263, 1627–1633.

Schorer, J., Cobley, S., Büsch, D., Bräutigam, H., & Baker, J. (2009). Influences of competition level, gender, player nationality, career stage and playing position on relative age effects. *Scandinavian Journal of Medicine and Science in Sports*, 19(5), 720–730.

Schorer, J., & Elferink-Gemser, M. (2013). How good are we at predicting athletes' futures? In D. Farrow, J. Baker, & C. MacMahon (Eds.), *Developing sport expertise: Researchers and coaches put theory into practice* (2nd ed.) (pp. 30–40). London: Routledge.

Schorer, J., Loffing, F., Hagemann, N., & Baker, J. (2012). Human handedness in interactive situations: negative perceptual frequency effects can be reversed!. *Journal of Sports Sciences*, 30, 507–513.

Simon, H. A., & Chase, W. H. (1973). Skill in chess. *American Scientist*, 61, 394–403.

Starkes, J., Deakin, J., Allard, F., Hodges, N., & Hayes, A. (1996). Deliberate practice in sports: what is it anyway? In K. A. Ericsson (Ed.), *The road to excellence: The acquisition of expert performance in the arts and sciences, sports and games* (pp. 81–106). Hillsdale, NJ: Erlbaum.

Sterkowicz, S., Lech, G., & Blecharz, J. (2010). Effects of laterality on the technical/tactical behavior in view of the results of judo fights. *Archives of Budo*, 6(4), 173–177.

Taylor, P. D., & Jonker, L. B. (1978). Evolutionary stable strategies and game dynamics. *Mathematical Biosciences*, 40(1), 145–156.

Tirp, J., Baker, J., Weigelt, M., & Schorer, J. (2014). Combat stance in judo – laterality differences between and within competition levels. *International Journal of Performance Analysis in Sport*, 14(1), 217–224.

Visnapuu, M., & Jürimäe, T. (2007). Handgrip strength and hand dimensions in young handball and basketball players. *Journal of Strength and Conditioning Research*, 21(3), 923–929.

Yilmaz, M. R., & Chatterjee, S. (2000). Patterns of NBA team performance from 1950 to 1998. *Journal of Applied Statistics*, 27(5), 555–566.

6

Perspectives From Sports Medicine

Todd S. Ellenbecker

Physiotherapy Associates Scottsdale Sports Clinic, Scottsdale, AZ, United States; Medical Services ATP World Tour, FL, United States

INTRODUCTION

The purpose of this chapter is to elaborate on the concept of laterality and unilateral dominance or selective sport-induced unilateral development and adaptation and discuss its relevance to the field of sports medicine. Critical to this chapter will be the specific use of data and examples from unilaterally dominant upper extremity athletes, and in particular, based on our research, an outline of the demands placed upon the elite tennis players' body in reference to the musculoskeletal adaptations that have been presented in the scientific literature. It is through the use of musculoskeletal profiling research that clinicians and researchers can learn more about the demands of a sport and better understand the stresses imparted on the body in athletes, which will allow for more effective interpretation of musculoskeletal testing for elite athletes in this population.

INTERPRETATION OF MUSCULOSKELETAL TESTING: THE NEED FOR UNDERSTANDING POPULATION-SPECIFIC LATERALITY IN SPORTS MEDICINE

One of the tenants in orthopedic and sports physical therapy and/or sports medicine in general is the use of range of motion (ROM), strength, and clinical tests to assess pain, function, and adaptation (Ellenbecker & Davies, 2000). It is imperative, however, that population-specific information is available regarding side-to-side variations and relationships to allow for high-level interpretation of these tests. For example, during the rehabilitation of an elite tennis player with lateral humeral epicondylitis on their dominant extremity, clinical testing of grip strength and isokinetic wrist extension and flexion strength may reveal equal strength between extremities on these important clinical tests. Upon initial review, one may interpret this similarly to what would be deduced for a patient from the general population that their strength has reached optimal, preinjury levels. This could lead to the conclusion that rehabilitation efforts can be discontinued and that the player can return to their sport through an interval return program (Ellenbecker, 1995). However, application of laterality-based research has established population-based descriptive data that can be used to better understand the musculoskeletal relationships between extremities in elite tennis players. Prior studies in this case show a dominance factor of 5–15% greater grip strength (Ellenbecker & Mattalino, 1997b) and significantly greater wrist flexion/extension strength (20–30%) (Ellenbecker, 1991; Ellenbecker, Roetert, & Riewald, 2006). In this example, the elite tennis player would not be ready for a full return to their sport and would not be considered for discharge from rehabilitative exercise programming. Application of this type of descriptive laterality research has significant implications on treatment and rehabilitation of injured athletes from specific populations.

Another example comes from the area of anatomical adaptation. Research (Ellenbecker, Mattalino, Elam, & Caplinger, 1998; Wright et al., 2006) has consistently shown anatomical adaptation in the dominant extremity of the throwing athlete and elite tennis player for elbow extension range of motion. The finding of 5–10 degrees of elbow flexion contracture on the dominant side would not be considered abnormal based on the adaptive research (Ellenbecker et al., 1998; Wright et al., 2006). Flexion contractures from bony hypertrophy or anterior capsular changes can limit full ulno-humeral (elbow) extension and are present in elite level performers in baseball and tennis. Knowledge of this finding is of critical importance to a treating clinician to best understand the degree or normal elbow extension expected in certain populations of athletes.

For the purposes of this chapter, three main divisions will be covered; upper extremity, lower extremity, and trunk. Each section will discuss, where applicable, examples of range of motion, muscular strength, and anatomical adaptations that have relevance to a treating clinician. The purpose of the presentation of these findings will be to provide a resource for clinicians to better understand the side-to-side variations in these parameters to enable high-level interpretation of both preventative and rehabilitative evaluation of the athlete.

UPPER EXTREMITY

Upper extremity injuries in tennis players have been extensively reported in epidemiological studies (Kibler, McQueen, & Uhl, 1988; Pluim, Staal, Windler, & Jayanthi, 2006; Reece, Fricker, & Maguire, 1986). The repetitive nature of tennis-specific movement patterns, as well as the explosive speed at which they are carried out, require precise acceleration of the arm to produce power and timely deceleration of the arm to prevent injury. Although the power generated to perform these actions comes from the kinetic chain or sequential activation of the body segments starting from the ground reaction forces up via the legs, hip, trunk, and finally through the shoulder and distal aspect of the arm, the upper extremity must serve as a conduit for the continued transmission of this energy to enable the kinetic chain activation to occur successfully for optimal performance. Stroke analysis in the modern game of tennis has estimated that 75% of the strokes hit during a match are forehands and serves (Roetert & Groppel, 2001). This means that 75% of the time, the dominant upper extremity is involved in high-level activation of shoulder internal rotation during the acceleration of the serve and forehand, and high levels of eccentric decelerative work during the follow-through phase of those two strokes. This can lead to preferential or selective muscular development in the upper extremity from these repetitive activation patterns. Similar sequential rotational activations are reported for throwing (Fleisig, Andrews, Dillman, & Escamilla, 1995) and volleyball spiking (Escamilla, 2009) and lead to upper extremity adaptations as well.

Range of Motion Profiling in the Upper Extremity

Flexibility patterns of the upper extremity in highly skilled tennis players and overhead athletes (baseball pitchers and softball players) have been extensively studied (Ellenbecker, Roetert, Bailie, Davies, & Brown, 2002; Ellenbecker, Roetert, Piorkowski, & Schulz, 1996; Kibler, Chandler, Livingston, & Roetert, 1996; Roetert, Ellenbecker, & Brown, 2000; Shanley et al., 2011; Wilk et al., 2011). This research consistently shows that shoulder internal rotation on the dominant extremity is less than the corresponding nondominant side. Not only is shoulder internal rotation limited on the dominant side in elite level tennis players, but this limitation begins in players as young as 11–12 years of age (Ellenbecker et al., 1996) and becomes progressively more limited (tighter) as players age and continue to play competitive tennis (Kibler et al., 1996; Roetert et al., 2000).

Recent research by Ellenbecker et al. (2002) measured the internal and external rotation range of motion with stabilization of the scapula

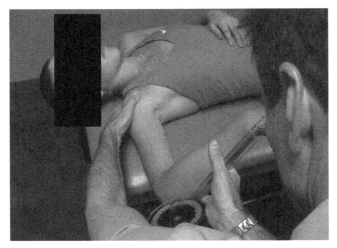

FIGURE 6.1   Measurement of shoulder internal rotation with 90 degrees of glenohumeral joint abduction with scapular stabilization.

in 90 degrees of abduction (Fig. 6.1) to determine bilateral differences in elite junior tennis players and professional baseball pitchers. They also measured and analyzed the total rotation (internal rotation measurement added to the external rotation measurement) range of motion of both the dominant and nondominant extremity. Their results found dominant arm internal rotation and dominant arm total rotation range of motion to be significantly less in the elite junior tennis players when compared to the nondominant arm. The 117 elite male junior tennis players tested averaged 45 degrees of internal rotation on the dominant arm versus 56 degrees on the nondominant arm. Total rotation range of motion values averaged 149 degrees on the dominant arm versus 158 degrees on the nondominant arm. The total rotation range of motion did differ between extremities as stated. This data can be used during musculoskeletal profiling and during rehabilitation to identify abnormal limitations in shoulder rotational range of motion and will be discussed in greater detail and through a case example later in this section.

By contrast, Ellenbecker et al. (2002) found no significant difference in shoulder total rotation range of motion in the professional baseball pitchers in their study. Significantly less internal rotation (42.5 dominant arm vs 52.4 degrees nondominant arm) was found in the baseball pitchers with significantly greater external rotation (103.2 dominant arm vs 94.5 degrees nondominant arm) on the dominant side. The total rotation range of motion measured in the asymptomatic baseball pitchers in this study was 145.7 degrees for the dominant extremity and only 1 degree different

(146.9) for the nondominant extremity. This finding has consistently been reported (equal bilateral total rotation) in throwing athletes and is now expected as an evaluation finding in throwing athletes (Shanley et al., 2011; Wilk et al., 2011). To further report on total rotation range of motion, Meister et al. (2005) tested young throwing athletes' shoulder internal and external rotation and found that between the ages of 8 and 16 years of age, absolute shoulder internal and external rotation changed significantly during development year over year. However, the consistent finding was that of total rotation range of motion of the glenohumeral joint. This total rotation range of motion remained essentially equal between extremities in this throwing population from age 8 to 16. Clinically, this means that the contralateral extremity can be used as the baseline extremity for establishing normal total rotation range of motion in young throwers despite the bilateral differences encountered in absolute shoulder internal or shoulder external rotation range of motion.

Interpretation of Shoulder Range of Motion: Why Knowledge of Laterality Is Needed to Aid in Proper Assessment in the Overhead Athlete

One common finding, as noted in the prior section, during the examination of the overhead athlete is the rather consistent finding of increased dominant arm external rotation (ER), as well as reduced dominant arm glenohumeral joint (GH) joint internal rotation (IR) (Brown, Niehues, Harrah, Yavorsky, & Hirshman, 1988; Ellenbecker, 1992, 1995; Ellenbecker et al., 1996). Ellenbecker et al. (1996) identified that this consistent relationship could occur only in a condition where GH joint rotation was measured with the scapula stabilized. Several proposed mechanisms have been discussed to attempt to explain this GH ROM relationship of increased ER and limited IR (Crockett et al., 2002; Ellenbecker, 1995; Meister et al., 2005). Tightness of the posterior capsule, tightness of the muscle tendon unit of the posterior rotator cuff, and humeral retroversion all have been described as structures that limit internal GH joint rotation. Crockett et al. (2002) and others (Chant, Litchfield, Griffin, & Thain, 2007; Osbahr, Cannon, & Speer, 2002; Reagan et al., 2002) have shown unilateral increases in humeral retroversion in throwing athletes, which would explain the increase in ER noted with accompanying IR loss.

Reinold et al. (2008) demonstrated the acute effects of pitching on GH ROM. Sixty-seven professional baseball pitchers were measured for GH joint rotational ROM with the use of scapular stabilization before and immediately after 50 to 60 pitches at full intensity. Results show a loss of 9.5 degrees of IR and 10.7 degrees of total rotation ROM on the dominant arm during this short-term response to overhead throwing. This study shows significant decreases in IR and total rotation ROM of the dominant GH joint in professional pitchers following an acute episode of throwing. Reinold et al. suggest that muscle tendinous adaptations from eccentric loading likely are implicated in this ROM adaptation following throwing (a term known as thixotropy). This musculotendinous adaptation may occur in addition to the osseous and capsular mechanisms previously reported (Reinold et al., 2008).

Careful measurement of GH rotational measurement using the total rotation concept (summing the external and IR measures together) guides the progression of stretching used in rehabilitation or the inclusion of specific mobilization techniques used to address capsular deficiencies. The total rotation ROM concept can be used by clinicians to guide the clinician during rehabilitation, specifically in the area of application of stretching and mobilization, to best determine which athlete's GH joint requires additional mobility and which extremity should not have additional mobility, because of the obvious harm induced by increases in capsular mobility and increases in humeral head translation during aggressive upper extremity exertion.

The Link and Definition of Glenohumeral Internal Rotation Deficiency, Total Rotation Range of Motion, and Shoulder Injuries

Wilk et al. (2011) have proposed the total range of motion (TROM) concept, where the amount of ER and IR at 90 degrees of abduction are added together and a TROM arc is determined (Ellenbecker et al., 2002). The authors reported the TROM in the throwing shoulders of professional baseball pitchers is within 5 degrees of the nonthrowing shoulder (Wilk et al., 2011). Furthermore, it is suggested that a TROM arc outside the 5 degrees range may be a contributing factor to shoulder injuries.

In a study by Wilk, Macrina, and Arrigo (2012), pitchers whose TROM comparison was outside the 5 degrees acceptable difference range exhibited a (2.5) times greater risk of sustaining a shoulder injury. Furthermore, 29 of the 37 injuries (78%) were sustained in throwers whose TROM was greater than 176 degrees. Stretching to increase IR passive range of motion (PROM), thereby treating the glenohumeral internal rotation deficiency (GIRD), may result in an increase of TROM greater than 176 degrees or outside the 5 degrees acceptable window compared to the contralateral shoulder. This may lead to an increased risk of injury due to the increased demands on the dynamic and static stabilizers surrounding the shoulder joint. Further research is needed to expose these effects on shoulder injuries. Wilk et al. (2012) believe TROM is a valuable assessment tool and an important component in PROM assessment of throwers' shoulders.

This should be incorporated in the thrower's shoulder examination to determine if an ROM discrepancy is present in the athlete.

External rotation deficiency (ERD) is defined as the difference between ER of the throwing shoulder and the nonthrowing shoulder of less than 5 degrees. Therefore, when comparing a baseball players' ER PROM from side-to-side, it would be expected to see an ER difference of greater than 5 degrees, indicating that a player's ER gain on his throwing side is significant enough to contribute to the demands of throwing, specifically during the late-cocking phase of the pitching motion. A pitcher with ER side-to-side differences that are less than 5 degrees may impart increased stresses on the static stabilizers, thereby contributing to an increased risk of injury over the career of the athlete (Wilk et al., 2012).

Normative Data

Population-specific normative data is an important consideration for the interpretation of ROM of the overhead athlete. As mentioned throughout this chapter, IR and ER ROM measures performed at 90 degrees of glenohumeral joint abduction are an essential part of the evaluation of the overhead athlete. Combined, these measures create the TROM (Wilk et al., 2012). For the purposes of this chapter, several key studies with large sport-specific subject populations are presented here, to provide a resource to enhance and facilitate the interpretation of ROM measures for the overhead athlete (Table 6.1).

In general, studies involving baseball pitchers show nearly symmetric total rotation ROM profiles, which are characterized by increased dominant arm ER and decreased dominant arm IR (Hurd et al., 2011; Wilk et al., 2012, 2011). This has been reported at the professional level (Ellenbecker et al., 2002; Wilk et al., 2012) as well as in high school and developmental age players (Hurd et al., 2011; Meister et al., 2005; Shanley et al., 2011). TROM in these studies with very large samples sizes are typically within 5 degrees when compared between the dominant and nondominant side. This is consistent with the recommendation of Wilk et al. (2012) that TROM in the baseball pitcher should be within the 5 degrees bilateral difference consistently reported in the literature (Wilk et al., 2011).

Ellenbecker et al. (2002, 1996) have reported decreases of 5–10 degrees on average in the dominant arm TROM parameter in uninjured elite level tennis players (Table 6.1). These differences in TROM are slightly larger than those reported in professional and developmental age throwing athletes (Table 6.1). Similarly, Reeser et al. (2010) reported decreases in dominant arm TROM in elite level volleyball players who were uninjured. These normative data profiles can assist clinicians in better interpreting the actual ROM measures from the overhead athlete in these populations.

TABLE 6.1   Glenohumeral Joint Rotational Range of Motion in Overhead Athletes

Dominant Arm	Nondominant Arm	N	Population/Age	Sources
ER: 132 + 11	127 + 11	369	Professional baseball pitchers/mean age: 25.6 years	Wilk et al. (2012)
IR: 52 + 12	63 + 12			
TR: 184	190			
ER: 125.6 + 11	117.8 + 11	143	High school baseball players/mean age: 15 years	Shanley et al. (2011)
IR: 53.4 + 11	61.4 + 9			
TR: 179	179			
ER: 123.8 + 13	121.1 + 14	103	High school softball/mean age: 15 years	Shanley et al. (2011)
IR: 60.2 + 13	66.8 + 12			
TR: 184	187			
ER: 143 + 13	136 + 12	294	Little league baseball players/age range: 8–16 years	Meister et al. (2005)
IR: 35.9 + 9	41.8 + 8			
TR: 178	178			
ER: 130	120	210	High school baseball pitchers/mean age: 16.1 years	Hurd et al. (2011)
IR: 60	75			
TR: 190	195			
ER: 103.9	99.1 + 9	150	Male elite junior tennis players	Ellenbecker et al. (2002)
IR: 39.4 + 9	52.2 + 9			
TR: 142	151			
ER: 105.6 + 7	101.3 + 7	149	Female elite junior tennis players	Ellenbecker et al. (2002)
IR: 41.5 + 8	52.1 + 7			
TR: 147	154			
ER: 89	87	276	Elite volleyball players	Reeser, Fleisig, Bolt, and Ruan (2010)
IR: 46	55			
TR: 135	154			

Summary of Current Recommendations for Interpreting GIRD and TROM Deficits

Historically, several definitions of GIRD have been used in the literature. Several operational definitions have been used to describe the pathologic condition that is defined as GIRD. GIRD is generally defined as the loss in degrees of glenohumeral IR of the dominant shoulder compared with the nondominant shoulder. Calculation of GIRD has been previously reported per Burkhart, Morgan, and Kibler (2003a, 2003b, 2003c) and others (Myers, Laudner, Pasquale, Bradley, & Lephart, 2006). Burkhart et al. report that an acceptable level of GIRD is defined as: (1) less than 20 degrees loss of shoulder IR comparing shoulders bilaterally or (2) greater than a 10% loss of the total rotation seen in the nonthrowing shoulder (Nondominant shoulder IR+ER ROM)×10%. Using this determination for example, assuming the nondominant shoulder has a total arc of motion of 160 degrees, the 10% rule would equate to only 16 degrees of loss being required for the determination of GIRD, rather than the standard 20 degrees loss typically needed. Burkhart et al. (2003a, 2003b, 2003c) have reported that as long as an athlete's GIRD is less than or equal to their ER gain (ERG), the throwing shoulder will have no abnormal rotational kinematics and will function properly.

To better understand the current recommendations for GIRD and TROM, the following definitions have been published in a detailed current concepts article by Manske, Wilk, Davies, Ellenbecker, and Reinold (2013). In this article the concepts of "anatomical" GIRD and "pathologic" GIRD were introduced. A loss of IR itself can be considered a normal variation observed in asymptomatic overhead athletes. Because of this common finding, it has been suggested that the term "anatomical GIRD" be used to describe this in the overhead athlete. Anatomical GIRD (A-GIRD) refers to a normal loss of IR alone with adequate ER gain. Despite this finding, the term GIRD has continued to have a negative connotation, implying that any side-to-side loss of IR may be pathological or may be a cause of future injury. Therefore a thorough clinical assessment of IR, ER, and total rotation range of motion is needed before stretching interventions are potentially applied, as in some athletes (i.e., those with A-GIRD) this is an expected and normal adaptation to repetitive overhead throwing.

A second term from the Manske et al. (2013) paper is pathologic GIRD (P-GIRD). A shoulder that has IR loss and a concomitant loss of TROM or an increase in ERD would be considered a pathologic glenohumeral internal rotation deficit. In determining clinically significant P-GIRD, one must also carefully evaluate ER, and thus TROM. Wilk et al. (2012) reported on 362 healthy throwers; TROM was within 5 degrees for all subjects. Ellenbecker et al. (2002) reported on asymptomatic professional baseball pitchers and asymptomatic elite tennis players, and reported that TROM was within 5 degrees for the baseball pitchers and within 10 degrees for the elite tennis players. Furthermore, Wilk et al. (2011) reported that a difference of greater than 5 degrees of TROM correlated with shoulder injuries.

Clinical Patient Example of Interpreting IR and TROM Measurements

Clinical application of the total rotation ROM concept is best demonstrated by a case presentation of a unilaterally dominant upper extremity athlete. If, during the initial evaluation of a high-level baseball pitcher, the clinician finds an ROM pattern of 120 degrees of external rotation and only 30 degrees of internal rotation, some uncertainty may exist as to whether this represents an ROM deficit in internal rotation that requires rehabilitative intervention via muscle tendon unit stretching and possibly via the use of specific glenohumeral joint mobilization. However, if measurement of that patient's nondominant extremity rotation reveals 90 degrees of external rotation and 60 degrees of internal rotation, the current recommendation based on the total rotation ROM concept would be to avoid extensive mobilization and passive stretching of the dominant extremity, because the total rotation ROM in both extremities is 150 degrees (120 degrees external rotation + 30 degrees internal rotation = 150 degrees dominant arm total rotation, and 90 degrees external rotation + 60 degrees internal rotation = 150 degrees total nondominant arm rotation). In elite level tennis players, the total active rotation ROM can be expected to be up to 10 degrees less on the dominant arm before clinical treatment to address internal rotation ROM restriction would be recommended or implemented.

This total rotation ROM concept can be used as illustrated to guide the clinician during rehabilitation, specifically in the area of application of stretching and mobilization, to best determine which glenohumeral joint requires additional mobility and which extremity should not have additional mobility, because of the obvious harm induced by increases in capsular mobility and increases in humeral head translation during aggressive upper extremity exertion.

Due to the findings of a consistent pattern of limited shoulder internal rotation, current strategies in rehabilitation and preventative conditioning utilize stretches for the muscles and shoulder joint capsule (posterior) that are responsible for limiting this important motion. Fig. 6.2A and B show two recommended self-stretches (sleeper stretch and cross-arm adduction stretch) for the shoulder in overhead athletes to address the limitations in internal rotation range of motion.

Additional upper extremity range of motion research has been performed to identify the normal profile of the overhead athlete and has relevance in this chapter on laterality for sports medicine. King, Brelsford, and Tullos (1969) initially reported on elbow range of motion in professional baseball pitchers. Fifty percent of the pitchers they examined were found to have a flexion contracture of the dominant elbow with 30% of subjects

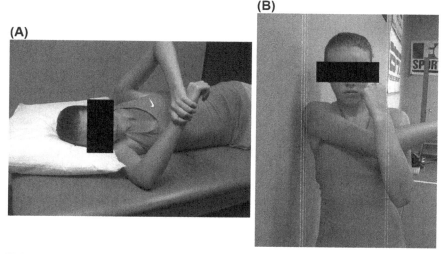

FIGURE 6.2 (A and B). Posterior shoulder stretches recommended to improve internal rotation range of motion in overhead athletes (A: sleeper stretch, and B: cross-arm stretch).

demonstrating a cubitus valgus deformity. A cubitus valgus deformity is a term used to describe an increase in the valgus angulation at the elbow that was found in the overhead athlete in this descriptive study on the dominant arm. Chinn, Priest, and Kent (1974) measured 84 world-class professional adult tennis players and reported significant elbow flexion contractures on the dominant arm, but no presence of a cubitus valgus deformity. Ellenbecker et al. (1998) measured elbow flexion contractures averaging 5 degrees in a population of 40 healthy professional baseball pitchers. Directly related to elbow function was wrist flexibility, which Ellenbecker et al. (1998) reported as significantly less in extension on the dominant arm due to tightness of the wrist flexor musculature, with no difference in wrist flexion range of motion between extremities.

Wright et al. (2006) reported on 33 throwing athletes prior to the competitive season. The average loss of elbow extension was 7 degrees, and the average loss of elbow flexion was 5.5 degrees. Ellenbecker and Roetert (1994) measured senior tennis players 55 years of age and older and found flexion contractures averaging 10 degrees in the dominant elbow, as well as significantly less wrist flexion range of motion. The higher utilization of the wrist extensor musculature is likely the cause of limited wrist flexor range of motion among the senior tennis players, as opposed to the reduced wrist extension range of motion from excessive overuse of the wrist flexor muscles inherent in baseball pitching (Fleisig et al., 1995; Morris, Jobe, Perry, Pink, & Healy, 1989).

A. LATERALITY – AN IMPORTANT AND OFTEN DISREGARDED TOPIC

Upper Extremity Muscular Strength Testing

One of the most important aspects in both rehabilitation and preventative conditioning programs for any athlete is muscular balance. Muscular imbalances occur in the upper extremity of the overhead athlete from selective activation of certain groups of muscles required to generate power for throwing, serving, and other tennis and sport-specific movement patterns. One of the primary muscular imbalances found in the overhead athlete is in the shoulder. Extensive research using isokinetic dynamometers to measure strength in elite tennis players has identified muscular imbalances between the shoulder internal and external rotators on the dominant, tennis playing extremity (Chandler, Kibler, Stracener, Ziegler, & Pace, 1992; Ellenbecker, 1991, 1992, 1995; Ellenbecker & Roetert, 2003a). The muscles that internally rotate the shoulder (pectoralis major, lattisimus dorsi, and subscapularis) become significantly stronger on the dominant arm from serving, hitting forehands, and other tennis movements. These large, powerful internal rotator muscles become so strong and dominant that an imbalance occurs between these muscles and their matching counterparts, the external rotators.

The external rotators (infraspinatus and teers minor) primarily function to stabilize the humeral head in the glenoid and to decelerate the shoulder during the follow-through phase of the tennis serve following ball contact. In contrast to the very large internal rotator muscles, the external rotator muscles that perform these vital stabilizing functions have very small relative cross-sectional areas through the shoulder joint (Matsen, Fu, & Hawkins, 1993), and are primarily located in the posterior aspect of the shoulder. Therefore a muscular imbalance occurs between the internal rotators and the external rotators.

The use of isokinetics in research has shown that the normal relationship between these important muscle groups is (2:3 or 66%) with the external rotators being the "2" and the internal rotators being the "3." However, in elite level tennis players, this relationship becomes more of a (1:2 or 50%) relationship where the internal rotators become twice as strong as the external rotators. Some sports scientists and physicians have lightheartedly referred to the internal rotators as "Cadillacs" and the external rotators as "Volkswagens" in describing the muscular imbalance in the overhead athlete's shoulder. This type of muscular imbalance can lead to injury and suboptimal performance.

Table 6.2 contains normative data from isokinetic testing of 147 elite junior tennis players by Ellenbecker and Roetert (2003a). Data presented are expressed as peak torque and work values relative to body weight. Additionally, data are presented for the external/internal rotation ratios of both the dominant tennis playing upper extremity and nondominant

TABLE 6.2 Isokinetic Peak Torque-to-Body Weight Ratios, Single Repetition Work-to-Body Weight Ratios, and External Rotation-to-Internal Rotation Ratios in Elite Junior Tennis Players[a]

	Dominant Arm		Nondominant Arm	
	Peak Torque (%)	Work (%)	Peak Torque (%)	Work (%)
External Rotation (ER)				
Male, 210 degrees/s	12	20	11	19
Male, 300 degrees/s	10	18	10	17
Female, 210 degrees/s	8	14	8	15
Female, 300 degrees/s	8	11	7	12
Internal Rotation (IR)				
Male, 210 degrees/s	17	32	14	27
Male, 300 degrees/s	15	28	13	23
Female, 210 degrees/s	12	23	11	19
Female, 300 degrees/s	11	15	10	13
ER/IR Ratio				
Male, 210 degrees/s	69	64	81	81
Male, 300 degrees/s	69	65	82	83
Female, 210 degrees/s	69	63	81	82
Female, 300 degrees/s	67	61	81	77

[a] *A Cybex 6000 series isokinetic dynamometer and 90 degrees of glenohumeral joint abduction were used. Data are expressed in foot-pounds per unit of body weight for ER and IR measures with ER/IR ratio representing the relative muscular balance between the external and internal rotators.*
Adapted from Ellenbecker, T., & Roetert, E.P. (2003a). Age specific isokinetic glenohumeral internal and external rotation strength in elite junior tennis players. Journal of Science and Medicine in Sport, 6(1), 63–70.

extremity. Testing is performed with the glenohumeral joint in 90 degrees of abduction with stabilization straps to prevent substitution.

Additional isokinetic data profiles can be found in the following references for professional baseball pitchers (Ellenbecker & Mattalino, 1997a; Wilk, Andrews, Arrigo, Keirns, & Erber, 1993) and show similar findings of greater dominant arm internal rotation and equal external rotation values. Lower dominant arm external/internal rotation ratios are reported in professional baseball pitcher data sets, similar to that reported in Table 6.2 for elite level tennis players (Ellenbecker & Mattalino, 1997a; Wilk et al., 1993).

A. LATERALITY – AN IMPORTANT AND OFTEN DISREGARDED TOPIC

Application of Isokinetic Profiling Data to Training and Rehabilitation Programming for the Overhead Athlete

Due to the presence of muscular imbalances in the overhead athlete, current strategies for performance enhancement and injury prevention/ rehabilitation focus on balancing these muscular imbalances. A great deal of emphasis is placed on the external rotators and muscles of the upper back that are, in most cases, underdeveloped in the tennis player and do not appear to be strengthened simply from repetitive overhead activity. The use of a supplemental set of exercises for the upper back and shoulder region is imperative to promote muscular balance and prevent injury. Ellenbecker and Roetert (2002) tested collegiate female tennis players immediately before and following a four-month season of college tennis competition. Despite competing and practicing on virtually a daily basis over the four-month time period, subjects did not show a significant increase in muscular strength development in the internal or external rotators measured with a Cybex isokinetic dynamometer in 90 degrees of glenohumeral joint abduction. This research supports the use of preventative rotator cuff strengthening programs since even high-level intense tennis play and competition does not appear to increase muscular strength in these important muscles. The application of specific exercises to strengthen the rotator cuff and scapular musculature is currently recommended (Ellenbecker & Cools, 2010; Ellenbecker & Roetert, 2002; Kibler, Sciascia, Uhl, Tambay, & Cunningham, 2008).

Isokinetic Muscular Endurance Testing in Elite Tennis Players

With specific reference to the upper extremity, muscular endurance is of paramount importance, and there has been some question about whether side-to-side variations in muscular endurance would parallel findings found for muscular strength. Research conducted by Ellenbecker and Roetert (1999) showed that the shoulder external rotators fatigued faster than the internal rotators in elite junior tennis players using a high-speed fatigue protocol on an isokinetic machine. Twenty repetitions of maximal effort concentric internal and external rotation with 90 degrees of glenohumeral joint abduction were performed at 300 degrees per second. Internal rotation strength showed a decline of only 15–20% over the 20 testing repetitions, while external rotation strength declined 30–38%. However, this finding was present bilaterally, with no dominant arm adaptation noted in muscular endurance in this unilaterally dominant upper extremity population. This finding of more rapid fatigue of the external rotators further exemplifies the importance of supplemental strength programming for the external rotators, since they are not only weaker than the internal rotators, but fatigue to both a greater extent and at a faster rate than the internal rotators of the shoulder in elite tennis players.

Postural Adaptations in the Upper Extremity of Overhead Athletes

Evaluation of the upper back and shoulder region of unilaterally dominant upper extremity overhead athletes reveals several important findings; the first is that the dominant arm is often lower than the nondominant side (Priest & Nagel, 1976). Additionally, the scapula is often protracted or further away from the spine on the dominant side. Kibler (1991) has devised a test called the lateral scapular slide test to measure the scapular position. Kibler has determined that on healthy uninjured persons less than a 1–1.5 cm difference should exist between sides. In tennis players, due to the repetitive stresses and eccentric loads placed on the muscles and structures in the posterior aspect of the shoulder and scapular region, scapular position often approaches or mimics the scapular position seen in persons with shoulder dysfunction (Kibler, 1998). The consistent finding of postural adaptations in tennis players has led to the development of the term "tennis shoulder" (Priest & Nagel, 1976). While this response is, in many cases, thought to be merely a response to the eccentric stresses and loads applied to the arm, exercises to enhance the muscular stabilization of this area are an important part of a comprehensive program for overhead athletes and provides an example of how knowledge of the kinetic link system can be applied in conditioning programs based on profiling research.

Laudner, Stanek, and Meister (2007) have measured scapular upward rotation on the dominant extremity in baseball pitchers and have compared that to position players in professional baseball players. Their study found that pitchers possess less dominant arm upward rotation than position players especially at 60 and 90 degrees of elevation. A follow-up study in 2013 by Laudner, Lynall, and Meister (2013) found that pitchers, when evaluated throughout a professional season, showed decreases in upward rotation at season end at 60 and 90 degrees with no change found in position players during the same time course of the season. These dominant arm changes in pitchers in scapular posture help to understand the muscular demands and stabilization needed on the dominant side in throwing athletes.

Oyama, Myers, Wassinger, Ricci, and Lephart (2008) tested 43 unilaterally dominant upper extremity collegiate athletes for resting scapular position and found that of those tested, tennis players had the most protracted dominant scapula as compared to the nondominant scapula.

This was compared to baseball and volleyball players. Additionally, all of the unilaterally dominant athletes presented with greater amounts of dominant scapular anterior tilt and scapular internal rotation. This is consistent with a seminal historical observation study by Priest and Nagel (1976) who defined tennis shoulder as one characterized by greater amounts of dominant arm scapular protraction, depression, and downward rotation.

Cools et al. (2010) measured 35 adolescent elite tennis players for scapular motion and strength bilaterally using a digital inclinometer and handheld dynamometer, respectively. They found that the dominant scapula had greater amounts of upward rotation at multiple angular positions compared to the nondominant side, a finding in contrast to what Laudner et al. (2013, 2007) have reported in baseball pitchers. Additionally, significantly great upper trapezius and serratus anterior strength was measured on the dominant side in the elite adolescent tennis players with no side-to-side differences or laterality effect for the middle and lower trapezius. Donatelli et al. (2000) measured professional baseball pitchers using a handheld dynamometer bilaterally and, in contrast to the work of Cools et al. (2010) found greater dominant arm middle and lower trapezius strength. These sport-specific differences in lateral dominance highlight the need for population-specific research to best understand the complex side-to-side interrelationships that are present in the overhead athlete. The important relationship of scapular stabilization and optimal scapular muscle strength has been detailed by Kibler (1991, 1998) for overhead functions and was also highlighted in a second study by Cools, Witvrouw, Mahieu, and Danneels (2005). Cools et al. tested healthy overhead athletes for isokinetic protraction and retraction strength and compared their strength relationships to a group of overhead throwing athletes diagnosed with impingement. The throwing athletes with impingement were found to have reduced scapular protraction strength measured with the isokinetic dynamometer as well as reduced electromyography (EMG) activity of the lower trapezius during retraction strength testing. The decrease in optimal function of dominant arm scapular stabilizers in overhead athletes with impingement would indicate the need for optimal scapular muscle strength and activation to allow for full overhead function in the unilaterally dominant upper extremity athlete.

Distal Upper Extremity Isokinetic Strength Profiling in Elite Tennis Players

Research using EMG demonstrates the consistently high activation levels in the wrist extensor muscles during nearly all phases of tennis strokes (Morris et al., 1989). Research has also shown that lesser skilled players and players with tennis elbow have higher activation levels in the forearm and wrist musculature and for longer durations than more accomplished, healthy tennis players (Kelley, Lombardo, Pink, Perry, & Giangarra, 1994). Isokinetic testing of the wrist flexors and extensors and forearm pronators and supinators has shown 20–30% greater strength on the dominant arm for the pronators, flexors, and extensors in highly skilled adult tennis players (Ellenbecker, 1991). Similar isokinetic research on elite junior tennis players has confirmed the presence of significantly greater dominant arm forearm pronation, as well as wrist flexion and extension strength in elite junior tennis players aged 12–17. This repeated finding of greater dominant arm distal muscular adaptation supports the inclusion of wrist and forearm strengthening and endurance exercise as an important part of a tennis player's program, due to the repeated reliance and activation of these important muscles with tennis play. Ellenbecker and Mattalino (1997b) have reported similar findings of unilateral dominance in professional baseball pitchers with 20–30% greater forearm pronation, wrist flexion, and wrist extension strength compared to the nondominant extremity. This consistent finding of increased distal upper extremity strength in both baseball and tennis players would have clinical ramifications during rehabilitation of overuse injury and following postsurgical cases as well, regarding return to play criterion.

Finally, Ellenbecker and Roetert (2003b) tested 38 elite junior tennis players in the pattern of elbow flexion extension strength using a Cybex 6000 isokinetic dynamometer. The goal of this research was to develop a similar profile for elbow flexion and extension strength and to compare strength levels between the dominant and nondominant extremity. Testing was performed in a supine position with stabilization straps with the shoulder in 45 degrees of abduction with the forearm in a neutral position during testing with a range of motion between (−10) degrees of extension to 125 degrees of elbow flexion. The results showed that male tennis players exhibited significantly greater dominant arm elbow extension strength and that no significant differences were found between extremities in elbow flexion muscular performance in both males and females. In elite junior tennis players, elbow extension strength on the dominant arm in both males and females was actually stronger than elbow flexion strength. This may be due to the high activation levels of triceps to generate elbow extension during the acceleration phase of the tennis serve (Morris et al., 1989).

Summary: Upper Extremity

Descriptive profiling research in overhead athletes has identified very specific muscular strength, range of motion, and postural adaptations to the unique unilateral demands of upper extremity dominant sports.

A. LATERALITY – AN IMPORTANT AND OFTEN DISREGARDED TOPIC

Information from these studies can enable clinicians to optimally interpret clinical tests from these populations of athletes for both rehabilitation and performance enhancement/injury prevention programs.

LOWER EXTREMITY

The lower extremity profiling research is far less prevalent in the literature as compared to published reports in the upper extremity. In contrast to the rather consistent upper extremity dominance reported in the literature in elite tennis players, a population featured significantly in this chapter, lower extremity profiling shows little side-to-side differences in function. Ellenbecker and Roetert (1995) tested elite junior players using a Cybex concentric dynamometer at speeds of 180 and 300 degrees per second to assess bilateral quadriceps and hamstring strength (Fig. 6.3). The testing protocol recommended is to utilize 5 repetitions at the 180 degrees per second speed, and 15 repetitions at the 300 degrees per second speed to test for the endurance capability of the quadriceps and hamstrings.

Results of testing showed that unlike the upper extremity in elite junior tennis players, the lower extremity quadriceps and hamstring strength parameters did not differ between extremities in this research. Hamstring/quadriceps ratios ranged between 55% and 65% at testing speeds of 180 and 300 degrees per second. This indicates a significant amount of relative quadriceps development relative to the hamstrings compared to other groups of athletes who have much higher hamstring/quadriceps ratios and greater relative hamstring development (Davies, 1992). This research

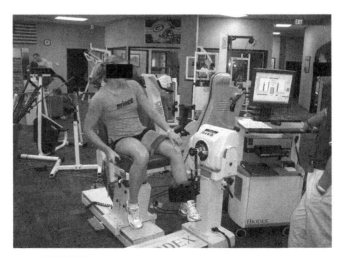

FIGURE 6.3   Knee extension/flexion testing set up.

shows that bilateral symmetry in hamstring and quadriceps strength is expected during the testing of healthy elite players.

In a follow-up study, Ellenbecker, Roetert, Sueyoshi, and Riewald (2007) published age-specific descriptive profiles of knee extension flexion strength in elite tennis players. Similar findings were reported showing symmetrical lower extremity strength values with isokinetic testing of the quadriceps and hamstrings.

In general, most lower extremity functional and isokinetic testing references (Davies, 1992; Reiman & Manske, 2009) utilize a bilateral comparison in both normal and athletic populations for strength, endurance, and functional testing. Bilateral symmetry is expected as a goal in tests such as the single leg hop test (De Carlo & Sell, 1997). DeCarlo and Sell reported bilateral symmetry by examining 889 healthy subjects in lower extremity functional tests. Goals set in physical therapy and rehabilitation assume bilateral symmetry in function for both open and closed chain lower extremity strength and functional testing with no lateral dominance effect expected (Davies, 1992; Reiman & Manske, 2009). The application of descriptive data in lower extremity functional tests often includes normalization for body height, body mass, and other factors; however, there is no allowance for significant side-to-side differences for data interpretation in normal uninjured subjects/athletes.

Lower Extremity Range of Motion

Similar to the plethora of upper extremity shoulder rotational range of motion data, there is a developing body of evidence regarding rotational range of motion in the hip in unilaterally dominant upper extremity athletes. Ellenbecker, Ellenbecker, et al. (2007) measured prone hip internal and external range of motion in 147 elite junior tennis players and 101 professional baseball pitchers. No significant differences were found in side-to-side comparisons of hip rotation range of motion, with only 8–15% of the elite tennis players showing more than a 10 degrees side-to-side difference. Hip external rotation differences among the baseball pitchers were more common (42% with greater than a 10 degrees side-to-side difference) but still not statistically significant side-to-side differences.

In a similar study measuring hip rotational range of motion, Sauers, Bliven, Johnson, Falsone, and Walters (2014) measured both professional baseball pitchers and position players to assess bilateral hip rotation range of motion. No clinically significant differences were measured in hip IR, ER, and total rotation range of motion in this population. Therefore in unilaterally dominant upper extremity athletes like elite tennis players and professional baseball players, hip rotation range of motion should be symmetrical. Significant bilateral differences measured in hip range of motion may therefore be suspicious for lower extremity injury based on the findings of these descriptive findings in these populations (Ellenbecker, Ellenbecker, et al., 2007; Sauers et al., 2014). In another study measuring passive range of motion in 19 professional baseball pitchers, Robb et al. (2010) found significantly less hip rotational range of motion in uninjured professional pitchers on the nondominant hip. A correlation was established between hip rotation range of motion in the nondominant hip and throwing velocity in this study. This study measured passive range of motion with overpressure exerted on the extremity, which might account for the difference between the studies of Ellenbecker, Ellenbecker, et al. (2007) and Sauers et al. (2014). Clearly, further research is needed to better define hip range of motion and other parameters in the lower extremity with regard to bilateral differences and laterality.

TRUNK

Descriptive profiling research among unilaterally dominant upper extremity athletes is very limited in the scientific literature at this time. The stresses placed upon the spine of the tennis player include repetitive extension with rotation during ground strokes, and the tennis serve can lead to overuse injury (Hainline, 1995). To prevent injury and enhance performance, the application of exercises and conditioning techniques to improve core stability has received increased attention in the physical training of nearly all athletes. Research profiling the strength of the muscles that dynamically stabilize the spine in athletes can provide valuable insight into the development of sport-specific training and rehabilitation programs. One of the main areas of laterality with respect to trunk strength would be in the analysis of trunk rotation strength. Rotational (left and right) movements are characteristically inherent in nearly all sports, with tennis and baseball containing large explosive arcs of rotational range of motion to generate angular momentum (Ellenbecker & Roetert, 2004).

Greater amounts of information on sagittal plane trunk extension flexion strength has been published in elite tennis players and in normal populations (Roetert, McCormick, Brown, & Ellenbecker, 1996; Timm, 1995). Research regarding trunk rotation strength is critically needed since all tennis strokes and other sport-specific movement patterns involve extensive acceleration and deceleration during trunk rotation. To increase the data base on trunk strength, Ellenbecker and Roetert (2004) tested 104 elite tennis players using an isokinetic trunk rotation device (Cybex TOR). Players were tested in the seated position and performed maximal trunk left and right rotation at two testing speeds, 60 and 120 degrees per second.

Results of testing showed no significant difference in left and right rotation of the trunk and generated torque and work to body weight ratios for normal uninjured players. Male elite players were able to rotate at levels ranging between 60% and 65% at 60 degrees per second, and 50–55% at 120 degrees per second. Females had torque to body weight ratios ranging between 45% and 50% at 60 degrees per second, and 40–45% at 120 degrees per second. Additionally, a standing medicine ball rotation functional test was used to determine the relationship between a more isolated measure of seated isokinetic torso rotation strength to a functional forehand and backhand simulation medicine ball throw. Results of this study showed significant correlations ($r = 0.7$–0.8) between the functional rotational medicine ball toss and the isokinetic torso rotation. Unlike the upper extremity, where unilateral differences in strength are commonplace, this study showed, in contrast, trunk rotational symmetry was the norm in elite tennis players. The use of rotational training methods is currently recommended based on the increased emphasis trunk rotation plays in the modern stances and stroke biomechanics in current players. It is hoped that increases in core stability and greater understanding of the specific muscular patterns in the trunk musculature in tennis players and other athletes will lead to the development of more specific training programs to both prevent injury and enhance performance. Further testing is clearly needed to further describe and identify side-to-side differences in rotational trunk strength to aid in interpretation of population-specific functional rotational testing.

SUMMARY

The discussion of side-to-side differences contained in this chapter provides a regional overview for clinicians and sport scientists to better understand the anatomical and physiologic demands placed on specific populations of athletes and how side-to-side differences in range of motion and muscular strength develop and occur. Further research will help to delineate critical levels of muscular imbalance or alteration to aid in both the postinjury rehabilitation and preventative evaluations of unilaterally dominant athletes such as those discussed in this chapter.

References

Brown, L. P., Niehues, S. L., Harrah, A., Yavorsky, P., & Hirshman, H. P. (1988). Upper extremity range of motion and isokinetic strength of the internal and external shoulder rotators in major league baseball players. *American Journal of Sports Medicine, 16*(6), 577–585.

Burkhart, S. S., Morgan, C. D., & Kibler, W. B. (2003). The disabled throwing shoulder: spectrum of pathology. Part I: pathoanatomy and biomechanics. *Arthroscopy, 19*(4), 404–420.

Burkhart, S. S., Morgan, C. D., & Kibler, W. B. (2003). The disabled throwing shoulder: spectrum of pathology. Part II: evaluation and treatment of SLAP lesions in throwers. *Arthroscopy*, *19*(5), 531–539.

Burkhart, S. S., Morgan, C. D., & Kibler, W. B. (2003). The disabled throwing shoulder: spectrum of pathology. Part III: the SICK scapula, scapular dyskinesis, the kinetic chain, and rehabilitation. *Arthroscopy*, *19*(6), 641–661.

Chandler, T. J., Kibler, W. B., Stracener, E. C., Ziegler, A. K., & Pace, B. (1992). Shoulder strength, power, and endurance in college tennis players. *American Journal of Sports Medicine*, *20*(4), 455–458.

Chant, C. B., Litchfield, R., Griffin, S., & Thain, L. M. F. (2007). Humeral head retroversion in competitive baseball players and its relationship to glenohumeral rotation range of motion. *Journal of Orthopaedic and Sports Physical Therapy*, *37*(9), 514–520.

Chinn, C. J., Priest, J. D., & Kent, B. E. (1974). Upper extremity range of motion, grip strength, and girth in highly skilled tennis players. *Physical Therapy*, *54*(5), 474–483.

Cools, A. M., Johansson, F. R., Cambier, D. C., Vande Velde, A., Palmans, T., & Witvrouw, E. E. (2010). Descriptive profile of scapulothoracic position, strength and flexibility variables in adolescent elite tennis players. *British Journal of Sports Medicine*, *44*(9), 678–684.

Cools, A. M., Witvrouw, E. E., Mahieu, N. N., & Danneels, L. A. (2005). Isokinetic scapular muscle performance in overhead athletes with and without impingement symptoms. *Journal of Athletic Training*, *40*(2), 104–110.

Crockett, H. C., Gross, L. B., Wilk, K. E., Schwartz, M. L., Reed, J., O'Mara, J., … Andrews, J. R. (2002). Osseous adaptation and range of motion at the glenohumeral joint in professional baseball pitchers. *American Journal of Sports Medicine*, *30*(1), 20–26.

Davies, G. J. (1992). *A compendium of isokinetics in clinical usage*. LaCrosse, WI: S & S Publishers.

De Carlo, M. S., & Sell, K. E. (1997). Normative data for range of motion and single-leg hop in high school athletes. *Journal of Sport Rehabilitation*, *6*(3), 246–255.

Donatelli, R., Ellenbecker, T. S., Ekedahl, S. R., Wilkes, J. S., Kocher, K., & Adam, J. (2000). Assessment of shoulder strength in professional baseball pitchers. *Journal of Orthopaedic and Sports Physical Therapy*, *30*(9), 544–551.

Ellenbecker, T. S. (1991). A total arm strength isokinetic profile of highly skilled tennis players. *Isokinetics & Exercise Science*, *1*(1), 9–21.

Ellenbecker, T. S. (1992). Shoulder internal and external rotation strength and range of motion of highly skilled junior tennis players. *Isokinetics & Exercise Science*, *2*(2), 65–72.

Ellenbecker, T. S. (1995). Rehabilitation of shoulder and elbow injuries in tennis players. *Clinics in Sports Medicine*, *14*(1), 87–110.

Ellenbecker, T. S., & Cools, A. (2010). Rehabilitation of shoulder impingement syndrome and rotator cuff injuries: an evidence-based review. *British Journal of Sports Medicine*, *44*(5), 319–327.

Ellenbecker, T. S., & Davies, G. J. (2000). The application of isokinetics in testing and rehabilitation of the shoulder complex. *Journal of Athletic Training*, *35*(3), 338–350.

Ellenbecker, T. S., Ellenbecker, G. A., Roetert, E. P., Silva, R. T., Keuter, G., & Sperling, F. (2007). Descriptive profile of hip rotation range of motion in elite tennis players and professional baseball pitchers. *American Journal of Sports Medicine*, *35*(8), 1371–1376.

Ellenbecker, T. S., & Mattalino, A. J. (1997). Concentric isokinetic shoulder internal and external rotation strength in professional baseball pitchers. *Journal of Orthopaedic and Sports Physical Therapy*, *25*(5), 323–328.

Ellenbecker, T. S., & Mattalino, A. J. (1997). *The elbow in sport*. Champaign, IL: Human Kinetics Publishers.

Ellenbecker, T. S., Mattalino, A. J., Elam, E. A., & Caplinger, R. A. (1998). Medial elbow joint laxity in professional baseball pitchers: a bilateral comparison using stress radiography. *American Journal of Sports Medicine*, *26*(3), 420–424.

Ellenbecker, T. S., & Roetert, E. P. (1994). *Unpublished data on distal upper extremity range of motion in elite tennis players – United States tennis association.*

Ellenbecker, T. S., & Roetert, E. P. (1995). Concentric isokinetic quadricep and hamstring strength in elite junior tennis players. *Isokinetics & Exercise Science, 5*(1), 3–6.

Ellenbecker, T. S., & Roetert, E. P. (1999). Testing isokinetic muscular fatigue of shoulder internal and external rotation in elite junior tennis players. *Journal of Orthopaedic and Sports Physical Therapy, 29*(5), 275–281.

Ellenbecker, T. S., & Roetert, E. P. (2002). Effects of a 4-month season on glenohumeral joint rotational strength and range of motion in female collegiate tennis players. *Journal of Strength and Conditioning Research, 16*(1), 92–96.

Ellenbecker, T., & Roetert, E. P. (2003). Age specific isokinetic glenohumeral internal and external rotation strength in elite junior tennis players. *Journal of Science and Medicine in Sport, 6*(1), 63–70.

Ellenbecker, T. S., & Roetert, E. P. (2003). Isokinetic profile of elbow flexion and extension strength in elite junior tennis players. *Journal of Orthopaedic and Sports Physical Therapy, 33*(2), 79–84.

Ellenbecker, T. S., & Roetert, E. P. (2004). An isokinetic profile of trunk rotation strength in elite tennis players. *Medicine and Science in Sports and Exercise, 36*(11), 1959–1963.

Ellenbecker, T. S., Roetert, E. P., Bailie, D. S., Davies, G. J., & Brown, S. W. (2002). Glenohumeral joint total rotation range of motion in elite tennis players and baseball pitchers. *Medicine and Science in Sports and Exercise, 34*(12), 2052–2056.

Ellenbecker, T. S., Roetert, E. P., Piorkowski, P. A., & Schulz, D. A. (1996). Glenohumeral joint internal and external rotation range of motion in elite junior tennis players. *Journal of Orthopaedic and Sports Physical Therapy, 24*(6), 336–341.

Ellenbecker, T. S., Roetert, E. P., & Riewald, S. (2006). Isokinetic profile of wrist and forearm strength in elite female junior tennis players. *British Journal of Sports Medicine, 40*(5), 411–414.

Ellenbecker, T. S., Roetert, E. P., Sueyoshi, T., & Riewald, S. (2007). A descriptive profile of age-specific knee extension flexion strength in elite junior tennis players. *British Journal of Sports Medicine, 41*(11), 5.

Escamilla, R. (2009). Electromyographic activity during upper extremity sports. In K. E. Wilk, M. M. Reinold, & J. R. Andrews (Eds.), *The athlete's shoulder* (2nd ed.) (pp. 385–400). Philadelphia: Churchill Livingstone Elsevier.

Fleisig, G. S., Andrews, J. R., Dillman, C. J., & Escamilla, R. F. (1995). Kinetics of baseball pitching with implications about injury mechanisms. *American Journal of Sports Medicine, 23*(2), 233–239.

Hainline, B. (1995). Low-back injury. *Clinics in Sports Medicine, 14*(1), 241–265.

Hurd, W. J., Kaplan, K. M., ElAttrache, N. S., Jobe, F. W., Morrey, B. F., & Kaufman, K. R. (2011). A profile of glenohumeral internal and external rotation motion in the uninjured high school baseball pitcher, part I: motion. *Journal of Athletic Training, 46*(3), 282–288.

Kelley, J. D., Lombardo, S. J., Pink, M., Perry, J., & Giangarra, C. E. (1994). Electromyographic and cinematographic analysis of elbow function in tennis players with lateral epicondylitis. *American Journal of Sports Medicine, 22*(3), 359–363.

Kibler, W. B. (1991). Role of the scapula in the overhead throwing motion. *Contemporary Orthopaedics, 22*(5), 525–532.

Kibler, W. B. (1998). The role of the scapula in athletic shoulder function. *American Journal of Sports Medicine, 26*(2), 325–337.

Kibler, W. B., Chandler, T. J., Livingston, B. P., & Roetert, E. P. (1996). Shoulder range of motion in elite tennis players: effect of age and years of tournament play. *American Journal of Sports Medicine, 24*(3), 279–285.

Kibler, W. B., McQueen, C., & Uhl, T. (1988). Fitness evaluation and fitness findings in competitive junior tennis players. *Clinics in Sports Medicine, 7*(2), 403–416.

A. LATERALITY – AN IMPORTANT AND OFTEN DISREGARDED TOPIC

Kibler, W. B., Sciascia, A. D., Uhl, T. L., Tambay, N., & Cunningham, T. (2008). Electromyographic analysis of specific exercises for scapular control in early phases of shoulder rehabilitation. *American Journal of Sports Medicine, 36*(9), 1789–1798.

King, J., Brelsford, H. J., & Tullos, H. S. (1969). Analysis of the pitching arm of the professional baseball pitcher. *Clinical Orthopaedics and Related Research, 67*, 116–123.

Laudner, K. G., Lynall, R., & Meister, K. (2013). Shoulder adaptations among pitchers and position players over the course of a competitive baseball season. *Clinical Journal of Sport Medicine, 23*(3), 184–189.

Laudner, K. G., Stanek, J. M., & Meister, K. (2007). Differences in scapular upward rotation between baseball pitchers and position players. *American Journal of Sports Medicine, 35*(12), 2091–2095.

Manske, R., Wilk, K. E., Davies, G., Ellenbecker, T. S., & Reinold, M. (2013). Glenohumeral motion deficits: friend or foe? *International Journal of Sports Physical Therapy, 8*(5), 537–553.

Matsen, F. A., Fu, F., & Hawkins, R. J. (1993). *The shoulder: A balance of mobility and stability.* Rosemont, IL: American Academy of Orthopaedic Surgeons.

Meister, K., Day, T., Horodyski, M., Kaminski, T. W., Wasik, M. R., & Tillman, S. (2005). Rotational motion changes in the glenohumeral joint of the adolescent/little league baseball player. *American Journal of Sports Medicine, 33*(5), 693–698.

Morris, M., Jobe, F. W., Perry, J., Pink, M., & Healy, B. S. (1989). Electromyographic analysis of elbow function in tennis players. *American Journal of Sports Medicine, 17*(2), 241–247.

Myers, J. B., Laudner, K. G., Pasquale, M. R., Bradley, J. P., & Lephart, S. M. (2006). Glenohumeral range of motion deficits and posterior shoulder tightness in throwers with pathologic internal impingement. *American Journal of Sports Medicine, 34*(3), 385–391.

Osbahr, D. C., Cannon, D. L., & Speer, K. P. (2002). Retroversion of the humerus in the throwing shoulder of college baseball pitchers. *American Journal of Sports Medicine, 30*(3), 347–353.

Oyama, S., Myers, J. B., Wassinger, C. A., Ricci, R. D., & Lephart, S. M. (2008). Asymmetric resting scapular posture in healthy overhead athletes. *Journal of Athletic Training, 43*(6), 565–570.

Pluim, B. M., Staal, J. B., Windler, G. E., & Jayanthi, N. (2006). Tennis injuries: occurrence, aetiology, and prevention. *British Journal of Sports Medicine, 40*(5), 415–423.

Priest, J. D., & Nagel, D. A. (1976). Tennis shoulder. *American Journal of Sports Medicine, 4*(1), 28–42.

Reagan, K. M., Meister, K., Horodyski, M. B., Werner, D. W., Carruthers, C., & Wilk, K. (2002). Humeral retroversion and its relationship to glenohumeral rotation in the shoulder of college baseball players. *American Journal of Sports Medicine, 30*(3), 354–360.

Reece, L. A., Fricker, P. A., & Maguire, K. F. (1986). Injuries of elite young tennis players at the Australian institute of sport. *Australian Journal of Science and Medicine in Sport, 18*(4), 11–15.

Reeser, J. C., Fleisig, G. S., Bolt, B., & Ruan, M. (2010). Upper limb biomechanics during the volleyball serve and spike. *Sports Health: A Multidisciplinary Approach, 2*(5), 368–374.

Reiman, M. P., & Manske, R. C. (2009). *Functional testing in human performance.* Champaign, IL: Human Kinetics Publishers.

Reinold, M. M., Wilk, K. E., Macrina, L. C., Sheheane, C., Dun, S., Fleisig, G. S., … Andrews, J. R. (2008). Changes in shoulder and elbow passive range of motion after pitching in professional baseball players. *American Journal of Sports Medicine, 36*(3), 523–527.

Robb, A. J., Fleisig, G., Wilk, K., Macrina, L., Bolt, B., & Pajaczkowski, J. (2010). Passive ranges of motion of the hips and their relationship with pitching biomechanics and ball velocity in professional baseball pitchers. *American Journal of Sports Medicine, 38*(12), 2487–2493.

Roetert, E. P., Ellenbecker, T. S., & Brown, S. W. (2000). Shoulder internal and external rotation range of motion in nationally ranked junior tennis players: a longitudinal analysis. *Journal of Strength and Conditioning Research, 14*(2), 140–143.

Roetert, E. P., & Groppel, J. L. (2001). Mastering the kinetic chain. In E. P. Roetert, & J. L. Groppel (Eds.), *World class tennis technique* (pp. 99–113). Champaign, IL: Human Kinetics.

Roetert, E. P., McCormick, T. J., Brown, S. W., & Ellenbecker, T. S. (1996). Relationship between isokinetic and functional trunk strength in elite junior tennis players. *Isokinetics & Exercise Science*, 6(1), 15–20.

Sauers, E. L., Bliven, K. C. H., Johnson, M. P., Falsone, S., & Walters, S. (2014). Hip and glenohumeral rotational range of motion in healthy professional baseball pitchers and position players. *American Journal of Sports Medicine*, 42(2), 430–436.

Shanley, E., Rauh, M. J., Michener, L. A., Ellenbecker, T. S., Garrison, J. C., & Thigpen, C. A. (2011). Shoulder range of motion measures as risk factors for shoulder and elbow injuries in high school softball and baseball players. *American Journal of Sports Medicine*, 39(9), 1997–2006.

Timm, K. E. (1995). Clinical applications of a normative database for the cybex TEF and TORSO spinal isokinetic dynamometers. *Isokinetics and Exercise Science*, 5(1), 43–49.

Wilk, K. E., Andrews, J. R., Arrigo, C. A., Keirns, M. A., & Erber, D. J. (1993). The strength characteristics of internal and external rotator muscles in professional baseball pitchers. *American Journal of Sports Medicine*, 21(1), 61–66.

Wilk, K. E., Macrina, L. C., & Arrigo, C. (2012). Passive range of motion characteristics in the overhead baseball pitcher and their implications for rehabilitation. *Clinical Orthopaedics and Related Research*, 470(6), 1586–1594.

Wilk, K. E., Macrina, L. C., Fleisig, G. S., Porterfield, R., Simpson, C. D., Harker, P., ... Andrews, J. R. (2011). Correlation of glenohumeral internal rotation deficit and total rotational motion to shoulder injuries in professional baseball pitchers. *American Journal of Sports Medicine*, 39(2), 329–335.

Wright, R. W., Steger-May, K., Wasserlauf, B. L., O'Neal, M. E., Weinberg, B. W., & Paletta, G. A. (2006). Elbow range of motion in professional baseball pitchers. *American Journal of Sports Medicine*, 34(2), 190–193.

A. LATERALITY – AN IMPORTANT AND OFTEN DISREGARDED TOPIC

MOTOR CONTROL AND LEARNING

7

What Can We Learn About Cognition From Studying Handedness? Insights From Cognitive Neuroscience

Jacqueline A. de Nooijer

Erasmus University Rotterdam, Rotterdam, The Netherlands

Roel M. Willems

Radboud University Nijmegen, Nijmegen, The Netherlands;
Max Planck Institute for Psycholinguistics, Nijmegen, The Netherlands

INTRODUCTION

Can we learn something about cognition by studying differences between left- and right-handers? This may seem a strange suggestion, given that left- and right-handers differ in how they perform actions, but why should they differ in how they think? In this chapter, we illustrate how studying differences between left- and right-handed participants has resulted in interesting insights concerning a variety of cognitive domains. Approximately 10% of the world population prefers to use their left hand over their right hand (Coren & Porac, 1977). There have been attempts to eliminate this "idiosyncrasy" by forcing left-handers to the use of their right hand for writing (e.g., Meng, 2007). Left-handedness has been associated with witchcraft and devil worship (Perelle & Ehrman, 2005) and considered a disease or "a neurotic symptom...one of the signs of an infantile psychoneurosis" (Blau, 1946, p. 182). Remnants of these ideas can still be found in our language. For example, we refer to someone as having "two left feet" when moving in an awkward manner, while being someone's "right-hand" means you are indispensable for this person. Where the word "right" in itself means "correct," the adjective "sinister" means "left" or "unlucky." Many expressions reflect this negative attitude toward the left hand. For example, "a left-handed diagnosis" is wrong, "a left-handed compliment" is an insult, "left-handed wisdom" is a collection of errors, and there are many more examples, not only in English, but in an array of languages (Coren, 2012).

Left-handers are regularly left out of scientific research samples in order to reduce heterogeneity of the participants. This is true for studies in neuroscience and neurogenetics (Willems, Van der Haegen, Fisher, & Francks, 2014), but also in psychology, linguistics, and human movement sciences such exclusions can occur. Left-handers might be a minority, but the differences between left- and right-handers might prove valuable in our understanding of cognition. In this chapter we, therefore, attempt to shed light on how cognition is influenced by handedness. What can we learn from left- versus right-handedness about how the brain functions (section: The Left-Handed Brain)? Can handedness influence the way we think (section: Left-Handed Language), and could it even influence the way we memorize and learn new information (section: Left-Handed Learners)? If so, can we use this information to influence left- and right-handers in their choices (section: Application of Results From Handedness Studies)? Lastly, we will conclude by summarizing what we have learned thus far from handedness studies on how we act and why (section: Conclusions and Summary). None of the sections give an exhaustive overview of the literature, but rather we want to illustrate the potential of studying left- and right-handers in cognitive neuroscience and psychology.

THE LEFT-HANDED BRAIN

In this section, we discuss what handedness can teach us about how the brain functions. Is there, for example, a difference in functional specialization of the two hemispheres between left- and right-handers and are there even differences in anatomical brain structures?

Cerebral Lateralization of Brain Function

The brain consists of two hemispheres that have functional specializations (i.e., lateralization). In the literature, many examples can be found of cognitive processes that are thought to take place in either the left or the right hemisphere. For example, right-hemisphere activation has been associated with emotional processing (e.g., Schwartz, Davidson, & Maer, 1975), creative thinking (e.g., Mihov, Denzler, & Förster, 2010), and face recognition (e.g., Ley & Bryden, 1979), while the left hemisphere is thought to be especially important for language processing (e.g., Frost et al., 1999; see Herve, Zago, Petit, Mazoyer, & Tzourio-Mazoyer, 2013; for a recent overview). Research on handedness and cerebral organization has mostly focused on differences between left- and right-handers in this functional specialization of the hemispheres, or lateralization.

Let us look at the case of lateralization of language in left- and right-handers. As mentioned before, language seems to be lateralized to the left hemisphere. Given that the left hemisphere controls the right side of the body, it was thought that there is a link between language lateralization and motor behavior. The reasoning was that if language is left-lateralized in right-handers, this must be the other way around in left-handers. This hypothesis turned out to be false. Indeed, in most right-handers (approximately 96%), language has a left-hemispheric dominance (Knecht et al., 2000), but the majority of left-handers (73%) also show left-hemispheric lateralization. The remainder of left-handers show bilateral or right-hemisphere lateralization for language (Pujol, Deus, Losilla, & Capdevila, 1999). Left-handers and ambidextrous people thus seem to show a reduction or reversal of functional asymmetries compared to right-handers. This is also the case in lateralization of language (see Carey & Johnstone, 2014; for an extensive meta-analysis).

Language therefore seems to be less lateralized to the left hemisphere in left- than in right-handers (Steinmetz, Volkmann, Jäncke, & Freund, 1991; Szaflarski et al., 2002; Tzourio, Crivello, Mellet, Nkanga-Ngila, & Mazoyer, 1998). This difference in lateralization might be strongest for speech production, given that most studies in this field have investigated language lateralization via a speech-production task, such as a word-generation task, where people are cued with a certain letter and then have to think of as many words that start with that letter as they can (e.g., Knecht et al., 2000). Of course, language is more complex than speech production and involves many more processes, such as language comprehension, that might paint a different picture when it comes to cerebral lateralization in left- and right-handers. Not many studies have been conducted to address this issue, although at least two studies have compared cerebral lateralization for language production (i.e., via a naming or word-generation task) and reading/comprehension (i.e., via a reading task or a lexical decision task). In one study, participants consisted of split-brain patients. In these patients the corpus callosum, the bridge between the two hemispheres, is severely damaged or completely disconnected. This results in an impairment of communication between the two hemispheres. For this reason the hemispheres can be studied in isolation in these patients, which can provide insight into the functional specialization of the two hemispheres. In these split-brain patients, speech production seemed to be more strongly left-lateralized than reading. When asked to read words that were presented in the left-visual field (reflecting right-hemisphere activity) the patients were able to do so, while producing (i.e., naming) the words presented in the left-visual field posed problems (Sperry, 1982). In the other study, left-handers were under investigation. Also here a difference in lateralization between speech production and comprehension was found. Fifty-seven left-handers participated, of which approximately half were shown to have left-hemispheric lateralization for speech production. Approximately 10% had bilateral dominance and 35% had right-hemisphere dominance, based on fMRI activation in the inferior temporal gyrus. When these participants performed a lexical decision task (i.e., indicate whether a string of letters forms an existing word or not), more than half of the participants showed activity in both the left and the right hemisphere. There was no clear dominance during this task for either of the hemispheres (Van der Haegen, Cai, & Brysbaert, 2012). This suggests that language lateralization depends on the language process that is under investigation, but also in part on handedness. Interestingly, having a left-handed family member (called "familial sinistrality") also influences the degree of language lateralization, and, according to some reports, more so than actual hand preference (Tzourio-Mazoyer, Petit, et al., 2010; Tzourio-Mazoyer, Simon, et al., 2010).

In areas other than language, handedness also seems to influence lateralization, for example, in the case of face perception, which is usually reported to show right-hemisphere dominance. In left-handers, however, both the left and right regions of the brain are activated when recognizing faces (Willems, Peelen, & Hagoort, 2010). In this respect, left-handers provide new insights as to how we thought the visual system works. Face processing was always thought to be strongly lateralized, but for left-handers this does not seem to be the case.

Brain Anatomy

In addition to a difference in left- and right-handers concerning the functional lateralization of the brain, there also seem to be differences in brain anatomy. The identification of brain structures that differ for right- and left-handers might be useful in studying the relationship between handedness, lateralization, and cognition (Guadalupe et al., 2014). As previously discussed, language seems to be mostly left-lateralized. Anatomically, this has been attributed to a larger planum temporale in the left hemisphere (a triangular area of the brain located on the superior temporal gyrus), which is associated with language processing (e.g., Geschwind & Levitsky, 1968).

It might be expected that because language is not as often left-lateralized in left-handers, there might be underlying anatomical reasons for this difference in lateralization. Indeed, asymmetry of the planum temporale has been found to differ for left- and right-handers, as measured with an in vivo method of magnetic resonance (Steinmetz et al., 1991).

Left-handers were found to have a lesser degree of leftward planum temporale asymmetry than right-handers. This might indicate a structural–functional relation in cerebral asymmetry. Also in the pars triangularis (i.e., part of the inferior frontal gyrus) a left-ward asymmetry for right-handers is found, but not for left-handers (Foundas, Leonard, & Heilman, 1995). Differences in anatomical correlates of cerebral lateralization might not only lie in the brain's gray, but also in its white matter, where volumetric analyses revealed a right-ward asymmetry that was not as clearly visible in left-handers as it was in right-handers (Herve, Crivello, Perchey, Mazoyer, & Tzourio-Mazoyer, 2006).

In addition, postmortem measurements suggest that the connection between the two hemispheres, the corpus callosum, is larger in left-handed and ambidextrous people than in right-handers. It is suggested that cognitive functions are represented more in both hemispheres in left- and mixed-handers (see section: Cerebral Lateralization of Brain Function). The anatomical connection between the hemispheres might, therefore, need to be stronger in left-handed and ambidextrous people (Witelson, 1985). Other cerebral cortical differences between left- and right-handers have been suggested, such as deeper left precentral sulci in right-handers (Amunts et al., 1996). However, these differences have not consistently been found (Good et al., 2001; Narr et al., 2007; Witelson & Kigar, 1992). A study with a large number of participants did not find any differences in bilateral cortical surface area in left-handers compared to right-handers (Guadalupe et al., 2014). It seems that any differences between cortical structures in left- and right-handers are, therefore, subtle.

LEFT-HANDED LANGUAGE

From the previous section, it seems that there are some differences in the brains of left- and right-handers. But does this affect people with a certain hand preference in any way in how they behave, think, or understand language? In this section, we will discuss whether handedness influences the way in which the world is viewed, by discussing one theory that is relevant in answering this question: *embodied cognition.*

Embodied Cognition

When we understand action words like "writing," we activate part of our brain that controls our movements, as though we were writing ourselves, at least according to theories of embodied cognition. According to this theory, cognitive processes like language, thought, and perception cannot be separated from how our body functions (Barsalou, 1999; Glenberg, 1997). This means that our body can influence cognition.

This influence of the motor system on cognition has been found in many cognitive domains, for example, in memory tasks where autobiographic memories are recalled faster when the participant is currently in the same body position as when the memory was created (i.e., when lying back in a chair it is easier to remember a visit to the dentist's office). These memories that are retrieved in congruent body positions are also remembered better after a two-week interval (Dijkstra, Kaschak, & Zwaan, 2007). Also when having to give estimations when unknowingly leaning to the left, lower estimations are given of, for instance, the height of the Eiffel Tower (Eerland, Guadalupe, & Zwaan, 2011). The idea here is that we represent numbers on a mental number line where lower numbers are represented on the left side of space, while larger numbers are positioned on the right side. Thus leaning to the left activates more small numbers than larger numbers, making our estimations smaller. Lastly, in processing emotions, the motor system also seems to play a role, as sentences describing a person that frowns are read more slowly when frowning muscles are paralyzed and the emotion can, therefore, not be simulated (Havas, Glenberg, Gutowski, Lucarelli, & Davidson, 2010).

The same influence of the motor system on cognition can be found in language processing. For example, when hearing action words (e.g., to kick, to throw, to write), this activates areas of the brain's motor and premotor areas. These are the same areas that are active when actually executing the action (e.g., Hauk, Johnsrude, & Pulvermüller, 2004; Tettamanti et al., 2005). In a similar vein, research has shown that action words that involve arm or leg movement (e.g., write, kick) can be recognized faster after arm or leg activation (Pulvermüller, Hauk, Nikulin, & Ilmoniemi, 2005). These studies suggest that the motor system influences language, but that language can also influence the motor system. Action (or the motor system) and language, therefore, seem to be tightly connected (e.g., Fischer & Zwaan, 2008; Willems & Casasanto, 2011; Willems & Hagoort, 2007).

As described above, the motor system is involved in processing language, which means that when we understand language, we activate our motor system. According to embodied cognition theories, this (pre)motor activation is reflected in mental representations or mental simulations that are created when we hear or read something. To illustrate, when participants read sentences in which the shape of a certain object was implied (e.g., the egg in the carton, where the egg is still in its shell) and then see a line drawing of the object mentioned in the sentence in which the shape either matched or mismatched the shape previously described (egg in the carton or egg in the pan; see Fig. 7.1), responses to the question whether the object appeared in the sentence were faster when the picture matched the shape implied by the sentence (Zwaan, Stanfield, & Yaxley, 2002). In a similar vein, when hearing a sentence such as "Close the drawer," (which

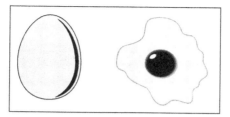

FIGURE 7.1 An example of the stimuli used by Zwaan et al. (2002), where objects were represented in different shapes. On the left, a drawing of what an egg looks like "in a carton" and on the right, the shape it has "in the pan." *Reproduced with permission from Zwaan, R. A., Stanfield, R. A., & Yaxley, R. H. (2002). Language comprehenders mentally represent the shapes of objects.* Psychological Science, 13, 168–171.

implies a movement away from the body) the denoted action interacts with the subsequent performance of an action, meaning that, in this example, a movement away from the body is facilitated (e.g., Glenberg & Kaschak, 2002). The findings described above suggest that we make mental simulations of what we read and hear.

The Body-Specificity Hypothesis

If we make mental simulations of what we read and see, then these mental simulations might be different for left- and right-handers, given that they perform actions differently. According to the body-specificity hypothesis, reading or hearing an action leads to the creation of a body-specific mental simulation of this action (Casasanto, 2009). For instance, when passively viewing the letters of the alphabet, right-handers activate part of the left premotor cortex (that is also active when writing with the right hand) (Longcamp, Anton, Roth, & Velay, 2003). When a similar study was conducted with left-handers, the right premotor area was activated (Longcamp, Anton, Roth, & Velay, 2005), suggesting that when merely viewing letters, mental simulations are made of writing those letters. In addition, when left- and right-handers are asked to imagine (simulate) executing a number of action verbs, such as "writing," right-handers activate left-premotor areas (congruent with activation of the right arm) while left-handers activate right-premotor areas (congruent with activation of the left arm) (Willems, Hagoort, & Casasanto, et al., 2010). There might even be a causal link between the premotor cortex and understanding of action verbs. This hypothesis seems to be supported by the finding that right-handers are faster to indicate that a given manual action (e.g., to write, to throw) or nonmanual action word (e.g., to earn, to wander) is an existing verb after stimulation of the left compared to the right premotor cortex (Willems, Labruna, D'Esposito, Ivry, & Casasanto, 2011; see Fig. 7.2). People seem to understand actions relative to how they would perform the action with their own body.

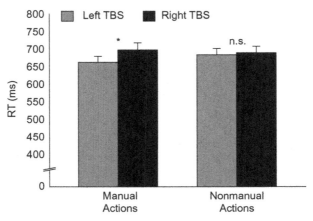

FIGURE 7.2   Results of Willems et al. (2011), in which reaction times reflect how fast a manual or nonmanual action was recognized after simulation of the left or right premotor cortex. Stimulation of the left premotor cortex selectively influenced reaction times (RT) to the manual action verbs, which is consistent with the hand preference of the right-handed participants that took part in this study. *Reproduced with permission from Willems, R. M., Labruna, L., D'Esposito, M., Ivry, R., & Casasanto, D. (2011). A functional role for the motor system in language understanding: evidence from theta-burst transcranial magnetic stimulation.* Psychological Science, 22, 849–854.

Left- and right-handers show the opposite pattern of motor activity not only when imagining executing actions, but also when merely listening to sounds of tools. When presented with sounds of tools that can be manipulated with one hand (i.e., hammer, saw, screwdriver) versus sounds that animals make, fMRI data showed that when hearing tool sounds, right-handers activate left-hemisphere motor-related areas, while left-handers activate right-hemisphere motor areas (Lewis, Phinney, Brefczynski-Lewis, & DeYoe, 2006). This difference did not exist for the sounds of animals. These results suggest that tool sounds are learned in the context of how they are used (with either the left or right hand). In this case, motor imagery might have facilitated the recognition of the tool sounds. These findings further suggest that manual experience acquired during tool manipulation can influence hemispheric representations of tools. Lateralization of tool representations can, therefore, not solely result from innate mechanisms, as no differences in the way tools are represented in the brain would be expected between left- and right-handers, if this were the case (for review see: Gainotti, 2015).

How Right is Right if You're Right-Handed

In the previous paragraphs, we illustrated how the processing of concrete actions is influenced by handedness. Bodily experiences can, however,

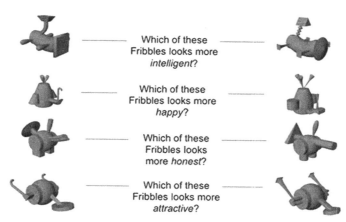

FIGURE 7.3   Stimuli used in Casasanto (2009), in which participants had to decide to which "fribble" they attributed the more positive attribute. *Reproduced from Casasanto, D. (2009). Embodiment of abstract concepts: good and bad in right- and left-handers.* Journal of Experimental Psychology: General, 138, 351–367.; Blackman, C. (2009). Lefty or righty? A new hold on how we think. *Stanford Report. Available at* http://news.stanford.edu/news/2009/august3/lefty-decision-study-080509.html.

also influence more abstract processes, such as the choices we make. For example, when having to make a choice between turning right or left in a "T-maze" task (i.e., a maze in which only a choice between left or right can be made), handedness was the best predictor for which direction participants would turn. In this study, right-handers turned right more often, while left-handers chose the left path (Scharine & McBeath, 2002).

Even our idea of what is good or positive seems to be influenced by handedness. This can, for instance, be seen when left- and right-handers are explicitly asked to draw "good" or "bad" animals in a box on the left or right side of space. Right-handers frequently drew the "good animal" in the box on the right, while left-handers associated the "good animal" with the box on the left (Casasanto, 2009). When presented with two boxes that were shown above each other, both left- and right-handers drew the "good animals" in the top box more often than in the bottom box. This is in the line with the "up is good" metaphor, as we can see in expressions as "Things are looking up" and "Being on top of the situation." Even though, as previously mentioned (in section: Introduction), there are many expressions that reflect the idea that "left is bad" and "right is good," this cultural notion does not prevent left-handers from associating the left side of space with positive valence.

The judgment of positive or negative characteristics to the left or right side of space is similar when done more implicitly, for example, when asked which of two nonsense figures (see Fig. 7.3) could be attributed a positive characteristic, such as intelligence, honesty, or attractiveness.

Right-handed participants indicated the figures on the right more often, while left-handers chose the figures on the left (Casasanto, 2009). Similar findings were found in children (Casasanto & Henetz, 2012).

Even though left- and right-handers treat the left and right side of space differently, it seems as though these views can be changed. Although right-handers associate good things with the right side, while left-handers associate good things with the left side, this association can be reversed. In right-handers who suffered a cerebrovascular accident, resulting in reduced motor fluency to the right arm/hand, seven out of eight patients indicated that the good animal should go to the left side of space (Casasanto & Chrysikou, 2011). In right-handers who experienced weakness in the left arm/hand, the "right is good" link still existed. In addition, when healthy right-handers' right hand was temporarily handicapped, a left-handers pattern also emerged. Here the natural right-handers associated "good" with the left side. These results suggest that motor fluency is an important factor in the bias toward the right or left side.

Although the bias toward the left or right side might be changed, it seems as though for right-handers, the left hemisphere is biased for processing positive things, while in left-handers, the right hemisphere processes positive things. This was suggested in the domain of music. If music is played only to either the left or the right ear, right-handers experience more positive effect when the music was presented to the right ear (i.e., left hemisphere), while left-handers experienced more positivity when music was played to the left ear (i.e., right hemisphere: McFarland & Kennison, 1989). This suggests that emotional valence is processed differently by left- and right-handers. In sum, we can conclude that left- and right-handers differ in how they mentally simulate actions, which can influence them in the choices they make and what they experience as being positive.

LEFT-HANDED LEARNERS

In the previous sections, we have seen that information might be processed differently by left- and right-handers. We will now have a closer look as to whether these differences in processing can also influence memory and learning.

Memory

In the previous section, we showed that left- and right-handers make different mental simulations of action words. Left-handers activate the right hemisphere when simulating these actions, while right-handers activate the left hemisphere. An interesting question is whether these different mental simulations, as proposed by embodied cognition theories, can then also influence our memory. So, does the way we interact with an object influence how well we can remember it? According to the body-specificity hypothesis (section: The Body-Specificity Hypothesis), word meanings are in part made up of the simulations of one's own actions. This might be reflected in how well these words are remembered. A recent study suggested that the experience people have with certain objects can influence how well they are remembered. For instance, words denoting objects that we can manipulate such as a camera are remembered better than words we do not interact with, such as a table (Madan & Singhal, 2012). If whether we interact with objects can influence how well we remember the object, then the way we interact with it (i.e., their affordances, e.g., Gibson, 1977) might also influence our memory. This, indeed, seems to be the case. The study that investigated this issue showed left- and right-handed participants a 3×3 grid with cups around the grid. The handles of these cups were pointed either toward the right or toward the left (see Fig. 7.4). Participants were then given instructions as to how to move the cups across the grid. Half of the participants executed the memorized actions with their dominant hand, the other half with their nondominant hand. Results showed that right-handers remembered more instructions when an object's handle was oriented to the right and actions had to be performed with the right hand. This suggests that motor simulation can support sequential memory for action and that memory is embodied, or at least that if the handle is oriented in congruence with the use by a right-hander, the mental simulation might be facilitated, enhancing memory performance. The same effect was not found for left-handers (Apel, Cangelosi, Ellis, Gosling, & Fischer, 2012). For an explanation of these differential findings for left- and right-handers see section "Influencing Right- but Not Left-Handers."

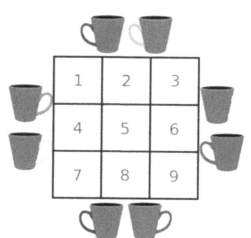

FIGURE 7.4 Example of the display that was used by Apel et al. (2012). When instructed to move the cups over the grid, right-handers remembered more instructions when the object's handle was oriented to the right and the actions had to be executed with the right hand. *Reproduced with permission from Apel, J. K., Cangelosi, A., Ellis, R., Goslin, J., & Fischer, M. H. (2012). Object affordance influences instruction span.* Experimental Brain Research, 223, *199–206.*

Learning

In the previous section, we presented some evidence for the hypothesis that if we see an object that is suitable for use (by right-handers), this can improve memory. We also saw that when we hear or read an action word, we create a mental simulation of this action. In addition, studies have shown that seeing a picture also automatically activates motor information (e.g., Borghi et al., 2007). Seeing a picture that mismatches the mental simulation created by verbal information might, therefore, hinder the consolidation of new information, as motor information is part of the word's meaning. Thus receiving contradictory motor information might hinder learning new information. So, if we hear a definition of a word and then see a picture that either matches (i.e., seeing a picture of a right-handed perspective as a right-hander) or mismatches (i.e., seeing a picture of a left-handed perspective as a right-hander; see Fig. 7.5) the mental simulation created, this might hinder word learning performance. Whether this is actually the case was recently investigated in a study in which novel action verbs from an artificial language were learned. Indeed, right-handers learned fewer word definitions when words were learned in combination with a mismatching left-handed perspective, compared to learning words with the right-handed perspective that matched the mental simulation created (de Nooijer, Van Gog, Paas, & Zwaan, 2013). The same effect was not found for left-handers. In right-handers, however, seeing a picture that mismatches the mental simulation created for that action can interfere with the consolidation of new information.

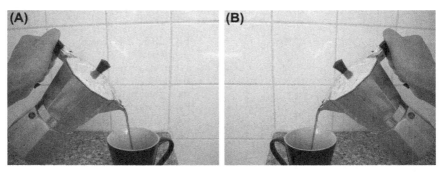

FIGURE 7.5   Example of the material used in the study by de Nooijer et al. (2013), where the pictures for the word "to pour" are shown for a first-person left-handed and right-handed perspective. *Reproduced with permission from de Nooijer, J. A., Van Gog, T., Paas, F., & Zwaan, R. A. (2013). When left is not right: handedness effects on learning object-manipulation words using pictures with left-or right-handed first-person perspectives.* Psychological Science, 24, 2515–2521.

Right-handers are not only influenced in how well they learn when they see a picture of an action that is performed by a left-hander while learning, but seeing a model with a different hand preference can also influence how well a task is learned. To illustrate, when right-handers were asked to learn a complex spatiotemporal task (i.e., learn a number of movement sequences), they performed better when observing a right-handed model, compared to seeing a left-handed model. This is true both when the model was observed from a first-person and a third-person perspective (Rohbanfard & Proteau, 2011).

Influencing Right- but Not Left-Handers

Thus far, it appears that handedness can have an influence on the way we judge things, how we memorize things, and how we learn new information. However, both when memorizing information and when learning new information, studies have found an influence on performance when right-handers are presented with the left-handed perspective (in the form of a picture, of a handle oriented to the left), but not when left-handers are presented with the right-handed perspective. Left-handers are not affected (or are less affected) by seeing the right-handed perspective (e.g., Apel et al., 2012; de Nooijer et al., 2013). Also in other studies similar results are obtained. For instance, when asked to press a button in a reaction time experiment with either the right or left index finger or both fingers, right-handers showed different brain activity (i.e., an increase of activity in dorsal premotor and right primary sensorimotor cortices) for making a unilateral versus a bilateral response, while left-handers did not. This suggests that there are differences in bimanual motor control related to handedness (Klöppel et al., 2007). Another study showed that perceived distance of objects varies when an object is in a difficult versus an easy to grasp position, but only in right-handers. Right-handers perceived tools as farther away when they are difficult to grasp, but left-handers did not (Linkenauger, Witt, Stefanucci, Bakdash, & Proffitt, 2009).

Why is this? Why do right-handers seem to behave differently when presented with a left-handed perspective (or left-handed action), but the opposite is not true for left-handers? One explanation might lie in the fact that right-handers outnumber left-handers by far. Left-handers, therefore live in a right-handed world. They use their right-hand more often than right-handers use their left hand and might therefore not have very strong hand-specific embodied connections (e.g., Stins, Kadar, & Costall, 2001). For this reason, left-handers might not have strong associations between objects and actions, as they need to be more flexible in the use of many objects.

APPLICATION OF RESULTS FROM HANDEDNESS STUDIES

Many of the scientific studies described here are very relevant for our understanding of the brain and cognitive processes. In this section, we will not so much focus on the theoretical relevance of these studies, but we will briefly discuss whether we can apply this knowledge outside of the scientific world.

We have already discussed how left- and right-handers can make different mental simulations of actions. We have also argued that if the mental simulation evoked by a picture matches the simulation the participant makes, this can improve memory and learning (in right-handers). This knowledge could be used for educational purposes, as the use of pictures while learning new information is not uncommon in the educational system. To illustrate, when learning a motor task, such as knot tying, it would be useful to use pictures showing a right-hander performing the action, as left-handers do not seem to be influenced by seeing a right-handed perspective. In addition, when a new (motor) task is learned, right-handers learn this task better when observing a right-handed model (Rohbanfard & Proteau, 2011). It would therefore be wise to have a right-hander teach another right-hander a new task. This knowledge can also be applied in the area of sports, where many new motor tasks have to be learned. For example, when in tennis a new move has to be learned, right-handers would benefit from having a right-handed trainer. As described earlier, left-handers do not seem to be hindered as much by seeing a right-handed perspective. Right-handers are used to seeing the right-handed perspective but are not familiar with the left-handed perspective. This could explain why left-handers seem to have a tactical advantage in several interactive sports (Hagemann, 2009). Another potential application of these results in the field of sports is based on the earlier described findings that right-handers prefer the right side of space, while left-handers prefer the left. During a sporting event, it might therefore be predicted to which side the opponent will move, when there are no obvious tactical reasons to choose either the left or right side.

In another field, knowledge about the influence of handedness might also be applicable, such as in the field of marketing. Handedness, namely, also seems to influence behavioral intentions. This was suggested by a study in which it was suggested that when orienting a product toward the dominant (right) hand of the participants (e.g., a mug with the handle to the right side), right-handers are sooner inclined to purchase the product presented in this advertisement. Probably because the product was presented in a way that is suitable for use, which facilitates simulation of the use of the product and can influence the behavioral intentions of the participants (Elder & Krishna, 2012).

In a very different area, namely politics, some application of handedness studies might also be found. The gestures politicians use can, for example, give us insightful information as to what they actually think. The gestures of four presidential candidates of whom two were right-handed (Kerry and Bush) and two left-handed (Obama and McCain) were analyzed for this purpose (Casasanto & Jasmin, 2010). Analyses of speeches by these candidates showed that left-handed gestures were more associated with positive valence in left-handers, while in right-handers this is true for right-handed gestures (see Fig. 7.6). Paying attention to the gestures politicians made might therefore provide information as to the valence politicians attribute to what they are saying. These findings could also be used to discover what valence teachers, trainers, coaches, or other people with authority attribute to what they are saying. In addition, as we already saw that right-handers, who made up 90% of the population, attribute more positive attributes to figures shown on the right side of space (Casasanto, 2009), voters might be influenced in their voting behavior when the desired candidate is shown on the right side of a billboard, while the undesired candidate is shown on the left (Casasanto & Jasmin, 2010).

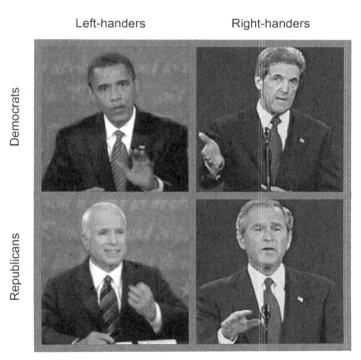

FIGURE 7.6   Examples of one-handed gestures in both left- and right-handed presidential candidates while talking about something with positive valence. *Reproduced with permission from Casasanto, D., & Jasmin, K. (2010). Good and bad in the hands of politicians: spontaneous gestures during positive and negative speech. PLoS One, 5, e11805.*

CONCLUSIONS AND SUMMARY

In this chapter, we have discussed an array of studies showing the influence of handedness on cognition. What have we learned from the studies discussed here? In section "The Left-Handed Brain," we discussed, among other things, some differences in cerebral organization between left- and right-handers. Here we saw that the functional specialization of the hemispheres might depend on handedness. These studies showed that for certain cognitive processes such as face perception, both hemispheres are capable of processing this information. While researchers used to think that some information could only be processed by one of the two hemispheres, studies with left-handers showed that both hemispheres might be capable of doing so. These studies, therefore, provide information on the flexibility of the brain.

Left-handers are also valuable in studies testing the role of motor activation on cognition. In sections "Left-Handed Language and Left-Handed Learners," we discussed how left- and right-handers differ in how they mentally simulate actions. This was found to influence them in the choices they make, what they experience as being positive, and how they memorize and learn new information. Lastly, in section "Application of Results From Handedness Studies," we suggested that the findings from studies that investigated the influence of handedness on cognition could be applied in the fields of education, marketing, and maybe even politics. In sum, whether it concerns cerebral lateralization, making choices, or learning new information, left-handers can contribute useful information about cognitive processes and help us understand a little bit better how we act and why.

References

Amunts, K., Schlaug, G., Schleicher, A., Steinmetz, H., Dabringhaus, A., Roland, P. E., & Zilles, K. (1996). Asymmetry in the human motor cortex and handedness. *NeuroImage*, *4*, 216–222.

Apel, J. K., Cangelosi, A., Ellis, R., Goslin, J., & Fischer, M. H. (2012). Object affordance influences instruction span. *Experimental Brain Research*, *223*, 199–206.

Barsalou, L. W. (1999). Perceptual symbol systems. *Behavioral & Brain Sciences*, *22*, 577–660.

Blackman, C. (2009). *Lefty or righty? A new hold on how we think*. Stanford Report. Available at http://news.stanford.edu/news/2009/august3/lefty-decision-study-080509.html.

Blau, A. (1946). *The master hand: A study of the origin and meaning of right and left sidedness and its relation to personality and language* (Vol. 5). New York: The American Orthopsychiatric Association, Research Monograph.

Borghi, A. M., Bonfiglioli, C., Lugli, L., Ricciardelli, P., Rubichi, S., & Nicoletti, R. (2007). Are visual stimuli sufficient to evoke motor information? Studies with hand primes. *Neuroscience Letters*, *411*, 17–21.

Carey, D. P., & Johnstone, L. T. (2014). Quantifying cerebral asymmetries for language in dextrals and adextrals with random-effects meta analysis. *Frontiers in Psychology*, *5*.

Casasanto, D. (2009). Embodiment of abstract concepts: good and bad in right- and left-handers. *Journal of Experimental Psychology: General, 138*, 351–367.

Casasanto, D., & Chrysikou, E. G. (2011). When left is "right": motor fluency shapes abstract concepts. *Psychological Science, 22*, 419–422.

Casasanto, D., & Henetz, T. (2012). Handedness shapes children's abstract concepts. *Cognitive Science, 36*, 359–372.

Casasanto, D., & Jasmin, K. (2010). Good and bad in the hands of politicians: spontaneous gestures during positive and negative speech. *PLoS One, 5*, e11805.

Coren, S. (2012). *The left-hander syndrome: The causes and consequences of left-handedness.* Simon and Schuster.

Coren, S., & Porac, C. (1977). Fifty centuries of right-handedness: the historical record. *Science, 198*, 631–632.

Dijkstra, K., Kaschak, M. P., & Zwaan, R. A. (2007). Body posture facilitates retrieval of autobiographical memories. *Cognition, 102*, 139–149.

Eerland, A., Guadalupe, T. M., & Zwaan, R. A. (2011). Leaning to the left makes the Eiffel Tower seem smaller: posture-modulated estimation. *Psychological Science, 22*, 1511–1514.

Elder, R. S., & Krishna, A. (2012). The "visual depiction effect" in advertising: facilitating embodied mental simulation through product orientation. *Journal of Consumer Research, 38*, 988–1003.

Fischer, M. H., & Zwaan, R. A. (2008). Embodied language: a review of the role of the motor system in language comprehension. *The Quarterly Journal of Experimental Psychology, 61*, 825–850.

Foundas, A. L., Leonard, C. M., & Heilman, K. M. (1995). Morphologic cerebral asymmetries and handedness: the pars triangularis and planum temporale. *Archives of Neurology, 52*, 501–508.

Frost, J. A., Binder, J. R., Springer, J. A., Hammeke, T. A., Bellgowan, P. S., Rao, S. M., & Cox, R. W. (1999). Language processing is strongly left lateralized in both sexes evidence from functional MRI. *Brain, 122*, 199–208.

Gainotti, G. (2015). The influence of handedness on hemispheric representation of tools: a survey. *Brain and Cognition, 94*, 10–16.

Geschwind, N., & Levitsky, W. (1968). Human brain: left-right asymmetries in temporal speech region. *Science, 161*, 186–187.

Gibson, J. J. (1977). The theory of affordances. In R. Shaw, & J. Bransford (Eds.), *Perceiving, acting, and knowing: Toward an ecological psychology* (pp. 67–82). Hillsdale, NJ: Lawrence Erlbaum.

Glenberg, A. M. (1997). What memory is for. *Behavioral & Brain Sciences, 20*, 1–55.

Glenberg, A. M., & Kaschak, M. P. (2002). Grounding language in action. *Psychonomic Bulletin & Review, 9*, 558–565.

Good, C. D., Johnsrude, I., Ashburner, J., Henson, R. N. A., Friston, K. J., & Frackowiak, R. S. (2001). Cerebral asymmetry and the effects of sex and handedness on brain structure: a voxel-based morphometric analysis of 465 normal adult human brains. *NeuroImage, 14*, 685–700.

Guadalupe, T., Willems, R. M., Zwiers, M. P., Arias Vasquez, A., Hoogman, M., Hagoort, P., … Francks, C. (2014). Differences in cerebral cortical anatomy of left- and right-handers. *Frontiers in Psychology, 5*.

Hagemann, N. (2009). The advantage of being left-handed in interactive sports. *Attention, Perception, & Psychophysics, 71*, 1641–1648.

Hauk, O., Johnsrude, I., & Pulvermüller, F. (2004). Somatotopic representation of action words in human motor and premotor cortex. *Neuron, 41*, 301–307.

Havas, D. A., Glenberg, A. M., Gutowski, K. A., Lucarelli, M. J., & Davidson, R. J. (2010). Cosmetic use of botulinum toxin-A affects processing of emotional language. *Psychological Science, 7*, 895–900.

Herve, P. Y., Crivello, F., Perchey, G., Mazoyer, B., & Tzourio-Mazoyer, N. (2006). Handedness and cerebral anatomical asymmetries in young adult males. *NeuroImage, 29*, 1066–1079.

Herve, P. Y., Zago, L., Petit, L., Mazoyer, B., & Tzourio-Mazoyer, N. (2013). Revisiting human hemispheric specialization with neuroimaging. *Trends in Cognitive Sciences, 17*, 69–80.

Klöppel, S., van Eimeren, T., Glauche, V., Vongerichten, A., Münchau, A., Frackowiak, R. S., … Siebner, H. R. (2007). The effect of handedness on cortical motor activation during simple bilateral movements. *NeuroImage, 34*, 274–280.

Knecht, S., Dräger, B., Deppe, M., Bobe, L., Lohmann, H., Flöel, A., … Henningsen, H. (2000). Handedness and hemispheric language dominance in healthy humans. *Brain, 123*, 2512–2518.

Lewis, J. W., Phinney, R. E., Brefczynski-Lewis, J. A., & DeYoe, E. A. (2006). Lefties get it "right" when hearing tool sounds. *Journal of Cognitive Neuroscience, 18*, 1314–1330.

Ley, R. G., & Bryden, M. P. (1979). Hemispheric differences in processing emotions and faces. *Brain and Language, 7*, 127–138.

Linkenauger, S. A., Witt, J. K., Stefanucci, J. K., Bakdash, J. Z., & Proffitt, D. R. (2009). The effects of handedness and reachability on perceived distance. *Journal of Experimental Psychology: Human Perception and Performance, 35*, 1649–1660.

Longcamp, M., Anton, J. L., Roth, M., & Velay, J. L. (2003). Visual presentation of single letters activates a premotor area involved in writing. *NeuroImage, 19*, 1492–1500.

Longcamp, M., Anton, J. L., Roth, M., & Velay, J. L. (2005). Premotor activations in response to visually presented single letters depend on the hand used to write: a study on left-handers. *Neuropsychologia, 43*, 1801–1809.

Madan, C. R., & Singhal, A. (2012). Encoding the world around us: motor-related processing influences verbal memory. *Consciousness and Cognition, 21*, 1563–1570.

McFarland, R. A., & Kennison, A. R. (1989). Handedness affects emotional valence asymmetry. *Perceptual and Motor Skills, 68*, 435–441.

Meng, L. F. (2007). The rate of handedness conversion and related factors in left-handed children. *Laterality: Asymmetries of Body, Brain and Cognition, 12*, 131–138.

Mihov, K. M., Denzler, M., & Förster, J. (2010). Hemispheric specialization and creative thinking: a meta-analytic review of lateralization of creativity. *Brain and Cognition, 72*, 442–448.

Narr, K. L., Bilder, R. M., Luders, E., Thompson, P. M., Woods, R. P., Robinson, D., … Toga, A. W. (2007). Asymmetries of cortical shape: effects of handedness, sex and schizophrenia. *NeuroImage, 34*, 939–948.

de Nooijer, J. A., Van Gog, T., Paas, F., & Zwaan, R. A. (2013). When left is not right: handedness effects on learning object-manipulation words using pictures with left-or right-handed first-person perspectives. *Psychological Science, 24*, 2515–2521.

Perelle, I. B., & Ehrman, L. (2005). On the other hand. *Behavior Genetics, 35*, 343–350.

Pujol, J., Deus, J., Losilla, J. M., & Capdevila, A. (1999). Cerebral lateralization of language in normal left-handed people studied by functional MRI. *Neurology, 52*, 1038.

Pulvermüller, F., Hauk, O., Nikulin, V. V., & Ilmoniemi, R. J. (2005). Functional links between motor and language systems. *European Journal of Neuroscience, 21*, 793–797.

Rohbanfard, H., & Proteau, L. (2011). Effects of the model's handedness and observer's viewpoint on observational learning. *Experimental Brain Research, 214*, 567–576.

Scharine, A. A., & McBeath, M. K. (2002). Right-handers and Americans favor turning to the right. *Human Factors, 44*, 248–256.

Schwartz, G. E., Davidson, R. J., & Maer, F. (1975). Right hemisphere lateralization for emotion in the human brain: interactions with cognition. *Science, 190*, 286–288.

Sperry, R. (1982). Some effects of disconnecting the cerebral hemispheres. *Science, 217*, 1223–1226.

Steinmetz, H., Volkmann, J., Jäncke, L., & Freund, H. J. (1991). Anatomical left–right asymmetry of language-related temporal cortex is different in left- and right-handers. *Annals of Neurology, 29*, 315–319.

Stins, J. F., Kadar, E. E., & Costall, A. (2001). A kinematic analysis of hand selection in a reaching task. *Laterality: Asymmetries of Body, Brain and Cognition, 6*, 347–367.

Szaflarski, J. P., Binder, J. R., Possing, E. T., McKiernan, K. A., Ward, B. D., & Hammeke, T. A. (2002). Language lateralization in left-handed and ambidextrous people fMRI data. *Neurology, 59*, 238–244.

Tettamanti, M., Buccino, G., Saccuman, M. C., Gallese, V., Danna, M., Scifo, P., & Perani, D. (2005). Listening to action-related sentences activates fronto-parietal motor circuits. *Journal of Cognitive Neuroscience, 17*, 273–281.

Tzourio, N., Crivello, F., Mellet, E., Nkanga-Ngila, B., & Mazoyer, B. (1998). Functional anatomy of dominance for speech comprehension in left handers vs right handers. *NeuroImage, 8*, 1–16.

Tzourio-Mazoyer, N., Petit, L., Razafimandimby, A., Crivello, F., Zago, L., Jobard, G., … Mazoyer, B. (2010). Left hemisphere lateralization for language in right-handers is controlled in part by familial sinistrality, manual preference strength, and head size. *The Journal of Neuroscience, 30*, 13314–13318.

Tzourio-Mazoyer, N., Simon, G., Crivello, F., Jobard, G., Zago, L., Perchey, G., … Mazoyer, B. (2010). Effect of familial sinistrality on planum temporale surface and brain tissue asymmetries. *Cerebral Cortex, 20*, 1476–1485.

Van der Haegen, L., Cai, Q., & Brysbaert, M. (2012). Colateralization of Broca's area and the visual word form area in left-handers: fMRI evidence. *Brain and Language, 122*, 171–178.

Willems, R. M., & Casasanto, D. (2011). Flexibility in embodied language understanding. *Frontiers in Psychology, 2*.

Willems, R. M., & Hagoort, P. (2007). Neural evidence for the interplay between language, gesture, and action: a review. *Brain and Language, 101*, 278–289.

Willems, R. M., Hagoort, P., & Casasanto, D. (2010). Body-specific representations of action verbs: neural evidence from right- and left-handers. *Psychological Science, 21*, 67–74.

Willems, R. M., Labruna, L., D'Esposito, M., Ivry, R., & Casasanto, D. (2011). A functional role for the motor system in language understanding: evidence from theta-burst transcranial magnetic stimulation. *Psychological Science, 22*, 849–854.

Willems, R. M., Peelen, M. V., & Hagoort, P. (2010). Cerebral lateralization of face-selective and body-selective visual areas depends on handedness. *Cerebral Cortex, 20*, 1719–1725.

Willems, R. M., Van der Haegen, L., Fisher, S. E., & Francks, C. (2014). On the other hand: including left-handers in cognitive neuroscience and neurogenetics. *Nature Reviews Neuroscience, 15*, 193–201.

Witelson, S. F. (1985). The brain connection: the corpus callosum is larger in left-handers. *Science, 229*, 665–668.

Witelson, S. F., & Kigar, D. L. (1992). Sylvian fissure morphology and asymmetry in men and women: bilateral differences in relation to handedness in men. *Journal of Comparative Neurology, 323*, 326–340.

Zwaan, R. A., Stanfield, R. A., & Yaxley, R. H. (2002). Language comprehenders mentally represent the shapes of objects. *Psychological Science, 13*, 168–171.

Laterality of Basic Motor Control Mechanisms: Different Roles of the Right and Left Brain Hemispheres

Robert L. Sainburg

Penn State College of Medicine, Hershey, PA, United States; Pennsylvania State University, University Park, PA, United States

INTRODUCTION

The ubiquitous nature of handedness across human populations is a striking effect of brain lateralization. Rogers and colleagues (MacNeilage, Rogers, & Vallortigara, 2009) have provided evidence that brain lateralization emerged early in animal evolution and is critical to ensure adaptive behavior because it allows the underlying neural processes to be performed in parallel, without interfering with one another. However, the neural processes that might underlie motor lateralization have not been well understood, and it has been unclear how handedness might fit into a broader context of brain lateralization. In this chapter, I will present evidence from studies of healthy individuals and stroke patients with specific lesions that have led to a fundamental framework for understanding the motor control processes that give rise to handedness. According to this hypothesis, the dominant hemisphere, left in right-handers, appears specialized for processes that predict the effects of limb and task dynamics in order to optimize costs, such as energy, speed, and smoothness. This type of predictive control, however, depends on the consistency of impending mechanical conditions, arising from within and external to the organism. The nondominant hemisphere, right in right-handers, appears specialized for impedance control processes that can stabilize performance and reduce errors in the face of unexpected mechanical conditions. This distinction of right and left hemisphere processes fits well into the broader hypothesis of brain lateralization proposed by Rogers and colleagues, which purports that the left hemisphere is specialized for well-established behaviors performed under familiar circumstances, and the right hemisphere for detecting and responding to unexpected stimuli. Our hypothesis for motor lateralization provides the mechanical equivalent to Roger's hypothesis, and thereby a framework for understanding the biology of handedness that is consistent with a broad and comparative body of literature. Most of the studies described or cited in this chapter address right-handed individuals, although some of the studies have addressed left-handers. In general, the findings in left-handers show a similar (reversed) pattern of asymmetries, although reduced in mean amplitude with greater variability in asymmetries between individuals. We address the neural and behavioral characteristics of left-handers in a later section of this chapter.

VERTEBRATE BRAIN LATERALIZATION

The division of labor between the two sides of the brain is a basic organizational feature of the vertebrate nervous system that appears to predate humans by half a billion years (Bisazza, Rogers, & Vallortigara, 1998). According to the work of Rogers and colleagues, a single organizing principle might account for the large array of emotional, language, perceptual, and cognitive asymmetries that have been described across an array of animals, including humans. While the left hemisphere is "specialized for control of well-established patterns of behavior, under ordinary and familiar circumstances," the right hemisphere is specialized for "detecting and responding to unexpected stimuli in the environment" (MacNeilage et al., 2009, p. 60). However, the role of handedness in this model has not been well elaborated. Our laboratory has developed a model of motor lateralization (Mutha, Haaland, & Sainburg, 2012, 2013; Sainburg, 2002, 2005), that we have termed *dynamic dominance*. This model proposes that the left hemisphere (in righties) is specialized for predictive processes that specify smooth and efficient movement trajectories under mechanically stable environmental circumstances, while the right hemisphere is specialized for impedance control mechanisms that confer robustness to movements performed under unpredictable and mechanically unstable environmental conditions. This corresponds with Roger's hypothesis and has been supported by a large array of experimental findings in healthy individuals and in patients with specific brain lesions, as well as by computational simulations. This may be the first explanation of handedness that is placed in the context of other neurobehavioral asymmetries across the animal kingdom and that is based on fundamental principles of control theory, neuroscience, and biomechanics.

HUMAN HANDEDNESS

More than a century of previous research has focused on identifying consistent performance characteristics that might define the motor asymmetry that we refer to as "handedness". The first quantitative study published by Woodworth in 1899 showed dominant hand advantages in rapid aiming movements made with a pencil that varied with the frequency of a metronome and with the availability of vision. Since this time, studies have attempted to distinguish arm performance asymmetries based on sensorimotor processing principles. This work has previously been summarized thoroughly by Carson (1993) and Carson, Goodman, Chua, and Elliott (1993). Overall, a large number of studies have focused on whether the use of sensory feedback might distinguish arm performance asymmetries. However, studies directly manipulating visual feedback (Carson, 1992; Shabbott & Sainburg, 2008) could not consistently distinguish between the arms. Another view was that the dominant system might be specialized for producing consistent movement initiation, or initial force amplitudes in isometric conditions, yet this hypothesis also did not hold up to experimental scrutiny (Carson, Elliott, et al., 1993). Reviewing this line of work, Carson (1993) expressed the difficulty in distinguishing whether manual asymmetries in target-aiming might result from right-hand advantages in movement planning or in responding to feedback. This issue was further complicated by a line of research characterizing ipsilesional motor deficits seen in unilateral stroke patients, which led to an opposite hypothesis about feedback, suggesting that the right hemisphere (and left hand, in righties) might be specialized for correcting errors during movement (Haaland & Harrington, 1989; Winstein & Pohl, 1995). Yet, another approach has been to differentiate performance asymmetries based on "task complexity." However, this is a difficult concept to define in relation to motor control and could reflect a plethora of underlying neural and mechanical processes in different tasks. It is therefore not surprising to find conflicting results of studies that explored manual asymmetries in task complexity (Hausmann, Kirk, & Corballis, 2004). While this research has been critical in demonstrating performance differences between the arms in different experimental contexts, it has not revealed fundamental control principles that might give rise to handedness. We will present evidence that Roger's fundamental hypothesis of brain lateralization might encompass the motor control differences that give rise to handedness.

TWO FUNDAMENTAL COMPONENTS OF MOTOR CONTROL

When considering the importance of energy conservation in the process of evolution, it is not surprising that humans seem to prefer coordination patterns that are optimized for energy efficiency (Alexander, 1997; Nishii & Taniai, 2009), even for movements that are not very energetically taxing, such as reaching. Predictive control can be efficient and can allow precise specification of trajectories that conform to different costs, including costs for accuracy, shape, velocity, direction, and energy, among others. For example, when pitching a ball, one might put a very high cost on deviations from maximum velocity and direction at ball release and a small cost on energy. However, when painting a house, energetic costs might prevail. Thus optimality is an important principle for predictive control (Todorov, 2004). However, optimal control requires predictions that do not take account of perturbations that might arise from the environment, or even within our own body. Therefore control of limb impedance through modulation of gains in feedback circuits is also an important component of biological movements (Mutha, Boulinguez, & Sainburg, 2008; Omrani, Diedrichsen, & Scott, 2013; Scott, 2004). Such control of impedance can be modulated through feedforward mechanisms that themselves can be modified during the course of motion. However, these two processes, while interactive, reflect independent aspects of motor control that have been well characterized.

In a study designed to explore how predictive and impedance control mechanisms might be combined during movements, Takahashi, Scheidt, and Reinkensmeyer (2001) examined how subjects adapt to two different force environments: a consistent field and a field that varied in magnitude from trial to trial but had the same mean magnitude as the consistent field. Both were "curl" fields, proportional to velocity and directed perpendicular to the targeted movements, and were imposed by a handheld robotic manipulandum (Fig. 8.1A). When initially exposed to the field, the forces induced large perpendicular errors (Fig. 8.1B, negative peak), but with practice, subjects learned to counter these errors. They might have done this by generating time-varying forces against the manipulandum that would exactly counter the applied forces, or by stiffening their arm as it moved along the intended straight trajectory. To examine these alternatives, the force field was removed following adaptation. In this "null" field, subjects showed errors that mirror imaged the initial errors (shaded region, Fig. 8.1B). Such aftereffects reflect prediction of and compensation for the applied forces (Hwang & Shadmehr, 2005; Lackner & DiZio, 1998; Wang, Dordevic, & Shadmehr, 2001). Thus the force field was compensated by using a predictive strategy that depended on an internal representation of the force field. When subjects were exposed to the inconsistent, or "noisy" field, they also adapted (Fig. 8.1C, positive peak), but following

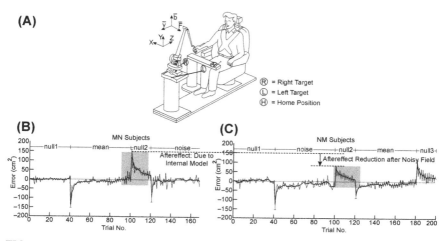

FIGURE 8.1   (A) Experimental Setup. Subjects held a robotic manipulandum while reaching to targets to the left and right of midline. (B) Perpendicular errors during the course of the session, in which subjects experienced the consistent field. (C) Perpendicular errors during the course of the session, in which subjects experienced the inconsistent (noisy) field. *From Takahashi, C. D., Scheidt, R. A., & Reinkensmeyer, D. J. (2001). Impedance control and internal model formation when reaching in a randomly varying dynamical environment. Journal of Neurophysiology, 86(2), 1047–1051.*

adaptation, the amplitude of the aftereffects were substantially reduced. The fact that subjects showed a reduced aftereffect amplitude pointed to the use of an impedance strategy that was implemented to deal with the unpredictability of the field variations. In addition, this impedance strategy allowed subjects to reduce the trial-to-trial errors that occurred both due to the inability to predict the field early in learning and due to the unpredictability of the field magnitude throughout learning. Therefore this study showed that subjects employ a hybrid control strategy, exploiting both predictive and impedance control mechanisms for efficient and robust coordination of arm movements, a phenomenon supported by a number of other studies (Ghez, Scheidt, & Heijink, 2007; Scheidt & Ghez, 2007; Yadav & Sainburg, 2014b).

DOMINANT ARM ADVANTAGES IN PREDICTIVE CONTROL

There has been substantial evidence that predictive and impedance control mechanisms are specialized in different cerebral hemispheres, imparting different control characteristics to each arm. In our laboratory, we have studied reaching movements made in the horizontal plane, with subjects' arms supported above the surface by an air sled that removes the fatiguing effects of gravity and friction during movements. A virtual reality interface is projected in a mirror, placed horizontally above the arm, and under a 55″ HDTV monitor. This allows projection of a virtual or veridical location for a cursor, representing hand position.

Fig. 8.2 shows examples of rapid horizontal plane-reaching movements, performed without visual feedback by each arm for a typical right-hander (Bagesteiro & Sainburg, 2002). As reflected by the graphs at the right, when dominant and nondominant arm movements were made at the same speed, dominant hand trajectories were substantially straighter, yet had slightly higher final position errors. Nondominant trajectories were initially deviated away from the target position and curved back toward the target at the end of motion. Fig. 8.2 (bottom) shows the elbow joint kinetics associated with these two movements. Note that the muscle torque profile remains near zero throughout the movement, while the elbow is accelerated by motion of the shoulder (interaction torque-dashed). The

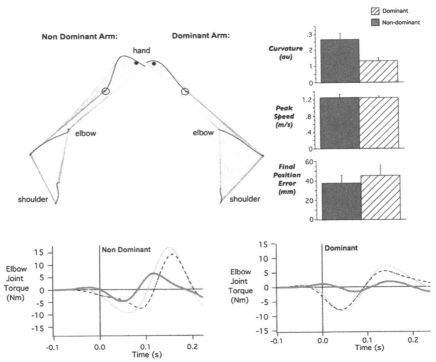

FIGURE 8.2   Shoulder, elbow, and hand trajectories from typical left (nondominant) and right (dominant) are movements toward a medial target. Bar plots show group means ±SE for curvature (minor/major axis), peak hand velocity, and final position error. Elbow joint torque profiles show computed muscle torque (*thick gray*), interaction torque (*dashed*), and net torque (*solid thin gray*). *From Bagesteiro, L. B., & Sainburg, R. L. (September 2003). Nondominant arm advantages in load compensation during rapid elbow joint movements. J Neurophysiol, 90(3), 1503–1513. Epub 2003 May 7.*

nondominant arm, however, generates excessive elbow muscle torque that deviates the hand laterally and increases the energetic cost to achieve the target. We have corroborated these findings in unsupported vertical reaching movements (Tomlinson & Sainburg, 2012) and in left-handers (Przybyla, Good, & Sainburg, 2012). We have also shown that both energetic costs and normalized muscle activities are higher in nondominant arm-reaching movements, while final position accuracies tend to be lower (Bagesteiro & Sainburg, 2003; Sainburg & Kalakanis, 2000).

Corroborating findings have been reported for different types of movements from other research groups. For example, Pigeon, DiZio, and Lackner (2013) reported interlimb differences in coordinated turn-and-reach movements performed while subjects were standing. Due to the rapid-trunk rotations that were required, substantial Coriolis torques were generated on the arm during movement. Subjects moved at two speeds and under two loading conditions (with and without a 1 lb weight), both of which manipulated the relative amplitude of the Coriolis torques. Dominant arm movements were performed straighter and were minimally affected by the speed and weight conditions, while nondominant arm movements were more curved and varied substantially with both load and speed conditions. Thus the dominant arm controller more accurately predicted and accounted for the effect of the Coriolis torques that were generated by trunk rotations, while the nondominant arm controller did not. Nevertheless, nondominant arm movements curved back toward the targets at the end of motion and were slightly more accurate with respect to radial errors. These findings are quite similar to our findings for reaching movements.

Hore and colleagues conducted a series of studies of overarm throwing in the dominant and nondominant arms, demonstrating asymmetries in controlling intersegmental dynamics during pitching motions. Dominant arm movements took advantage of the whipping actions of interaction torques to generate accurate high speed motions of the hand at ball release (Debicki, Gribble, Watts, & Hore, 2004, 2011; Hore, O'Brien, & Watts, 2005; Hore, Watts, & Tweed, 1996, 1999). As such, dominant interjoint coordination patterns were different between slow and fast throws. However, the nondominant arm did not exploit these interactions and simply scaled interjoint coordination patterns for different speed motions.

We conclude that the dominant control system is specialized for coordinating limb and task dynamics. We have previously shown that this process relies on feedforward use of vision and proprioception for predictive control (Ghez, Gordon, & Ghilardi, 1995; Ghez, Gordon, Ghilardi, Christakos, & Cooper, 1990; Ghez, Gordon, Ghilardi, & Sainburg, 1994; Ghez & Sainburg, 1995; Gordon, Ghilardi, Cooper, & Ghez, 1994; Sainburg, Poizner, & Ghez, 1993). However, regardless of large trajectory deviations, the nondominant system often makes movements of similar or greater final position accuracy, suggesting that this controller might be specialized for the control of steady-state position through impedance control mechanisms.

NONDOMINANT ARM ADVANTAGES IN IMPEDANCE CONTROL

Schabowsky, Hidler, and Lum (2007) examined interlimb asymmetries in adaptation to novel curl fields (such as those described above), while Duff and Sainburg (2007) examined asymmetries in adaptation to novel inertial loads. Both studies showed that while the nondominant arm adapted to the applied force conditions, aftereffects were small and inconsistent. In contrast, dominant arm adaptation to the same conditions was characterized by large aftereffects that mirrored the initial errors introduced by exposure to the forces. In addition, we have shown that the nondominant arm responds to unexpected inertial loading with greater final position accuracy than the dominant arm, through both short and long latency proprioceptive responses (Bagesteiro & Sainburg, 2003). These findings suggest that the nondominant controller might be advantaged for impedance control mechanisms. Such an advantage is consistent with Goble's findings that the nondominant arm is more accurate at proprioceptive matching tasks (Goble & Brown, 2008; Goble, Lewis, & Brown, 2006; Goble, Noble, & Brown, 2009). Indeed, this might be the basis for observations that the nondominant arm tends to achieve more accurate final positions, when reaching movements are made without visual feedback of the hand, toward a large number of targets distributed throughout the workspace (Przybyla, Coelho, Akpinar, Kirazci, & Sainburg, 2013). Based on evidence for a nondominant arm specialization for impedance control and a dominant arm specialization for predictive control of limb dynamics, we recently proposed a hybrid control scheme, in which each hemisphere contributes its specialization to the control of each arm. According to this view, manual asymmetry results from the predominant influence of the mechanism associated with the contralateral hemisphere (Coelho, Przybyla, Yadav, & Sainburg, 2013; Yadav & Sainburg, 2011, 2014a).

THE EFFECTS OF HYBRID CONTROL ON MOTOR PERFORMANCE AND ADAPTATION

According to our hybrid control hypothesis, the asymmetry in performance associated with handedness emerges from different specializations of each hemisphere's motor control system: the dominant arm controller is specialized for predictive control of dynamics, while the nondominant arm controller is specialized for impedance control. If this is the case, then certain task conditions should present advantages to the dominant arm, while others should advantage the nondominant arm. This perspective is a unique view of handedness, in that we predict that the nondominant system can be advantaged over the dominant system for certain aspects of control. As a direct test of this hypothesis, we designed a study in which each arm should be advantaged by a given type of force field, while the other arm is disadvantaged by that field (Yadav & Sainburg, 2014b).

Each of two alternative force fields were applied by a robotic manipulandum attached to an arm support. The field designed to advantage the predictive controller had a consistent magnitude between trials that varied with the square of hand velocity. The field designed to advantage the impedance controller had an inconsistent magnitude between trials that varied linearly with hand velocity. The rationale for using a velocity square field to advantage the dynamic controller was that limb dynamics normally include terms that vary with the square of velocities and so should be consistent with the characteristics of the dynamic controller, while the impedance controller should not be well adapted to counter such force fields. Alternatively, we designed an inconsistent and unpredictable velocity-dependent curl field that varied in magnitude from trial to trial. We expected that this field should be most compatible with an impedance controller but incompatible with a predictive controller that would be unable to anticipate trial-to-trial variations in force field magnitudes. Therefore we predicted an arm X field interaction, such that the dominant arm should perform best within the consistent field and the nondominant arm in the inconsistent field, as illustrated in Fig. 8.3. In this figure, the terms "good" and "bad" refer to measures of performance in the two different fields. We expect performance of the dominant arm to be best in the predictable field, while performance of the nondominant arm should be best in the unpredictable field.

Fig. 8.4 shows the unequivocal results of this experiment, with two measures of movement quality: mean squared jerk, a measure that varies

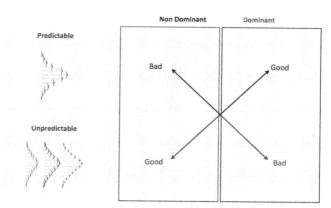

FIGURE 8.3 Force field structure is shown at left: Fields were generated perpendicular to the direction of the target and varied with either the square of velocity (predictable field) or linearly with velocity (unpredictable). The unpredictable field could be one of three amplitudes. Right: We predicted a hand X field interaction for performance and adaptation within each field, such that the nondominant arm should perform better (good) in the unpredictable field, while the dominant arm should perform better (good) in the predictable field.

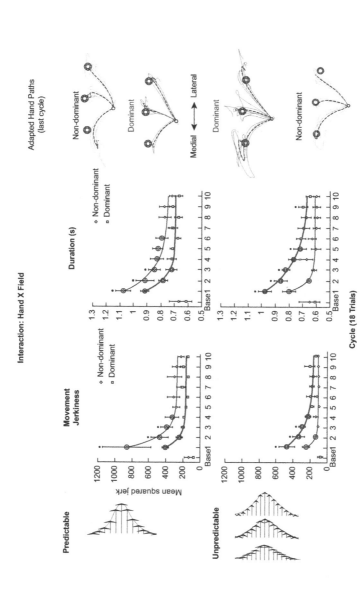

FIGURE 8.4 Force fields were generated perpendicular to the direction of the target and varied with either the square of velocity (predictable field) or linearly with velocity (unpredictable). Group mean ±SE for mean squared jerk (left) and movement duration (right) are shown across all 180 movements (10 cycles). Baseline performance is shown at the left of each plot. Example hand paths for the last cycle of adaptation are shown for each arm and each field. Example individual paths (*dashed*) and mean (*solid*) paths are shown for each condition. *From Yadav, V., & Sainburg, R. L. (2014). Limb dominance results from asymmetries in predictive and impedance control mechanisms. PLoS One, 9(4).*

inversely with movement smoothness, and movement duration. The right-most column of the figure shows the last cycle (18 trials) of the 180 trial adaptation session, when each arm was exposed to each field. Clearly, the dominant arm trials (average hand path is shown as a dotted line) were straighter and more accurately directed than the nondominant paths in the predictable field (top). In contrast, the nondominant arm movements were advantaged in the unpredictable field. The plots in the center of the graph show data from all subjects, as subjects adapted to the two fields over 18 cycles (180 trials). The dominant arm was advantaged throughout adaptation in the predictable field, while the nondominant arm was disadvantaged in this field. In contrast the nondominant arm was advantaged by the unpredictable field, while the dominant arm showed poorer performance throughout adaptation in this field. These results were quite unique in demonstrating a condition in which the nondominant arm showed an unequivocal and substantial advantage in performance over the dominant arm. The importance of these findings is that the experiment was based on a hypotheses about each arm's control specialization. These findings provide strong support for the hypothesis that each arm controller is specialized for different control algorithms. Our next question is whether these specializations are localized in each hemisphere.

HEMISPHERIC SPECIALIZATIONS FOR CONTROL OF LIMB DYNAMICS AND LIMB IMPEDANCE

The previous sections detailed evidence that predictive control of limb and task dynamics and impedance control reflect two distinct components of motor control that are, nevertheless, seamlessly integrated into unilateral arm performance. This is exemplified by the experiment of Takahashi et al. (2001), demonstrating the combination of mechanisms to adapt to a noisy force field using the dominant arm. However, we have also presented evidence that these control processes are localized to each hemisphere. The logical interpretation of these two lines of evidence is that both hemispheres are exploited during unilateral arm movements, but that the contribution of the contralateral hemisphere predominates in the control process for each arm. According to this idea, one would expect that a lesion to one hemisphere should produce sensorimotor deficits in both arms. In fact, those deficits should reflect the nature of the control associated with the damaged hemisphere. We directly tested this hypothesis in a series of experiments focused on ipsilesional arm performance in patients with unilateral stroke that resulted in substantial paresis of the contralateral arm. While testing the contralateral arm was precluded by paresis, the ipsilesional arm experiments provided a strong test of our hypothesis.

Indeed, as early as 1967, it has been recognized that unilateral hemisphere damage can result in ipsilesional performance deficits (Chestnut & Haaland, 2008; Haaland, Prestopnik, Knight, & Lee, 2004; Haaland et al., 2009; Hermsdorfer, Ulrich, Marquardt, Goldenberg, & Mai, 1999; Sainburg & Duff, 2006; Schaefer, Haaland, & Sainburg, 2007, 2009; Swinnen, Debaere, Puttemans, Vangheluwe, & Kiekens, 2002; Wetter, Poole, & Haaland, 2005; Winstein & Pohl, 1995; Wyke, 1967; Yarosh, Hoffman, & Strick, 2004). Our hypothesis of hybrid control has clear predictions for unilateral brain lesions that affect sensorimotor function. Because we hypothesize that both hemispheres contribute different mechanisms to each arm, unilateral hemisphere lesions should produce hemisphere-specific deficits in the ipsilesional arm of stroke patients. We limited our analysis to patients with right-handedness because of restrictions in recruitment of stroke patients. In order to ensure that any potential differences in ipsilesional performance were due to the side of the lesion, rather than other factors, such as intrahemispheric lesion location, size of the lesion, age, and contralesional impairment level, we matched our groups for impairment level, a number of demographic factors including age and gender, and most importantly for intrahemispheric lesion location and volume, as characterized by structural MRI analysis (see Fig. 8.5).

Chronic stroke patients with either left or right hemisphere damage (LHD or RHD) used their ipsilesional arm, and the control subjects used either their left or right arm (LHC or RHC) to perform targeted reaching movements in different directions within the workspace ipsilateral to their reaching arm. The results of this study are depicted in Fig. 8.6A, which shows variability in performance at two points in the movement: at peak velocity or at the final position. The ellipses reflect 95% confidence intervals around the cloud of hand path points for representative LHD and RHD patients. LHD patients had greater variabilities early in movement and significantly worse initial direction accuracies and greater trajectory curvatures than both age-matched control subjects and RHD patients. In contrast, RHD patients showed lower initial trajectory variabilities and trajectory deviations, but greater final position variances and errors than both their control group and LHD patients. These variabilities were quantified as a ratio between each subject's variable errors, calculated at the time of peak velocity divided by the variable error, calculated at the end of movement (Fig. 8.6B). In addition, measures of mean final position error and mean peak velocity for each direction of movement, across all groups is shown in Fig. 8.6C and D. While peak velocities were substantially lower for LHD patients, compared to all other groups, final position errors were higher for RHD patients.

We conclude that LHD produced deficits in controlling the ipsilesional arm trajectory, but not the final steady state position of movements. In contrast, RHD produced deficits in ipsilesional final position

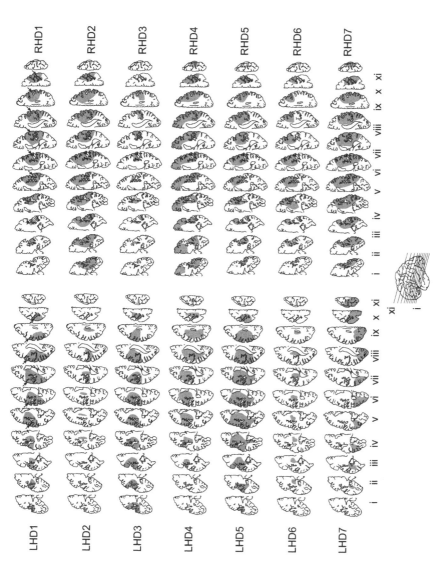

FIGURE 8.5 Lesion locations were traced on 11 axial slices (see insert for slice level) from MRI or CT scans for each LHD (1–7) and RHD (1–7) patient. Slices are displayed left-to-right from inferior to superior (i–xi) for both groups of patients. *Arrows in the top row indicate location of central sulcus. From Schaefer, S. Y., Haaland, K. Y., & Sainburg, R. L. (November 2009). Hemispheric specialization and functional impact of ipsilesional deficits in movement coordination and accuracy. Neuropsychologia. 47(13), 2953–2966. http://dx.doi.org/10.1016/j.neuropsychologia.2009.06.025. Epub 2009 Jun 30.*

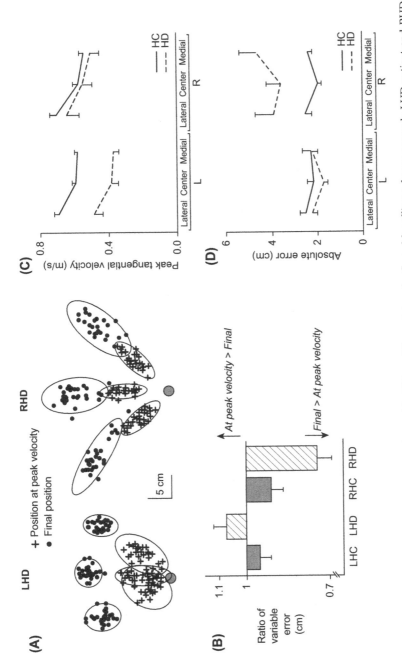

FIGURE 8.6 (A) Sample positional variation plots, with 95% confidence interval reflected by ellipses for an example LHD patient and RHD patient. (B) Group data reflecting ratio of positional variation at peak velocity divided by positional variation at end of movement for LHD, RHD, left hemisphere control (LHC), and right hemisphere control (RHC) groups. (C) Mean ±SE for peak velocity and (D) absolute final position error for all four groups (LHD, LHC, RHD, RHC) for movements to each target. *From Schaefer, S. Y., Haaland, K. Y., & Sainburg, R. L. (November 2009). Hemispheric specialization and functional impact of ipsilesional deficits in movement coordination and accuracy. Neuropsychologia, 47(13), 2953–2966. http://dx.doi.org/10.1016/j.neuropsychologia.2009.06.025. Epub 2009 Jun 30.*

accuracy, but not the speed or variability of the trajectory. These results provided evidence that each hemisphere contributes different control mechanisms to both arms and were corroborated by a study of single joint movements in RHD and LHD (Schaefer et al., 2007). They have also been extended to the contralesional arm in patients with mild hemiparesis (Mani et al., 2013).

MOTOR ASYMMETRIES IN LEFT-HANDERS

The rationale for studying right-handers to understand motor lateralization is that right-handedness reflects a fairly homogenous population, with respect to both behavioral and neurophysiological measures (Dassonville, Zhu, Ugurbil, Kim, & Ashe, 1997; Perelle & Ehrman, 1982, 1994). In contrast, left-handers represent a much more diverse and heterogeneous group. Thus, left-handedness should not be considered an opposite condition to right-handedness, nor should one predict that left-handers should show opposite patterns of behavior and neural activity. As stated by Perelle and Ehrman (1982, p. 1256), "Left handed individuals do not fit into a single, neat, phenotypic or genotypic classification. They are different from right-handers, but more important, they are different from other left-handers and should not be lumped into a single category." The degree of lateralization of left-handers, measured as a laterality quotient, is on average significantly lower than that of right-handers, while the variability of that measure is substantially higher than that of right-handers (Chatagny et al., 2013). Thus left-handedness seems to represent individuals with a range between those that show completely mixed patterns of hand use, with no particular bias for one hand, and those that appear mirror imaged to right-handers, behaviorally (Chatagny et al., 2013; Perelle & Ehrman, 1982). In light of these differences, the fact that left-handers also show substantially different patterns of neural activation during unimanual tasks should not be surprising. In fact, left-handers tend to show greater activation of ipsilateral cortex during unilateral unimanual tasks when compared to right-handers performing the same tasks (Dassonville et al., 1997; Kim et al., 1993). This pattern of activation suggests that the tendency for left-handers to show a greater degree of behavioral symmetry is not due to a more symmetric (less lateralized) brain, but rather to a difference in recruitment of a lateralized brain. That is, left-handed individuals display motor behavior that is more symmetric because of bilateral hemisphere recruitment, which allows each hand to benefit from the specialization of each hemisphere. If, on the other hand, left-hander's brains were more symmetric, each hemisphere would reflect a mirror image in structure and function to the other hemisphere. Symmetry in behavior would be associated with greater contralateral hemisphere recruitment, regardless of which arm was used. The fact that recruitment of ipsilateral cortex is greater in left-handers than right-handers is consistent with the requirement for left-handers to adapt to a right-handed environment, and thus use the nondominant right arm in dominant arm tasks, such as opening doors and using scissors.

Evidence that ipsilateral hemisphere recruitment during nondominant arm use can be increased with experience has been demonstrated by Philip and Frey (2014). In this study, right-handed individuals with partial or complete dominant hand amputations were studied, after the individuals had largely switched dominance functions to the unimpaired left hand. The improved performance of the previously nondominant arm in activities, such as rapid tracing tasks, was associated with greater activation of the ipsilateral (left) hemisphere. Thus the experience-dependent improvement in left arm function, associated with dominance retraining, occurred through recruitment of the lateralized functions of the left, ipsilateral hemisphere, rather than by rewriting the lateralized functionality of the contralateral-right hemisphere. Taken together, these findings suggest that left-handers are a heterogeneous group of individuals who do not represent the neural or behavioral mirror image of right-handers.

APPLICATION TO SPORTS AND ATHLETICS

The evidence presented above that left-handers show greater recruitment of ipsilateral cortex during dominant arm use, and that this recruitment appears to be dependent on experience, has potential implications for understanding the role of handedness in sports. Previous studies have reported an increased incidence of left-handers in fencing and racquet sports (Bisiacchi, Ripoll, Stein, Simonet, & Azémar, 1985). A prominent rationale for the higher incidence of left-handers in such sports is a game theory-based negative frequency effect (Loffing, Hagemann, & Strauss, 2012). That is, because of the higher incidence of right-handers, players learn a bias through training with right-handed opponents. However, given the findings reported in this chapter and a recent study that we published on right-handed elite fencers, we propose an alternative explanation. Motor lateralization, or handedness, emerges from an inherent asymmetry in the functional organization of the left and right hemispheres. The hemisphere contralateral to the dominant arm is specialized for predictive control of limb and task dynamics that allows the specification of motions that can be optimized for maximum speed, trajectory parameters, power, or even efficiency. In contrast, the other hemisphere is specialized for impedance control that is important for robust performance in the face of unexpected environmental conditions. Whereas most bilateral activities are specialized for distributing these functions across the hands, such as when cutting bread or hammering nails, performance of many sports could be improved by exploiting both aspects of control for a single arm. In fact, all healthy individuals exploit both hemispheres for control of each arm (Yadav & Sainburg, 2014a), which is why lesions of one hemisphere produce deficits in both the contralesional and the ipsilesional arms of stroke survivors (Chestnut & Haaland, 2008; Haaland et al., 2004, 2009; Hermsdorfer et al., 1999; Sainburg & Duff, 2006; Schaefer et al., 2007, 2009; Swinnen et al., 2002; Wetter et al., 2005; Winstein & Pohl, 1995; Wyke, 1967; Yarosh et al., 2004). The fact that dominant arm amputees retrain their nondominant arm by recruiting greater ipsilateral cortex demonstrates that such bilateral recruitment patterns can be experience- and practice-dependent (Philip & Frey, 2014). We now propose that many sports offer such practice through elite use of a single arm for complex and high-level function. For example, in fencing, the dominant arm is used both for thrusting-type motions that are expected to recruit the left hemisphere in right-handers and blocking motions that impede forces imposed by the opponent and are expected to recruit the right hemisphere in right-handers. Nevertheless, the sport is almost entirely focused on the use of the dominant arm.

Our hypothesis predicts that fencers should recruit both hemispheres more symmetrically than nonfencers and should exhibit greater behavioral symmetry, even though fencing extensively practices unilateral arm movements. This prediction emerges from the hypothesis that the type of practice involved in fencing should elicit bilateral hemispheric recruitment, and this pattern of recruitment should result in more symmetric behavior. We verified this prediction in a recent study, in which we compared arm selection patterns in eight healthy college age fencers to eight age-matched healthy volunteers, who did not engage in organized sports (Akpinar, Sainburg, Kirazci, & Przybyla, 2015). In this study, 32 targets were presented in random order across the entire reachable horizontal workspace. Our findings showed that fencers tended to use the nondominant (nonpracticed) arm to reach to midline targets, as well as to reach targets across the body midline more than nonfencers. Overall, fencers displayed greater symmetry in their use of both arms than did nonfencers. We propose that this increased behavioral symmetry results from bilateral hemispheric recruitment during fencing practice and performance. This hypothesis might explain the tendency for greater representation of left-handers in fencing and racquet sports: many left-handers have learned to recruit ipsilateral cortex to a greater degree than their right-handed counterparts, simply through practice of daily activities performed in a right-handed world. These left-handers would likely have an inherent advantage in learning to recruit both hemispheres for fencing. However, this does not indicate that all left-handers have an inherent advantage for any sport. Instead, athletically talented lefties might have a greater tendency to self-select for racquet sports and fencing because of the relative ease of recruiting both hemispheres for dominant arm use during initial exposure to the sport.

SUMMARY AND CONCLUSIONS

Rogers and colleagues proposed a single organizing principle for the large array of emotional, language, perceptual, and cognitive asymmetries that have been described across the evolutionary spectrum of animals. According to this idea, the left side of the brain is specialized for control of well-established patterns of behavior under familiar and predictable circumstances, while the right side is specialized for detecting and responding to unexpected environmental events. Whereas more than a century of research has focused on identifying consistent performance characteristics that might define motor asymmetry in humans, this line of research has not revealed fundamental motor control mechanisms that might give rise to handedness. Studies of motor coordination in healthy individuals and of hemisphere-specific deficits in stroke patients have provided evidence for an explanation of handedness that is based on fundamental motor control processes: the dominant hemisphere, left in right-handers, appears specialized for predictive control processes that account for the effects of limb and task dynamics to optimize costs that might depend on task conditions. This type of control, however, depends on the predictability and consistency of the mechanical environment. The nondominant hemisphere, right in right-handers, appears specialized for impedance control processes that can stabilize performance and reduce errors in the face of unexpected mechanical conditions. These two aspects of control have been well studied and established for unimanual movements of the dominant arm. We have reviewed substantial evidence, demonstrating that these two aspects of control are specialized in different cerebral hemispheres, imparting different control characteristics to each arm. This has been shown across a range of movements, including horizontal and vertical reaching movements, turn and reach movements, overhand throwing, and through studies of adaptation to novel force environments.

Based on the aforementioned evidence, we have proposed a hybrid control scheme, in which each hemisphere contributes its specialization to control of each arm, while asymmetry results from the predominant influence of the mechanism associated with the contralateral hemisphere. According to this scheme, a lesion to a single hemisphere should produce sensorimotor deficits in both arms. In addition, those deficits should reflect the nature of the control associated with the damaged hemisphere. We reviewed evidence for hemisphere-specific ipsilesional arm deficits in patients with unilateral stroke, which confirms the predictions of our hybrid model. Recent evidence has emphasized the functional importance of ipsilesional deficits, suggesting the need to address the ipsilesional arm in rehabilitation for stroke.

We conclude that handedness results from lateralization of predictive and impedance control mechanisms, which are integrated into unilateral movements of each arm, in order to ensure both optimality and robustness against unpredictable mechanical conditions. Handedness appears to emerge due to the predominant influence of the contralateral hemisphere. Rogers and colleagues have shown that lateralization is essential for efficient parallel performance of the lateralized processes, emphasizing the importance of lateralization for optimal and adaptive behavior. This view of handedness fits Roger's more global hypothesis of brain lateralization and provides a fundamental explanation of the motor control mechanisms that result in the emergence of motor performance asymmetries.

Most of the studies described or cited in this chapter addressed right-handed individuals. I expect that either right- or left-handedness should be viewed from the same perspective. However, the extent of handedness might represent very different neural phenomenon. Lack of establishment of handedness might reflect a nonlateralized system, which is likely to result in poor integration of predictive with impedance processes for movement control. For example, MacNeilage et al. (2009) showed that when chicks do not establish lateralization in their visual systems, the visual processes that are normally lateralized are not performed well when they must be implemented simultaneously. In terms of handedness, lack of lateralization might result in ineffective prediction of limb dynamics and poor ability to stabilize against unpredicted perturbations. The results might be incoordination, which could account for the fact that children with developmental coordination disorder have lower laterality indices (Hill & Bishop, 1998). However, simply measuring limb preference or even performance might not provide a good indication of whether subjects are well lateralized, because it is likely that practice can lead to more symmetrical behaviors by developing better access to ipsilateral hemispheric processes. In fact, an fMRI study demonstrated that use of the nondominant arm in chronic amputees with dominant arm amputation demonstrated that these individuals increased nondominant arm proficiency, in part, by accessing ipsilateral hemisphere motor regions (Philip & Frey, 2014). Thus one might expect that high-level practice of a skill with one arm, such as fencing, or persistent practice of the nondominant arm in a sport, such as lacrosse, might lead to more symmetrical performance, and thus lower laterality scores but with improvements, rather than decrements, in function.

References

Akpinar, S., Sainburg, R. L., Kirazci, S., & Przybyla, A. (2015). Motor asymmetry in elite fencers. *Journal of Motor Behavior*, 47(4), 302–311.

Alexander, R. M. (1997). A minimum energy cost hypothesis for human arm trajectories. *Biological Cybernetics*, 76(2), 97–105.

Bagesteiro, L. B., & Sainburg, R. L. (2002). Handedness: dominant arm advantages in control of limb dynamics. *Journal of Neurophysiology*, 88(5), 2408–2421.

Bagesteiro, L. B., & Sainburg, R. L. (2003). Nondominant arm advantages in load compensation during rapid elbow joint movements. *Journal of Neurophysiology*, 90(3), 1503–1513.

Bisazza, A., Rogers, L. J., & Vallortigara, G. (1998). The origins of cerebral asymmetry: a review of evidence of behavioural and brain lateralization in fishes, reptiles and amphibians. *Neuroscience and Biobehavioral Reviews, 22*(3), 411–426.

Bisiacchi, P. S., Ripoll, H., Stein, J. F., Simonet, P., & Azémar, G. (1985). Left-handedness in fencers: an attentional advantage? *Perceptual and Motor Skills, 61,* 507–513.

Carson, R. G. (1992). Visual feedback processing and manual asymmetries: an evolving perspective. In L. Proteau, & D. Elliot (Eds.), *Vision and motor control* (pp. 49–65). Amsterdam: North-Holland.

Carson, R. G. (1993). Manual asymmetries: old problems and new directions. *Human Movement Science, 12*(5), 479–506.

Carson, R. G., Elliott, D., Goodman, D., Thyer, L., Chua, R., & Roy, E. A. (1993). The role of impulse variability in manual-aiming asymmetries. *Psychological Research, 55*(4), 291–298.

Carson, R. G., Goodman, D., Chua, R., & Elliott, D. (1993). Asymmetries in the regulation of visually guided aiming. *Journal of Motor Behavior, 25*(1), 21–32.

Chatagny, P., Badoud, S., Kaeser, M., Gindrat, A. D., Savidan, J., Fregosi, M., ... Rouiller, E. M. (2013). Distinction between hand dominance and hand preference in primates: a behavioral investigation of manual dexterity in nonhuman primates (macaques) and human subjects. *Brain and Behavior, 3*(5), 575–595.

Chestnut, C., & Haaland, K. Y. (2008). Functional significance of ipsilesional motor deficits after unilateral stroke. *Archives of Physical Medicine and Rehabilitation, 89*(1), 62–68.

Coelho, C. J., Przybyla, A., Yadav, V., & Sainburg, R. L. (2013). Hemispheric differences in the control of limb dynamics: a link between arm performance asymmetries and arm selection patterns. *Journal of Neurophysiology, 109*(3), 825–838.

Dassonville, P., Zhu, X. H., Ugurbil, K., Kim, S. G., & Ashe, J. (1997). Functional activation in motor cortex reflects the direction and the degree of handedness. *Proceedings of the National Academy of Sciences of the United States of America, 94*(25), 14015–14018.

Debicki, D. B., Gribble, P. L., Watts, S., & Hore, J. (2004). Kinematics of wrist joint flexion in overarm throws made by skilled subjects. *Experimental Brain Research, 154*(3), 382–394.

Debicki, D. B., Gribble, P. L., Watts, S., & Hore, J. (2011). Wrist muscle activation, interaction torque and mechanical properties in unskilled throws of different speeds. *Experimental Brain Research, 208*(1), 115–125.

Duff, S. V., & Sainburg, R. L. (2007). Lateralization of motor adaptation reveals independence in control of trajectory and steady-state position. *Experimental Brain Research, 179*(4), 551–561.

Ghez, C., Gordon, J., & Ghilardi, M. F. (1995). Impairments of reaching movements in patients without proprioception. II. Effects of visual information on accuracy. *Journal of Neurophysiology, 73*(1), 361–372.

Ghez, C., Gordon, J., Ghilardi, M. F., Christakos, C. N., & Cooper, S. E. (1990). Roles of proprioceptive input in the programming of arm trajectories. *Cold Spring Harbor Symposia on Quantitative Biology, 55,* 837–847.

Ghez, C., Gordon, M. F., Ghilardi, M. F., & Sainburg, R. (1994). Contributions of vision and proprioception to accuracy in limb movements. In M. S. Gazzaniga (Ed.), *The cognitive neurosciences* (pp. 549–564). Cambridge, MA: MIT Press.

Ghez, C., & Sainburg, R. (1995). Proprioceptive control of interjoint coordination. *Canadian Journal of Physiology and Pharmacology, 73*(2), 273–284.

Ghez, C., Scheidt, R., & Heijink, H. (2007). Different learned coordinate frames for planning trajectories and final positions in reaching. *Journal of Neurophysiology, 98*(6), 3614–3626.

Goble, D. J., & Brown, S. H. (2008). Upper limb asymmetries in the matching of proprioceptive versus visual targets. *Journal of Neurophysiology, 99*(6), 3063–3074.

Goble, D. J., Lewis, C. A., & Brown, S. H. (2006). Upper limb asymmetries in the utilization of proprioceptive feedback. *Experimental Brain Research, 168*(1–2), 307–311.

Goble, D. J., Noble, B. C., & Brown, S. H. (2009). Proprioceptive target matching asymmetries in left-handed individuals. *Experimental Brain Research, 197*(4), 403–408.

Gordon, J., Ghilardi, M. F., Cooper, S. E., & Ghez, C. (1994). Accuracy of planar reaching movements – II. Systematic extent errors resulting from inertial anisotropy. *Experimental Brain Research, 99*(1), 112–130.

Haaland, K. Y., & Harrington, D. L. (1989). Hemispheric control of the initial and corrective components of aiming movements. *Neuropsychologia, 27*(7), 961–969.

Haaland, K. Y., Prestopnik, J. L., Knight, R. T., & Lee, R. R. (2004). Hemispheric asymmetries for kinematic and positional aspects of reaching. *Brain, 127*(5), 1145–1158.

Haaland, K. Y., Schaefer, S. Y., Knight, R. T., Adair, J., Magalhaes, A., Sadek, J., & Sainburg, R. L. (2009). Ipsilesional trajectory control is related to contralesional arm paralysis after left hemisphere damage. *Experimental Brain Research, 196*(2), 195–204.

Hausmann, M., Kirk, I. J., & Corballis, M. C. (2004). Influence of task complexity on manual asymmetries. *Cortex, 40*(1), 103–110.

Hermsdorfer, J., Ulrich, S., Marquardt, C., Goldenberg, G., & Mai, N. (1999). Prehension with the ipsilesional hand after unilateral brain damage. *Cortex, 35*(2), 139–161.

Hill, E. L., & Bishop, D. V. M. (1998). A reaching test reveals weak hand preference in specific language impairment and developmental co-ordination disorder. *Laterality: Asymmetries of Body, Brain and Cognition, 3*(4), 295–310.

Hore, J., O'Brien, M., & Watts, S. (2005). Control of joint rotations in overarm throws of different speeds made by dominant and nondominant arms. *Journal of Neurophysiology, 94*(6), 3975–3986.

Hore, J., Watts, S., & Tweed, D. (1996). Errors in the control of joint rotations associated with inaccuracies in overarm throws. *Journal of Neurophysiology, 75*(3), 1013–1025.

Hore, J., Watts, S., & Tweed, D. (1999). Prediction and compensation by an internal model for back forces during finger opening in an overarm throw. *Journal of Neurophysiology, 82*(3), 1187–1197.

Hwang, E. J., & Shadmehr, R. (2005). Internal models of limb dynamics and the encoding of limb state. *Journal of Neural Engineering, 2*(3), S266–S278.

Kim, S. G., Ashe, J., Hendrich, K., Ellermann, J. M., Merkle, H., Ugurbil, K., & Georgopoulos, A. P. (1993). Functional magnetic resonance imaging of motor cortex: hemispheric asymmetry and handedness. *Science, 261*(5121), 615–617.

Lackner, J. R., & DiZio, P. (1998). Adaptation in a rotating artificial gravity environment. *Brain Research Reviews, 28*(1–2), 194–202.

Loffing, F., Hagemann, N., & Strauss, B. (2012). Left-handedness in professional and amateur tennis. *PLoS One, 7*(11), e49325.

MacNeilage, P. F., Rogers, L. J., & Vallortigara, G. (2009). Origins of the left & right brain. *Scientific American, 301*(1), 60–67.

Mani, S., Mutha, P. K., Przybyla, A., Haaland, K. Y., Good, D. C., Sainburg, R. L. (April 2013). Contralesional motor deficits after unilateral stroke reflect hemisphere-specific control mechanisms. *Brain, 136*(Pt 4), 1288–1303.

Mutha, P. K., Boulinguez, P., & Sainburg, R. L. (2008). Visual modulation of proprioceptive reflexes during movement. *Brain Research, 1246*, 54–69.

Mutha, P. K., Haaland, K. Y., & Sainburg, R. L. (2012). The effects of brain lateralization on motor control and adaptation. *Journal of Motor Behavior, 44*(6), 455–469.

Mutha, P. K., Haaland, K. Y., & Sainburg, R. L. (2013). Rethinking motor lateralization: specialized but complementary mechanisms for motor control of each arm. *PLoS One, 8*(3).

Nishii, J., & Taniai, Y. (2009). Evaluation of trajectory planning models for arm-reaching movements based on energy cost. *Neural Computation, 21*(9), 2634–2647.

Omrani, M., Diedrichsen, J., & Scott, S. H. (2013). Rapid feedback corrections during a bimanual postural task. *Journal of Neurophysiology, 109*(1), 147–161.

Perelle, I. B., & Ehrman, L. (1982). What is a lefthander? *Experientia, 38*(10), 1256–1258.

Perelle, I. B., & Ehrman, L. (1994). An international study of human handedness: the data. *Behavior Genetics, 24*(3), 217–227.

Philip, B. A., & Frey, S. H. (2014). Compensatory changes accompanying chronic forced use of the nondominant hand by unilateral amputees. *Journal of Neuroscience, 34*(10), 3622–3631.

Pigeon, P., DiZio, P., & Lackner, J. R. (2013). Immediate compensation for variations in self-generated Coriolis torques related to body dynamics and carried objects. *Journal of Neurophysiology, 110*(6), 1370–1384.

Przybyla, A., Coelho, C. J., Akpinar, S., Kirazci, S., & Sainburg, R. L. (2013). Sensorimotor performance asymmetries predict hand selection. *Neuroscience, 228*, 349–360.

Przybyla, A., Good, D. C., & Sainburg, R. L. (2012). Dynamic dominance varies with handedness: reduced interlimb asymmetries in left-handers. *Experimental Brain Research, 216*(3), 419–431.

Sainburg, R. L. (2002). Evidence for a dynamic-dominance hypothesis of handedness. *Experimental Brain Research, 142*(2), 241–258.

Sainburg, R. L. (2005). Handedness: differential specializations for control of trajectory and position. *Exercise and Sport Sciences Reviews, 33*(4), 206–213.

Sainburg, R. L., & Duff, S. V. (2006). Does motor lateralization have implications for stroke rehabilitation? *Journal of Rehabilitation Research and Development, 43*(3), 311–322.

Sainburg, R. L., & Kalakanis, D. (2000). Differences in control of limb dynamics during dominant and nondominant arm reaching. *Journal of Neurophysiology, 83*(5), 2661–2675.

Sainburg, R. L., Poizner, H., & Ghez, C. (1993). Loss of proprioception produces deficits in interjoint coordination. *Journal of Neurophysiology, 70*(5), 2136–2147.

Schabowsky, C. N., Hidler, J. M., & Lum, P. S. (2007). Greater reliance on impedance control in the nondominant arm compared with the dominant arm when adapting to a novel dynamic environment. *Experimental Brain Research, 182*(4), 567–577.

Schaefer, S. Y., Haaland, K. Y., & Sainburg, R. L. (2007). Ipsilesional motor deficits following stroke reflect hemispheric specializations for movement control. *Brain, 130*(8), 2146–2158.

Schaefer, S. Y., Haaland, K. Y., & Sainburg, R. L. (2009). Hemispheric specialization and functional impact of ipsilesional deficits in movement coordination and accuracy. *Neuropsychologia, 47*(13), 2953–2966.

Scheidt, R. A., & Ghez, C. (2007). Separate adaptive mechanisms for controlling trajectory and final position in reaching. *Journal of Neurophysiology, 98*(6), 3600–3613.

Scott, S. H. (2004). Optimal feedback control and the neural basis of volitional motor control. *Nature Reviews Neuroscience, 5*(7), 532–544.

Shabbott, B. A., & Sainburg, R. L. (2008). Differentiating between two models of motor lateralization. *Journal of Neurophysiology, 100*(2), 565–575.

Swinnen, S. P., Debaere, F., Puttemans, V., Vangheluwe, S., & Kiekens, C. (2002). Coordination deficits on the ipsilesional side after unilateral stroke: the effect of practice on nonisodirectional ipsilateral coordination. *Acta Psychologica, 110*(2–3), 305–320.

Takahashi, C. D., Scheidt, R. A., & Reinkensmeyer, D. J. (2001). Impedance control and internal model formation when reaching in a randomly varying dynamical environment. *Journal of Neurophysiology, 86*(2), 1047–1051.

Todorov, E. (2004). Optimality principles in sensorimotor control. *Nature Neuroscience, 7*(9), 907–915.

Tomlinson, T., & Sainburg, R. (2012). Dynamic dominance persists during unsupported reaching. *Journal of Motor Behavior, 44*(1), 13–25.

Wang, T., Dordevic, G. S., & Shadmehr, R. (2001). Learning the dynamics of reaching movements results in the modification of arm impedance and long-latency perturbation responses. *Biological Cybernetics, 85*(6), 437–448.

Wetter, S., Poole, J. L., & Haaland, K. Y. (2005). Functional implications of ipsilesional motor deficits after unilateral stroke. *Archives of Physical Medicine and Rehabilitation, 86*(4), 776–781.

Winstein, C. J., & Pohl, P. S. (1995). Effects of unilateral brain damage on the control of goal-directed hand movements. *Experimental Brain Research, 105*(1), 163–174.

Woodworth, R. S. (1899). The accuracy of voluntary movement. *Psychological Review, 3*(Suppl. 2).

Wyke, M. (1967). Effect of brain lesions on the rapidity of arm movement. *Neurology, 17*(11), 1113–1120.

Yadav, V., & Sainburg, R. L. (2011). Motor lateralization is characterized by a serial hybrid control scheme. *Neuroscience, 196,* 153–167.

Yadav, V., & Sainburg, R. L. (2014). Handedness can be explained by a serial hybrid control scheme. *Neuroscience, 278,* 385–396.

Yadav, V., & Sainburg, R. L. (2014). Limb dominance results from asymmetries in predictive and impedance control mechanisms. *PLoS One, 9*(4).

Yarosh, C. A., Hoffman, D. S., & Strick, P. L. (2004). Deficits in movements of the wrist ipsilateral to a stroke in hemiparetic subjects. *Journal of Neurophysiology, 92*(6), 3276–3285.

9

Effector Transfer

Charles H. Shea

Texas A&M University, TX, United States

Stefan Panzer

Saarland University, Saarbrücken, Germany

Deanna M. Kennedy

Texas A&M University, TX, United States

Movements play an important role in our everyday life. When we reach to pick up a cup of coffee, sign our name on a document, or shift gears in our car, we take for granted our ability to accurately produce the desired pattern of movement. Indeed, many everyday movements appear to be planned and executed with little or no cognitive effort when the dominant limb is used. However, if we are required to do these tasks with the nondominant limb, for example, as when a right-handed driver attempts to shift gears in a British automobile for the first time with their nondominant hand/arm, we find the task not only requires more attention, effort, and/or time, but performance still can be appreciably diminished. In the case of a more complex movement sequence, like writing your signature with the nondominant limb, the difficulties seem to substantially increase. In the following sections, we will review the effector transfer literature related to simple and more complex movement sequences. Clearly the learning and transfer of learned movements are important in our everyday life as well as in sports and work. However, the transfer of these tasks also has special theoretical importance because the transfer of these tasks provides a unique window into how movements are coded, planned, structured, and executed as well as providing hints as to the role that hand dominance and hemispheric asymmetry play in the production of learned movements. In addition, a better understanding of how movements are affected by transfer has the potential to provide information key to understanding various movement disorders as well as designing learning and relearning therapies after stroke, traumatic brain injury, or other hemispherical trauma that forces an individual to use the nondominant or previously unpracticed limb (e.g., Tangeman, Banaitis, & Williams, 1990; Winstein, Merians, & Sullivan, 1999).

THE STRUCTURE, CONTROL, AND EFFECTOR TRANSFER OF MOVEMENT SEQUENCES

The manner in which movement sequences are coded, processed, and transferred has garnered a great deal of experimental and theoretical attention over the last 30 years. Seminal work by Lashley (1951) on the serial order issue in behavior has stimulated research on sequential learning. He proposed that sequential movements were controlled by central plans, and that the plans were hierarchically organized such that the order of the movement elements (segments comprising the sequence) was determined independent of the characteristics of the individual movement elements (see also Rosenbaum, Cohen, Jax, Weiss, & van der Wel, 2007). The notion of hierarchical control of movement sequences was later refined as a result of a series of important experiments and theoretical models by Rosenbaum (1990), Rosenbaum, Hindorff, and Munro (1986), Rosenbaum, Kenny, and Derr (1983), Rosenbaum and Saltzman (1984), Rosenbaum, Saltzman, and Kingman (1984) in the 1980s and early 1990s. The models described the hierarchical control of movement sequences in terms of an inverted tree/branch metaphor such that higher levels (nodes), which were thought to process sequence information, branched into lower levels, where specific element/effector information was stored (also see Povel & Collard, 1982; Restle, 1970). The codes containing this information were thought to be retrieved, unpacked, edited, and/or parameterized prior to execution so as to meet the specific task demands. The model accounted fairly well for at least some of the time delays between the executions of the discrete individual and/or grouped elements in the sequence.

The research on movement sequences has led to a number of theoretical models (e.g., Henry & Rogers, 1960; Keele, Jennings, Jones, Caulton, & Cohen, 1995; Klapp, 1996; Rosenbaum, 1990; Rosenbaum, Inhoff, & Gordon, 1984; Rosenbaum & Saltzman, 1984; Schmidt, 1975) designed to account for the unique characteristics of specific movement classes and the associated demands on memory and control mechanisms resulting from linkages among individual movement elements. One result of this research suggests that movement sequences are hierarchically structured and that the processing of the sequence is relatively independent of the processing of the elements composing the sequence (e.g., Keele et al., 1995; Klapp, 1995, 1996; for discussions, see Keele, Cohen, & Ivry, 1990; MacKay, 1982; Park & Shea, 2002; Sternberg, Knoll, & Turock, 1990).

Keele et al. (1995; see also Keele, Ivry, Mayr, Hazeltine, & Heuer, 2003), for example, proposed a modular theory of sequence processing with a cognitive and motor processing modules. They proposed that the processing conducted by the models were independent. The cognitive processing module was responsible for computing successive spatial locations and organization of the elements in the sequence. The motor processing module was responsible for selecting specific effectors and computing activation patterns to achieve these locations. Similarly, Verwey (1995, 2003) proposed that movement sequences were represented in memory in two coding schemes, which he also labeled cognitive and motor. The cognitive representation stored information on how the individual elements in the sequence were ordered and organized into chunks (termed subsequences by Kovacs, Muehlbauer, & Shea, 2009). The motor representation (which was stored in a motor buffer) maintained information related to the selection and activation pattern of the various effectors.

Using a different conceptual approach, Hikasoka et al. (1999) and Bapi, Doya, and Harner (2000) proposed a model of sequence control that is similar in some ways with that of both Keele et al. and Verwey's models, but differs in some important ways, especially in terms of effector transfer. Hikosaka et al. (1999) proposed that sequence learning involves both a fast developing, effector-independent component represented in visual–spatial coordinates (e.g., spatial locations of end effectors and/or sequential target positions) and a slower developing, effector-dependent motor component that is represented in motor coordinates (e.g., activation patterns of the agonist/antagonist muscles and/or the sequence of joint angles). The Hikosaka model, at least on the surface, also seems to have many similarities to theoretical perspectives that propose intrinsic and extrinsic coordinate or coding systems (e.g., Criscimagna-Hemminger, Donchin, Gazzaniga, & Shadmehr, 2003; Krakauer, Ghilardi, & Ghez, 1999). The intrinsic coordinates are thought to be represented in terms of an internal model of joint representations (Criscimagna-Hemminger et al., 2003), musculoskeletal forces and dynamics (Krakauer et al., 1999), and/or orientation of body segments relative to each other (Lange, Godde, & Braun, 2004). This type of coordinate system is thought to be effector dependent to the extent that biomechanical, neurological, and dynamic properties of the effectors used on the transfer test are dissimilar to those used during practice. The extrinsic coordinates are thought to reflect Cartesian coordinates of the task space with respect to the body and/or visual display. Thus this type of coordinate system is thought to be effector independent when the extrinsic coordinates are reinstated during an effector transfer test even though intrinsic characteristics of the required transfer movement may have been altered. Each of these theoretical perspectives argues that two types of processing modules, representations, or coordinate systems, depending on the theoretical perspective, are developed independently at different rates during practice and can limit effector transfer, depending on the degree to which they are reinstated.

Hikosaka Perspective

As noted above, Hikosaka et al. (1999) and Hikosaka, Nakamura, Sakai, and Nakahara (2002) proposed that the processing of a movement sequence is distributed in the brain in independent visual-spatial and motor coordinate systems with different neural substrates subserving the production of movements based on the two coordinate systems. According to this perspective the learning of movement sequences involves both a fast developing, effector-independent component represented in visual–spatial coordinates, and a slower developing effector-dependent component that is represented in motor coordinates. In our opinion, the Hikosaka perspective has the potential to provide, with some modifications, a unifying way to understand the various factors that influence coding and transfer of movement sequences and perhaps even inform us related to the effector transfer of aiming movements.

In terms of the neural substrate, the Hikosaka et al. (1999) model proposed that intracortical bidirectional (loop circuits) connections develop over practice between the association cortices, motor cortex, basal ganglia, and cerebellum. Visual–spatial processing is supported by circuits formed between the prefrontal and parietal cortices, anterior basal ganglia (head of the caudate), and posterior lobe of the cerebellum, while motor processing is supported by the motor cortex, midposterior basal ganglia (putamen), anterior lobe of the cerebellum, and dentate nucleus circuits. The mechanisms based on spatial and motor coordinates are capable of operating independently, and thus, through practice, an individual acquires a given sequence in visual–spatial and motor coordinates. For successful completion of the sequential task the two mechanisms must interact. This interaction is facilitated in two ways: a translation mechanism relying predominantly on the premotor area and a coordination or switching mechanism relying predominantly on the presupplementary motor area (pre-SMA). The role of the translation mechanism during the initial stages of practice is to transform the information from visual into motor coordinates while the role of the coordinative mechanism is to suppress the output of the motor sequence mechanism if this output conflicts with that of the spatial sequence mechanism. The imaging work suggests the association cortex, anterior basal ganglia circuits, and parietal-prefrontal cortical loops are more active early in learning. During this early stage of learning, explicit knowledge related to the visual–spatial characteristics of the sequence seem to be available to consciousness, and attention requirements are relatively high. On the other hand, the circuits within the motor system appear to develop more slowly and at a more implicit level.

Hikosaka proposed that eventually practice results in a shift from loops specific to visual–spatial coordinate processing to loops associated with motor coordinate processing. According to this perspective the two sequential processes are developed in parallel, each coded in a different coordinate system. Initially, a sequence is coded in visual–spatial coordinates that rely on attention, explicit knowledge, and working memory. The visual–spatial representation is thought to be transferable to unpracticed effectors, resulting in relatively good performance of a novel task variation that has the same visual/spatial characteristics. Simultaneously, another code represented in motor coordinates (e.g., sequential pattern of muscle activation and/or joint angles) develops. Motor representations are more effector-specific (Hikosaka et al., 2002), given that anatomical and neurological properties of the specific effector used during practice are being exploited to improve performance (Jordan, 1995; Park & Shea, 2005), and thus transfer to other effectors based on this code could be limited.

Experiments Involving the Production of Key Press Sequences

The model proposed by Hikosaka et al. (1999, 2002) was developed based largely on findings from multielement key pressing tasks (e.g., 2×5, 2×10 tasks). The 2×5 and 2×10 tasks were originally devised to test sequence learning in monkeys (Hikosaka, Rand, Miyachi, & Miyashita, 1995) and later humans (e.g., Bapi et al., 2000; Hikosaka et al., 1996; Sakai et al., 1998). The 2×10 task in the Bapi et al. (2000) experiment, for example, required participants to complete trials (termed hypersets) composed of 10 sets where each set involves sequentially depressing two keys on the key pad of the computer keyboard. The trial started with the illumination of two squares on a 3×3 grid and the participant sequentially "hits" the corresponding keys on the 3×3 keyboard (see Fig. 9.1, normal). For the top panel, the first finger was to be used to depress the keys on the left column, the middle finger for the keys in the center column, and the ring finger for the keys on the right column. If the participant depressed the keys in the wrong order (where the correct order was learned by trial and error), the correct keys were not depressed, and/or the response was not entered in 1.2 s, the same set was repeated. If the set was responded to correctly and within the "time out window," the next set was presented. The trial was completed when the participant performed the 10 sets without an error. With practice, participants performed the task with increasing precision and speed. Two effector transfer tests were administered; spatial and motor effector transfer tests. In the effector transfer tests the same hand was used but was positioned differently with respect to the keyboard (Fig. 9.1). In the spatial effector transfer test the position and order of the illuminated keys remained the same but because of the positioning of the hand, different fingers

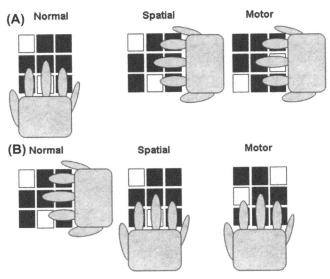

FIGURE 9.1   Illustration of the A and B tasks used by Hikosaka et al. (1999, 2002). Note that the spatial test condition used the same visual–spatial display as in the normal condition, but different effectors were required while the display was rotated on the motor test requiring the same pattern of effector responses.

had to be used to depress the key. Thus if the task was coded in visual spatial coordinates, the participants should respond similarly to that in the normal practice conditions. In the motor effector transfer test the position and order of the illuminated keys was rotated 90 degrees from that observed during acquisition, but the hand was also positioned 90 degrees from the original position. Because of the positioning of the hand and the rotation of the keys the same fingers as used during practice had to be used to depress the keys. Thus if the task was coded in motor coordinates the participants should respond similarly to that in the normal practice conditions.

Data from experiments using the above protocol (Hikosaka et al., 1999; see also Bapi et al., 2000) have provided evidence that movement sequence learning involves both a fast developing, effector-independent component represented in visual–spatial coordinates (e.g., spatial locations of end effectors and/or sequential target positions) and a slower developing, effector-dependent motor component that is represented in motor coordinates (e.g., activation patterns of the agonist/antagonist muscles/joint angles). That is, performance on the spatial transfer test is similar to performance on the original task relatively early in practice, but as practice progressed, performance on the motor transfer test increased and eventually exceeded that on the spatial transfer test.

Effector Transfer of Dynamic Movement Sequences

Research involving key press tasks has provided great insight into the ways in which movement sequences are coded, structured over practice, and transferred, but research using key press tasks may provide limited insight into the impact of a number of factors that often play important roles in the control of movement sequences. Note that in key press tasks, measurement of the movement outcome is limited to the time required to respond (element duration). Thus, only one point in the key press movement of the finger is recorded: the time at which the movement of the finger is sufficient for the computer to sense the switch closure. We consider key press responses as very simple movements because the spatial precision of the movement is minimal in that often the finger rests on the key to be pressed and force does not have to be regulated or controlled as long as the force is sufficient to depress the key. It should also be noted that there are a number of examples where principles developed through the study of relatively simple tasks do not generalize to more complex skill learning (for review see Wulf & Shea, 2002). While key press responses require the selection and activation of different end effectors, they do not require (1) the delicate control of agonist and antagonist forces, (2) storage and utilization of forces stored in and generated from the stretch of parallel and serial elastic components of muscles/tendons, (3) the management of the momentum generated by the ongoing movement, (4) the ability to accelerate and decelerate the movement in attempts to correct an ongoing movement trajectory to achieve a target location, and (5) the selection of control strategies as movement difficulty or movement parameters are increased or decreased. In addition, key press tasks do not afford the researcher the opportunity to more continually monitor the progress of the movement. Thus it is important to determine if more dynamic movement sequences follow similar principles as key press tasks.

Shea and colleagues (e.g., Braden, Panzer, & Shea, 2008; Ellenbuerger et al., 2012; Gruetzmacher, Panzer, Blandin, & Shea, 2011; Kovacs, Han, & Shea, 2009; Kovacs, Muehlbauer, et al., 2009; Panzer, Krueger, Muehlbauer, & Shea, 2010; Park & Shea, 2002, 2003, 2005; for review see Shea, Kovacs, & Panzer, 2011) have investigated effector transfer using a variety of static force production and dynamic movement sequence tasks. Park and Shea (2002), for example, conducted a series of effector transfer experiments where participants attempted to reproduce a goal waveform by producing two sequential force pulses in one second, with the second peak requiring 77% of the force required to produce the first peak. Since the experiment was based on Schmidt's (1975) notion of schema theory, the authors used error measures that separated relative (also termed invariant feature) from absolute (also termed variant feature) characteristics. In Experiment 1, right-handed participants were provided 200 trials of practice producing the goal waveform. To signal the start of each trial, the computer displayed the goal waveform for that trial. Participants were then instructed to exert force against the load cell in an attempt to produce a continuous pattern of force that resembled, as closely as possible, the goal waveform displayed on the computer monitor. During acquisition, one group used the right limb (dominant) triceps and the other group used the left limb (nondominant) triceps to produce the force pattern (see Fig. 9.2A). Following 20 blocks of 10 trials of practice on the respective task, a delayed retention test using the muscle group used during acquisition and an effector transfer test using the homologous muscles of the contralateral limb were administered.

In Experiment 2 (Fig. 9.2B), the same practice and transfer schedule was used, but the participants only used their right limb. One group practiced the task using primarily the bicep (flexion), and effector transfer was assessed using the triceps, while the other group used the triceps (extension) during acquisition with effector transfer assessed using the biceps.

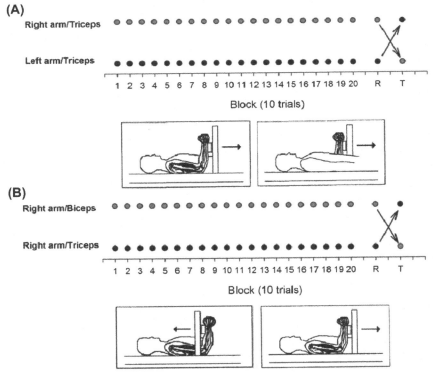

FIGURE 9.2 Illustration of the design of the Park and Shea (2002): Experiments 1 (A) and 2 (B). Note that Experiment 1 involved transfer to the contralateral limb while Experiment 2 involved transfer to a different muscle group on the same limb. *Modified from Park, J.-H., Shea, C. H. (September 1, 2002). Effector independence. Journal of Motor Behavior, 34(3).*

Thus this experiment required transfer to an ipsilateral effector and not to the homologous muscle of the contralateral limb. Across the two experiments the researchers could determine if differences existed between contralateral and ipsilateral effector transfer.

The analysis indicated essentially the same pattern of results for the contralateral and ipsilateral effector transfer. That is, residual root mean square error (*RMSE*), a measure of the errors in the response structure, and timing errors, a measure of the scaling of the response with respect to time, were unaffected by the switch in the muscle group. However, total *RMSE*, an overall measure of performance, and force errors, a measure of errors in scaling force, were negatively affected by both contralateral and ipsilateral effector transfer. The data suggested that the effector independence of task structure and time scaling are quite robust. Further, the findings suggested that the ability to scale force is dependent on the muscles, but not necessarily on the activation pattern of the response used during practice. It is interesting to note that the effector independence of the force parameter remained even though the same limb was used. Hemispheric asymmetries (e.g., Henningsen, Ende-Henningsen, & Gordon, 1995) have been proposed as a possible reason for the difficulty in scaling forces across limbs. However, force parameterization was also poorer when a new muscle group from the same limb was required.

Using a similar but different task, Panzer, Krueger, Muehlbauer, Kovacs, and Shea (2009) asked participants to produce a waveform similar to that in Park and Shea (2002). However, instead of a static force, their task required elbow flexion and extension (see Fig. 9.3). They tested the notion proposed by Hikosaka et al. (1999) that movement sequences were represented early in practice using codes based in visual-spatial coordinates, which were thought to be effector independent, while later in practice the dominate code is based in motor coordinates, which are thought to be effector dependent (Bapi et al., 2000; Hikosaka et al., 1999). To test this notion Panzer et al. (2009) asked participants to practice a relatively simple movement sequence that involved three movement reversals with a movement duration of 1300 ms. At the beginning of each acquisition trial the goal waveform was displayed, however, as soon as the participant began to move, the goal waveform disappeared. Approximately 2 s following the completion of the response knowledge of results was provided by overlaying the participant's performance trace on the goal waveform. Following only 99 practice trials using the left or the right limb, a retention test and two effector transfer tests were administered (Fig. 9.3B–D, respectively). Motor coordinates were reinstated on the "motor" effector transfer test and the visual spatial coordinates were reinstated on the "spatial" effector transfer test. Note that the retention test was conducted with the same limb as used during acquisition, and the effector transfer tests were conducted using the contralateral limb.

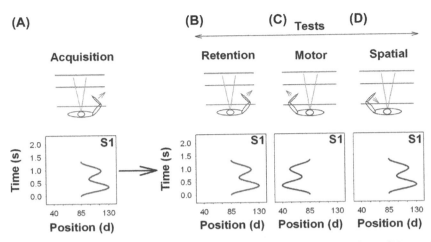

FIGURE 9.3   Illustration of the participant position (top) in the right limb condition and the displays (bottom). Columns A and B represent conditions during acquisition and retention. Columns C and D represent the position of the participant and displays for the motor and visual–spatial effector transfer tests, respectively.

The results indicated that performance on the "motor" transfer test was significantly better than on the spatial transfer test. In fact, performance on the motor transfer test, regardless of the limb used during acquisition, was as effective as on the retention test. These findings are particularly interesting because they indicated, contrary to the earlier findings, that effective codes in motor coordinates can be developed following relatively little practice for rapid movement sequences. Note that in this experiment, participants were encouraged to preplan the movement because extrinsic feedback was not provided during the trial. This manipulation may have played a role in determining the control processes used to produce the movement and the development of the codes in motor coordinates.

Kovacs, Boyle, Gruetzmatcher, and Shea (2010) conducted an additional series of experiments aimed at determining if the control processes rather than the difficulty of the movement play a role in determining the pattern of effector transfer. They asked participants to produce a slightly more difficult movement sequence (Fig. 9.4) than that used by Panzer et al. (2009) and then manipulated the control processes used to produce the movement. To do this, one group was provided online feedback during the production of the response, and the other was not provided feedback until the completion of the response, as in Panzer et al. (2009). The thinking was that the online feedback would encourage the participant to utilize online (closed loop) control processes, while withholding the online feedback until the completion of the response would encourage preplanned control (open loop). The results indicated that when concurrent visual feedback was provided during

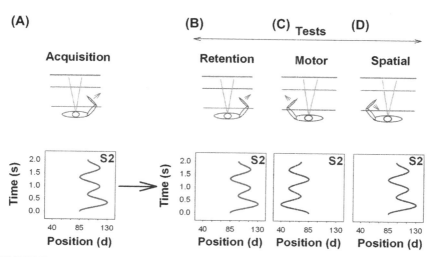

FIGURE 9.4   Illustration of the participant position (top) and the display (bottom). Columns A and B represent conditions during acquisition and retention. Columns C and D represent the position of the participant and displays for the motor and visual–spatial effector transfer tests, respectively. *Modified from Kovacs, A. J., Boyle, J., Grutmacher, N., Shea, C. H. (2010). Coding of on-line and pre-planned movement sequences, Acta Psychologica, 133, 119-126.*

the production of the movement, which was thought to encourage online control, the participants performed transfer tests with the contralateral limb significantly better when the visual–spatial coordinates were reinstated than when the motor coordinates were reinstated. When concurrent visual feedback was not provided, which was thought to encourage preplanned control, the opposite was observed. The data are consistent with the hypothesis that the mode of control plays a role in determining the coordinate system used to code the movement sequence rather than determined solely on the basis of sequence difficulty or stage of practice as has been proposed.

Kovacs et al. (2010) hypothesized, based on the findings of Panzer et al. (2009), that while relatively simple motor tasks may be coded, even following relatively little practice, in motor coordinates, the dominant code for more complex movement sequences would be in spatial coordinates. To test this notion, Kovacs et al. (2010) asked participants to practice either a simple or a slightly more complex movement sequence for one practice session (99 trials). The simpler movement sequence (S1) involved three movement reversals with a movement duration of 1300ms, and the more complex movement sequence (S2) involved five movement reversals with a movement duration of 2000ms (see Fig. 9.5). Interestingly, the first 1300ms of the longer sequences was the same as the shorter duration sequence. While it was not possible to precisely manipulate movement difficulty or complexity, Kovacs et al. (2010) hypothesized that the increased

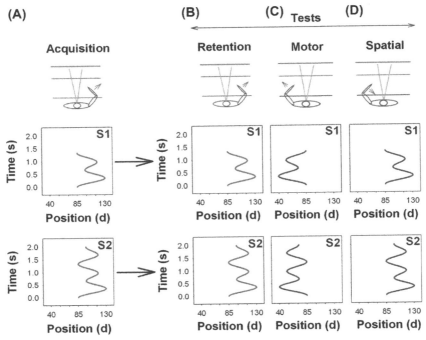

FIGURE 9.5 Illustration of the participant position (top) and the displays for the simple (S1) and more complex (S2) tasks (bottom). Columns A and B represent conditions during acquisition and retention. Columns C and D represent the position of the participant and displays for the motor and visual–spatial effector transfer tests, respectively.

movement duration and number of reversals (functional difficulty) of S2 may result in participants more effectively coding the sequence using spatial coordinates following only 99 trials of practice, while S1 may be coded at this stage of practice in motor coordinates.

The results confirmed these predictions. Participants that practiced S1 performed the motor transfer test with the contralateral limb as effectively as they performed the retention test, which was conducted under the same conditions and with the same limb as during practice. Alternatively, participants that practiced S2 performed the spatial transfer test, where the spatial coordinates were reinstated, as well as the retention test. These findings provide strong support for the notion that the coordinate system used to code movement sequences and the manner in which participants respond on effector transfer tests is influenced by the characteristics of the movement and the way in which feedback is provided.

In the previously discussed force and limb movement tasks, chunking processes were minimized. To increase the opportunity for participants to group a number of relatively independent elements together during the course of practice and to bridge the gap between the more traditional sequence-learning literature (see Verwey, Shea, & Wright, 2015 for a review) and the Hikosaka perspective, another task was used. Kovacs, Muehlbauer, et al. (2009) conducted three experiments with 1, 4, and 12 days of practice, respectively, looking at effector transfer of a 14-element dynamic movement sequence. The transfer conditions were designed based on the Hikosaka perspective to determine if reinstating the visual–spatial coordinates on the effector transfer test, which required movements to the same spatial locations utilized during acquisition, resulted in better effector transfer than reinstating the motor coordinates, which required the same pattern of homologous muscle activation. The manipulation of the number of days of practice was important because Hikosaka proposed that the development of the codes in visual-spatial coordinates is thought to occur relatively early in practice with the development of codes in motor coordinates requiring additional practice especially if the movement sequences were relatively complex.

A continuous, dynamic (14 elements) arm movement sequence was utilized in the Kovacs, Muehlbauer, et al. (2009) experiments. In essence, the task required the participant to move the lever from one illuminated target to the next (see Fig. 9.6A). When the pointer attached to the lever crossed the target boundary, the illumination for that target was turned off, and the next target in the sequence was illuminated. Note, participants were not informed that the targets were illuminated in a fixed order (14 elements). Participants were simply told to move from one target to the next as quickly and smoothly as possible. However, as practice continued, participants produced the sequence faster and faster. Indeed, the speed with which the elements were produced clearly indicated that they had learned the sequence and were not dependent on the pattern of illuminations. Following each of the practice periods a delayed retention test (Fig. 9.6B) and two effector transfer tests (Fig. 9.6C and D) were administered. On one effector transfer test the motor coordinates were reinstated such that the participant was

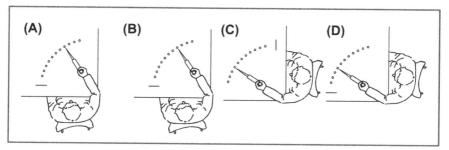

FIGURE 9.6 Illustration of the participant position and target display during acquisition trials (A), retention test (B), motor effector transfer test (C), and spatial effector transfer test (D). The start position is indicated by the horizontal/vertical line at the bottom left/top right in (A, B, D)/(C).

required to produce the same pattern of muscle action with the contralateral limb (homologous muscles) as was utilized during acquisition, but the visual display was changed (mirror image). On the other transfer test the spatial positions of the targets were the same as experienced during acquisition, but because of the change in the position of the participant, a new pattern of activation of the muscles of the contralateral limb was required to achieve the target positions.

Using similar movement sequences, Park and Shea (2005), Shea, Park, and Braden (2006), and Wilde and Shea (2006) have demonstrated that participants, relatively early in practice in an attempt to learn and manage the many elements in the sequence, begin to impose an organization on the elements in the sequence. The organization included chunking elements together into relatively intact subsequences and passing through intermediate targets in the sequence, thus functionally reducing the number of elements. The subsequence structure was evident by the pattern of element durations and location of zero crossing on the acceleration record. Later in practice, participants appeared to optimize the utilization of the specific effectors used to produce the movement and optimize movement dynamics (Dean, Kovacs, & Shea, 2008; Jordan, 1995; Muehlbauer, Panzer, & Shea, 2007). The structure imposed on the elements in the optimization processes occurring later in practice are thought to occur in motor coordinates, while the development of the sequence structure is thought to occur in visual–spatial coordinates.

Results demonstrated better transfer when visual–spatial coordinates were reinstated than when motor coordinates where reinstated regardless of the amount of practice (1, 4, or 12 days; experiments 1–3, respectively). Transfer (left to right and right to left) was symmetric when visual–spatial coordinates were reinstated but not when motor coordinates were reinstated. When motor coordinates were reinstated after 12 days of practice and vision was occluded, transfer was better from right limb to left than vice versa. The data are also consistent with the notion that multiple codes (visual, spatial, and motor) are developed over practice, with each code contributing to transfer performance when the respective coordinates are reinstated. Further, the results indicate a disruption of the linkage (concatenation) between subsequences when one or more coordinates are changed on the transfer test.

EFFECTOR TRANSFER CAN DISRUPT SEQUENCE CONCATENATION

One of the most interesting and consistent findings in the Kovacs, Muehlbauer, et al. (2009) set of experiments was that much of the performance decrement observed in element duration on both the motor and spatial transfer tests relative to the retention test could be accounted for by an increased duration of a few elements in the sequence while other element durations were essentially unchanged. In fact, for both the motor and spatial transfer tests the three largest increases in element durations occurred for Elements 1, 6, and 11. It is interesting that the elements preceding Elements 6 and 11 were virtually unchanged on the transfer tests relative to the retention test. In addition, Verwey (1999, 2001, 2003) has suggested, and Park and Shea (2002, 2003, 2005) have provided evidence, that the motor buffer has a limited capacity of five or fewer items, effectively restricting the size of movement subsequences. Together these pieces of information are consistent with the notion that participants, over the course of practice, created a structure for the 14-element sequence consisting of three subsequences (Elements 1–5, 6–10, and 11–14). Our previous research (e.g., Braden et al., 2008; Park & Shea, 2005; Wilde & Shea, 2006), using similar sequences, has consistently highlighted the finding that participants structure or chunk (Verwey, 1999, 2003) elements that make up complex sequences in similar ways. Generally subsequences have been operationally defined as a relatively long movement time to a target (beginning of subsequence) followed by relatively short movement times to one or more of the following targets (see Nissen & Bullemer, 1987; Povel & Collard, 1982; Verwey, 1994). The delay prior to the first item in a subsequence was thought to occur because the subsequence had to be retrieved, programmed, and/or otherwise readied for execution. The following elements in the subsequence are produced more rapidly than the first because processing related to their production was completed prior to or during the production of the first element in the subsequence. The end result would be a faster, more fluent response. Later in practice, the time required to produce the first element in the subsequence is also reduced by a process known as "concatenation" (Verwey, 1999) or "coarticulation" (Jordan, 1995), in which subsequences become interassociated (e.g., Brown & Carr, 1989). This parallel processing notion suggests that the processes involved in preparing the next subsequence are begun during the execution of the current subsequence, as opposed to carrying out these processing steps after the completion of the previous subsequence. However, on transfer tests, the linkages between subsequence, cues for initiating the next subsequence, and/or an increased processing load associated with producing the subsequence with an unpracticed limb could disrupt the transition from one subsequence to the next. The result would be the reemergence of relatively long element durations for those elements at or near the start of each subsequence. This is precisely what was observed by Kovacs, Muehlbauer, et al. (2009). It is interesting that Park and Shea (2005) (also see Wilde & Shea, 2006) have provided evidence that the markers indicating the transition between subsequences observed earlier in practice, but lost after additional practice, reappeared in the delayed retention and transfer tests. On the delayed retention test, response variability increased at the same points where transitions were seen earlier in practice. When Park and Shea asked participants to produce the response with their left hand (effector transfer test), the markers associated with the transitions between subsequences were even more pronounced. This was thought to occur not only because of the added processing load required to translate the response pattern to a new set of effectors but also because the stimuli that trigger the next subsequence was somehow tied to specific motor or visual–spatial information not available on the transfer test. If this is the case, the visual–spatial information is more important to the concatenation process than motor information as indicated by a greater disruption on the mirror transfer test than on the spatial transfer test.

MULTIPLE REPRESENTATIONS

Numerous theoretical perspectives discussed earlier have proposed that independent codes, representations, coordinate systems, and/or processing modules contribute to sequence production. Further, these perspectives often argue that the development of and reliance on these codes change over practice. These movement codes have been variously labeled relative and absolute (e.g., Schmidt, 1975), invariant and variant (Schmidt, 1985, 1988), structural and metrical (Kelso, 1981), higher and lower order (e.g., Fowler & Turvey, 1978), essential and nonessential (Gelfand & Tsetlin, 1971; Kelso, Putnam, & Goodman, 1983; Langley & Zelaznik, 1984), extrinsic and intrinsic (e.g., Criscimagna-Hemminger et al., 2003; Lange et al., 2004), visual–spatial and motor (Bapi et al., 2000; Hikosaka et al., 1999), and cognitive and motor (Keele et al., 1995; Shea & Wulf, 2005; Verwey, 1995). These distinctions imply that one set of codes is more abstract, develops more quickly, and is more available to consciousness (e.g., extrinsic, visual–spatial, cognitive) than the other (e.g., intrinsic, motor). Thus, it was important to assess the saliency of the different codes on effector transfer tests following various amounts of practice. Kovacs, Muehlbauer, et al. (2009) used an effector transfer paradigm to determine how well a learned sequence could be performed when one set of cues (visual–spatial or motor) was available during transfer but the other was altered. In very general terms, the results indicated that visual–spatial cues developed relatively early in practice and continued to be refined across 12 days of practice. Alternatively, the motor code did not appear to develop until much later in practice and appeared to be less effectively transferred from the nondominant to the dominant limb than vice versa. However, in other experiments (e.g., Kovacs et al., 2009; Panzer et al., 2009) where the sequence was comprised of relative few elements and online feedback was withheld during the production of the movement, performance on the transfer tests indicated greater reliance on motor codes after relatively little practice. These findings suggest that not only practice, but also the manner in which the response is controlled play a role in determining the effectiveness of transfer to an unpracticed limb.

It is important to note that the present data are consistent with a multiple code explanation for sequence production. A multiple coding explanation would argue that each code potentially adds to retention and transfer performance. This is different from that proposed by Hikosaka et al. (1999), where the reliance on codes was thought to shift from visual–spatial to motor over practice. After 1 and 4 days of practice the spatial transfer test was performed more efficiently than the mirror transfer test. However, the motor transfer test had only one valid code (motor) on which to base transfer performance. Alternatively, the spatial transfer condition provided both the same visual display of the targets and the same spatial positions as those used in practice. These two codes (visual and spatial) resulted in better performance than one code (motor). Indeed, when the visual information was not provided on the no-vision spatial test after 12 days of practice, performance was reduced to the level observed for the motor code alone. Consistent with this logic, performance on the mirror transfer test, where the visual display was altered, was unaffected by the withdrawal of the visual display. In fact, on the retention test, where all codes were valid, removal of the visual display resulted in reduced performance. These data are consistent with the notion that retention and transfer performance are determined by multiple codes that act together to enhance performance rather than the pure dominance of a single, most salient code.

These results have the potential to shed light on the reasons for differences across experiments on transfer tests. For example, using a key-press task, Bapi et al. (2000) found that when visual and motor codes were valid, transfer performance was better than when visual and spatial codes were available. Alternatively, Willingham, Wells, Farrell, and Stemwedel (2000), also using a key-press task, found that transfer was better when location (visual and spatial cues) was valid than when only motor cues were valid. However, in the Willingham et al. experiment, visual and spatial cues were available in the location condition, whereas only motor cues were valid in the motor condition. Thus the benefit for the location condition may have been due to the availability of two codes. At any rate, the present data suggest that it is important to consider the number of cues that are valid on transfer tests so that appropriate comparisons can be made.

IMPLICIT VERSUS EXPLICIT CODING

An additional goal of many of the effector transfer experiments was to determine the extent to which sequential movements are implicitly learned and whether or not the number of items in the sequence and/or the amount of practice was related to the extent to which the sequence knowledge was available at an explicit level. To assess the implicit/explicit nature of the sequence information an interview and three post experiment tests were administered (Park & Shea, 2005; also see Shea et al., 2006). The authors hypothesized that when the sequence was initially composed of more elements, it would be more likely to be learned implicitly than when the movement pattern was originally presented as fewer elements. They also hypothesized that as the result of additional practice (Experiment 2), where the distinction between elements might fade, and the movement was structured into subsequences, participants may also experience difficulty in explicitly identifying the arrangement of these elements in the sequence. Each of these post hoc tests as well as the more open-ended interviews with the participants indicated that the movement sequence was clearly represented in an explicit way in both experiments. Participants without exception could complete the sequence when it was interrupted, produce the sequence without the aid of the stimuli, and precisely describe the order of the elements. There was some anecdotal evidence after extended practice, however, that participants in describing the sequence engaged in what has been termed "inverse cognition." That is, they had to think about producing the movement in order to construct the target sequence. In fact, 5 of 10 participants in the 10-element condition in Experiment 1 described the sequence as composed of more than 10 elements. These elements, however, accurately described the movement path. Thus the sequence information could be described in terms of the movement path in much the same way that a skilled typist might determine the location of a particular letter on the keyboard. To find the "s" key, for example, they might think about typing an "s" and realize that the ring finger of their left hand would be used. By considering the base position of the left hand, the typist could identify the specific "s" key. A similar procedure appeared to be used by participants when asked to describe the sequence of targets. It is also interesting to note that 7 of 10 participants in the four-day group in Experiment 2, when asked to describe the sequence, did so initially by making arm movements that appeared to represent the sequence and only after prompting reverted to descriptions using the target designations. Interestingly, it has been argued that effector transfer specifically, and abstractness of memory states in general, is associated with explicit sequence knowledge and not implicit knowledge. This notion would be consistent with the present findings of strong explicit knowledge and strong effector transfer after 1 day of practice (Experiments 1 and 2). However, after 4 days of practice, effector transfer performance, where the contralateral limb was used, was poorer than retention performance, where the limb used during practice was used, and yet participants were able to generate strong explicit knowledge related to the repeated sequence. As noted earlier, however, there appeared to be subtle, but perhaps important, differences in what might be called the accessibility of the explicit knowledge between the one- and four-day practice groups. After 1 day of practice, participants in the interview phase readily described the movement sequences in terms of the targets and elements composing the sequence. After 4 days of practice, participants were able to construct this information, but initially volunteered sequence information in terms of the movement pattern itself and not the targets/elements. Indeed, participants after 4 days of practice readily provided sequence information by moving their arm through the movement pattern rather than using word or spatial designations to describe the movement sequence. Clearly, these participants were able upon request to generate other descriptions, including those that involved the targets, but this seemed to require additional processing on their part. The finding that participants after 4 days of practice could demonstrate relatively strong explicit knowledge of the sequence does not negate the argument that strong implicit knowledge had also developed. It is entirely possible that after 1 day of practice participants relied more on the abstract explicit knowledge they had acquired to produce the movement sequence. The consequence was that the movement performance was effector independent. After 4 days of practice, however, implicit memory for the task, which is thought to be more specific, may have developed to the extent that it was relied on for the retention and transfer tests. The consequence was effector-dependent performance. This scenario is consistent with the notion of dual-memory systems (e.g., Willingham, 1997, 1998), with one system supporting performance at early stages of practice and the other supporting more automated performance after more extensive practice. Future studies may wish to design post experiment tests to more directly and more quantitatively characterize this form of implicit/explicit distinction. Indeed, the post experiment interview and tests were designed to determine the degree of explicit knowledge and not the extent to which implicit knowledge might have developed over practice.

HANDEDNESS, HEMISPHERIC ASYMMETRIES, AND EFFECTOR TRANSFER

Previous research has provided evidence that effector transfer is asymmetric (e.g., Criscimagna-Hemminger et al., 2003; Hicks, 1975; Laszlo, Baguley, & Bairstow, 1970; Sainburg & Wang, 2002; Schulze, Lüders, & Jäncke, 2002; Taylor & Heilmann, 1980). To account for the asymmetry associated with effector transfer, four theoretical models have been proposed. The first, termed the Callosal Access model (Hicks, 1974; Taylor & Heilmann, 1980), proposes one motor representation is stored in the dominant hemisphere regardless of the limb used for practice. According to the model, the dominant limb has direct access to key information stored in the dominant hemisphere, whereas the nondominant limb has only indirect access to the same information via the corpus callosum (Taylor & Heilmann, 1980). As such, it is predicted that the dominant limb will benefit more from practice with the nondominant limb than the nondominant limb from practice with the dominant limb.

Alternatively, the Proficiency model (Laszlo et al., 1970) as well as the Cross-Activation model (Parlow & Kinsbourne, 1989), propose that effector transfer occurs from the dominant to the nondominant limb. More specifically, the Proficiency model (Laszlo et al., 1970) is based on the notion that a motor representation is created and stored in the hemisphere contralateral to the limb used for practice. When the dominant limb is used for practice the motor representation is created and stored in the dominant hemisphere, whereas practice with the nondominant limb results in the motor representation created and stored in the nondominant hemisphere. It is believed there is a general advantage for motor representations created and stored in the dominant hemisphere. The Cross-Activation model (Parlow & Kinsbourne, 1989) proposes that two motor representations are generated when the dominant limb is used for practice: one stored in the dominant hemisphere and another weaker version in the nondominant hemisphere. However, when the nondominant limb is used for practice, only one motor representation is generated in the nondominant hemisphere (Parlow & Kinsbourne, 1989). Without a motor representation stored in the dominant hemisphere, it is predicted that the nondominant limb will benefit more from practice with the dominant limb than the dominant limb will from practice with the nondominant.

A limitation associated with each of these models, however, is they cannot account for the conflicting results reported in the literature (e.g., Laszlo et al., 1970; Parlow & Kinsbourne, 1989) regarding the direction of effector transfer (i.e., dominant to nondominant or nondominant to dominant). More recently, however, Sainburg and Wang (2002), Wang and Sainburg (2004, 2006), and Mutha, Haaland, and Sainburg (2012) proposed a fourth model, the Dynamic Dominance model, that emphasized effector transfer was associated with asymmetry of the cerebral hemispheres and hemispheric specialization (e.g., Mutha et al., 2012). For example, Sainburg and Wang (2002) demonstrated that the information transferred between the limbs was specific to each limb. Using a visuomotor perturbation task, participants were required to adapt to a 30 degrees visual rotation of the target with either the right or left limb. After practice with one limb, participants performed the visual rotation task with the contralateral limb. The results indicated improved performance related to trajectory information on the test trials with the right dominant arm after practice with the left nondominant limb, whereas the nondominant limb improved performance on measures related to accuracy of the final position after the practice with the right dominant arm. As such, Sainburg and Kalakanis (2000) and Sainburg and Wang (2002) reported that for right-handed participants the dominant limb was more effective in trajectory control, whereas the nondominant limb is more proficient at tuning spatial locations of the end effector.

According to the Dynamic Dominance model, information related to trajectory and end point position is stored in two different memory resources in each hemisphere (Wang & Sainburg, 2004). Both limbs have symmetric (equal) access to the stored information; however, the arm used during practice determines the type of information transferred for each effector. More specifically, the Dynamic Dominance model would predict that the trajectory information transfers from the nondominant to the dominant limb while information related to the end effector position transfers from the dominant to the nondominant limb (Sainburg & Wang, 2002).

Given this information, researchers and practitioners designing effector transfer training programs to acquire new skills or to maintain skills while one limb is injured should consider the dominant and nondominant hemispheres/limb systems responsible for different features of the task and plan accordingly. Practitioners should also consider the nature of the task to be learned and then consider which hemispheres/limb system should to be trained first and what might be the best practice conditions.

SUMMARY

Current research has isolated handedness and the coordinate system used to code movement information as important factors in determining the effectiveness of effector transfer to the contralateral limb. When relatively simple movement sequences are preplanned or more complex movement sequences have been extensively practiced, effector transfer to conditions where the motor coordinates are reinstated result in enhanced transfer relative to when the visual–spatial coordinates are reinstated. When complex movement sequences have not been extensively practiced and/or the production of the sequence relies on online feedback to produce the response, effector transfer is enhanced when the visual–spatial coordinates are reinstated relative to when the motor coordinates are reinstated. In most situations, performance is further enhanced when both coordinate systems are reinstated, although this may be difficult to achieve with many effector transfer tasks. When aiming movements are utilized and visual information is manipulated, it appears that the dominant limb/hemisphere system is best suited for initial (preplanned) direction control and load compensation, while the nondominant limb/hemisphere system was more effective in positional control. Following practice of movement sequences the differences in effector transfer performance for the dominant and nondominant limbs is, in general, relatively small, with the transfer performance dependent on the degree to which the coordinate systems have been reinstated.

References

Bapi, R. S., Doya, K., & Harner, A. M. (2000). Evidence for effector independent and dependent representations and their differential time course of acquisition during motor sequence learning. *Experimental Brain Research*, *132*, 149–162.

Braden, H., Panzer, S., & Shea, C. H. (2008). The effects of sequence difficulty and practice on proportional and non-proportional transfer. *Quarterly Journal of Experimental Psychology*, *61*, 1321–1339.

Brown, T. L., & Carr, T. H. (1989). Automaticity in skill acquisition: mechanisms for reducing interference in concurrent performance. *Journal of Experimental Psychology: Human Perception and Performance*, *15*, 686–700.

Criscimagna-Hemminger, S. E., Donchin, O., Gazzaniga, M. S., & Shadmehr, R. (2003). Learned dynamics of reaching movements generalize from dominant to nondominant arm. *Journal of Neurophysiology*, *89*, 168–176.

Dean, N., Kovacs, A. J., & Shea, C. H. (2008). Transfer of movement sequences: bigger is better. *Acta Psychologica*, *127*, 355–368.

Ellenbuerger, T., Panzer, S., Boutin, A., Blandin, Y. L., Fischer, L., Schorer, J., & Shea, C. H. (2012). Observational training in visual half-fields and the coding of movement sequences. *Human Movement Science*, *31*, 1436–1448.

Fowler, C. A., & Turvey, M. T. (1978). Concept of command neurons in explanations of behavior. *Behavioral and Brain Sciences*, *1*, 20–22.

Gelfand, I. M., & Tsetlin, M. (1971). Mathematical modeling of mechanisms of the central nervous system. In I. M. Gelfand, V. Gurfinkel, S. Fomin, & M. Tsetlin (Eds.), *Models of the structural-functional organization of certain biological systems* (pp. 1–22). Cambridge, MA: MIT Press.

Gruetzmacher, N., Panzer, S., Blandin, Y., & Shea, C. H. (2011). Observation and physical practice: coding of simple motor sequences. *Quarterly Journal of Experimental Psychology*, *64*, 1111–1123.

Henningsen, H., Ende-Henningsen, B., & Gordon, A. M. (1995). Asymmetric control of bilateral isometric finger forces. *Experimental Brain Research*, *105*, 304–311.

Henry, F. M., & Rogers, D. E. (1960). Increased response latency for complicated movements and a "memory drum" theory of neuromotor reaction. *Research Quarterly*, *31*, 448–458.

Hicks, R. E. (1974). Asymmetry of bilateral transfer. *The American Journal of Psychology*, *87*, 667–674.

Hicks, R. E. (1975). Intrahemispheric response competition between voval and unimanual performances in normal adult human males. *Journal of Comparative and Physiological Psychology*, *89*, 50–60.

Hikosaka, O., Nakahara, H., Rand, M. K., Sakai, K., Lu, X. F., Nakamura, K., … Doya, K. (1999). Parallel neural networks for learning sequential procedures. *Trends in Neurosciences*, *22*, 464–471.

Hikosaka, O., Nakamura, K., Sakai, K., & Nakahara, H. (2002). Central mechanisms of motor skill learning. *Current Opinion in Neurobiology*, *12*, 217–222.

Hikosaka, O., Rand, M. K., Miyachi, S., & Miyashita, K. (1995). Learning of sequential movements in the monkey: process of learning and retention of memory. *Journal of Neurophysiology*, *74*, 1652–1661.

Hikosaka, O., Sakai, K., Miyauchi, S., Takino, R., Sasaki, Y., & Putz, B. (1996). Activation of human presupplementary motor area in learning of sequential procedures: a functional MRI study. *Journal of Neurophysiology*, *76*, 617–621.

Jordan, M. I. (1995). The organization of action sequences: evidence from a relearning task. *Journal of Motor Behavior*, *27*, 179–192.

Keele, S. W., Cohen, A., & Ivry, R. (1990). Motor programs: concepts and issues. In M. Jeannerod (Ed.), *Attention and performance XIII* (pp. 77–110). Hillsdale, NJ: Erlbaum.

Keele, S. W., Ivry, R., Mayr, U., Hazeltine, E., & Heuer, H. (2003). The cognitive and neural architecture of sequence representation. *Psychological Review*, *110*, 316–339.

Keele, S. W., Jennings, P., Jones, S., Caulton, D., & Cohen, A. (1995). On the modularity of sequence representation. *Journal of Motor Behavior, 27*, 17–30.

Kelso, J. A. S. (1981). Contrasting perspectives on order and regulation in movement. In J. Long, & A. Baddeley (Eds.), *Attention and performance IX* (pp. 437–457). Hillsdale, NJ: Erlbaum.

Kelso, J. A., Putnam, C. A., & Goodman, D. (1983). On the nature of human interlimb coordination. *Quarterly Journal of Experimental Psychology, 35A*, 347–375.

Klapp, S. T. (1995). Motor response programming during simple and choice reaction time: the role of practice. *Journal of Experimental Psychology: Human Perception and Performance, 21*, 1015–1027.

Klapp, S. T. (1996). Reaction time analysis of central motor control. In H. N. Zelaznik (Ed.), *Advances in motor learning and control* (pp. 13–35). Champaign, IL: Human Kinetics.

Kovacs, A. J., Boyle, J., Gruetzmatcher, N., & Shea, C. H. (2010). Coding of on-line and pre-planned movement sequences. *Acta Psychologica, 133*, 119–126.

Kovacs, A. J., Han, D.-W., & Shea, C. H. (2009). The representation of movement sequences is related to task characteristics. *Acta Psychologica, 132*, 54–61.

Kovacs, A. J., Muehlbauer, T., & Shea, C. H. (2009). The coding and effector transfer of movement sequences. *Journal of Experimental Psychology: Human Perception and performance, 35*, 390–407.

Krakauer, J. W., Ghilardi, M. F., & Ghez, C. (1999). Independent learning of internal models for kinematic and dynamic control of reaching. *Nature Neuroscience, 2*, 1026–1031.

Lange, R. K., Godde, B., & Braun, C. (2004). EEG correlates of coordinate processing during intermanual transfer. *Experimental Brain Research, 159*, 161–171.

Langley, D. J., & Zelaznik, H. N. (1984). The acquisition of time properties associated with a sequential motor skill. *Journal of Motor Behavior, 16*, 275–301.

Lashley, K. S. (1951). The problem of serial order in behavior. In L. A. Jeffress (Ed.), *Cerebral mechanisms in behavior* (pp. 112–136). New York: Wiley.

Laszlo, H. G., Baguley, R. A., & Bairstow, P. J. (1970). Bilateral transfer in tapping skill in the absence of peripheral information. *Journal of Motor Behavior, 2*, 261–271.

MacKay, D. G. (1982). The problem of flexibility and fluency in skilled behavior. *Psychological Review, 89*, 483–506.

Muehlbauer, T., Panzer, S., & Shea, C. H. (2007). The transfer of movement sequences: effects of decreased and increased load. *Quarterly Journal of Experimental Psychology, 60*, 770–778.

Mutha, P. K., Haaland, K. Y., & Sainburg, R. (2012). The effects of brain lateralization on motor control and adaptation. *Journal of Motor Behavior, 44*, 455–469.

Nissen, M. J., & Bullemer, P. (1987). Attentional requirements of learning: evidence from performance measures. *Cognitive Psychology, 19*, 1–32.

Panzer, S., Krueger, M., Muehlbauer, T., Kovacs, A., & Shea, C. H. (2009). Inter-manual transfer and practice: coding of simple motor sequences. *Acta Psychologica, 131*, 99–109.

Panzer, S., Krueger, M., Muehlbauer, T., & Shea, C. H. (2010). Asymmetric effector transfer of complex movement sequences: effects of increased and decreased loads. *Human Movement Science, 29*, 62–72.

Park, J. H., & Shea, C. H. (2002). Effector independence. *Journal of Motor Behavior, 34*, 253–270.

Park, J. H., & Shea, C. H. (2003). Effect of practice on effector independence. *Journal of Motor Behavior, 35*, 33–40.

Park, J. H., & Shea, C. H. (2005). Sequence learning: response structure and effector transfer. *Quarterly Journal of Experimental Psychology A: Human Experimental Psychology, 58A*, 387–419.

Parlow, S. E., & Kinsbourne, M. (1989). Asymmetrical transfer of training between hands: implications for interhemispheric communication in normal brain. *Brain and Cognition, 11*, 98–113.

Povel, D., & Collard, R. (1982). Structural factors in patterned finger tapping. *Acta Psychologica, 52*, 107–123.

Restle, F. (1970). Theory of serial pattern learning: structural trees. *Psychological Review, 77*, 481–495.

Rosenbaum, D. A. (1990). On choosing between movement sequences: comments on rose (1988). *Journal of Experimental Psychology: Human Perception and Performance, 16*, 439–444.

Rosenbaum, D. A., Cohen, R. G., Jax, S. A., Weiss, D. J., & van der Wel, R. (2007). The problem of serial order in behavior: lashley's legacy. *Human Movement Science, 26*, 525–554.

Rosenbaum, D. A., Hindorff, V., & Munro, E. M. (1986). Programming of rapid finger sequences. In H. Heuer, & C. Fromm (Eds.), *Generation and modulation of action patterns* (pp. 64–71). Berlin: Springer.

Rosenbaum, D. A., Inhoff, A. W., & Gordon, A. M. (1984). Choosing between movement sequences: a hierarchical editor. *Journal of Experimental Psychology: General, 113*, 372–393.

Rosenbaum, D. A., Kenny, S., & Derr, M. A. (1983). Hierarchical control of rapid movement sequences. *Journal of Experimental Psychology: Human Perception and Performance, 9*, 86–102.

Rosenbaum, D. A., & Saltzman, E. (1984). A motor-program editor. In W. Prinz, & A. Sanders (Eds.), *Cognition and motor processes* (Vol. VIII) (pp. 93–106). Berlin: Springer.

Rosenbaum, D. A., Saltzman, E., & Kingman, A. (1984). Choosing between movement sequences. In S. Kornblum, & J. Requin (Eds.), *Preparatory states and processes* (pp. 119–134). Hillsdale, NJ: Erlbaum.

Sainburg, R. L., & Kalakanis, D. (2000). Differences in control of limb dynamics during dominant and nondominant arm reaching. *Journal of Neurophysiology, 83*, 2661–2675.

Sainburg, R. L., & Wang, J. S. (2002). Interlimb transfer of visuomotor rotations: independence of direction and final position information. *Experimental Brain Research, 145*, 437–447.

Sakai, K., Hikosaka, O., Miyauchi, S., Takino, R., Sasaki, Y., & Putz, B. (1998). Transition of brain activation from frontal to parietal areas in visuomotor sequence learning. *Journal of Neuroscience, 18*, 1827–1840.

Schmidt, R. A. (1975). Schema theory of discrete motor skill learning. *Psychological Review, 82*, 225–260.

Schmidt, R. A. (1985). The search for invariance in skilled movement behavior. *Research Quarterly for Exercise and Sport, 56*, 188–200.

Schmidt, R. A. (1988). *Motor control and learning*. Champaign, IL: Human Kinetics.

Schulze, K., Lüders, E., & Jäncke, L. (2002). Intermanual transfer in a simple motor task. *Cortex, 38*(5), 805–815.

Shea, C. H., Kovacs, A. J., & Panzer, S. (2011). The coding and inter-manual transfer of movement sequences. *Frontiers in Psychology, 2*.

Shea, C. H., Park, J. H., & Braden, H. W. (2006). Age-related effects in sequential motor learning. *Physical Therapy, 86*, 478–488.

Shea, C. H., & Wulf, G. (2005). Schema theory: a critical appraisal and reevaluation. *Journal of Motor Behavior, 37*, 85–101.

Sternberg, S., Knoll, R. L., & Turock, D. L. (1990). Hierarchical control in the execution of action sequences: tests of two invariance properties. In M. Jeannerod (Ed.), *Attention and performance XIII* (pp. 3–55). Hillsdale, NJ: Erlbaum.

Tangeman, P. T., Banaitis, D. A., & Williams, A. K. (1990). Rehabilitation of chronic stroke patients: changes in functional performance. *Archives of Physical Medicine and Rehabilitation, 71*, 876–880.

Taylor, H. G., & Heilmann, K. M. (1980). Left hemisphere motor dominance in right-handers. *Cortex, 16*, 587–603.

Verwey, W. B. (1994). Evidence for the development of concurrent processing in a sequential keypressing task. *Acta Psychologica, 85*, 245–262.

Verwey, W. B. (1995). A forthcoming key press can be selected while earlier ones are executed. *Journal of Motor Behavior, 27*, 275–284.

Verwey, W. B. (1999). Evidence for a multistage model of practice in a sequential movement task. *Journal of Experimental Psychology: Human Perception and Performance, 25*, 1693–1708.

Verwey, W. B. (2001). Concatenating familiar movement sequences: the versatile cognitive processor. *Acta Psychologica, 106,* 69–95.

Verwey, W. B. (2003). Effect of sequence length on the execution of familiar keying sequences: lasting segmentation and preparation? *Journal of Motor Behavior, 35,* 343–354.

Verwey, W. B., Shea, C. H., & Wright, D. L. (2015). A cognitive framework for explaining serial processing and sequence execution strategies. *Psychonomics Bulletin and Review, 22,* 54–77.

Wang, J., & Sainburg, R. L. (2004). Interlimb transfer of novel inertial dynamics is asymmetrical. *Journal of Neurophysiology, 92,* 349–360.

Wang, J., & Sainburg, R. L. (2006). Interlimb transfer of visuomotor rotations depends on handedness. *Experimental Brain Research, 175,* 223–230.

Wilde, H., & Shea, C. H. (2006). Proportional and nonproportional transfer of movement sequences. *Quarterly Journal of Experimental Psychology, 59,* 1626–1647.

Willingham, D. B. (1997). Systems of memory in the human brain. *Neuron, 18,* 5–8.

Willingham, D. B. (1998). A neuropsychological theory of motor skill learning. *Psychological Review, 105,* 558–584.

Willingham, D. B., Wells, L. A., Farrell, J. M., & Stemwedel, M. E. (2000). Implicit motor sequence learning is represented in response locations. *Memory & Cognition, 28,* 366–375.

Winstein, C. J., Merians, A. S., & Sullivan, K. J. (1999). Motor learning after unilateral brain damage. *Neuropsychologia, 37,* 975–987.

Wulf, G., & Shea, C. H. (2002). Principles derived from the study of simple skills do not generalize to complex skill learning. *Psychonomics Bulletin and Review, 9,* 185–211.

10

Near Misses and the Effect of Attentional Asymmetries on Sporting Performance

Owen Churches, Michael E.R. Nicholls
Flinders University, Adelaide, SA, Australia

ATTENTION

The human sensory system is constantly bombarded by a welter of incoming information from the surrounding environment. The sheer volume of this information makes it impossible for the human brain to attend to all of this information at once. As a consequence, the brain has developed mechanisms that allow it to attend selectively to information that is deemed to be biologically important to the organism. This selective processing was originally likened to a processing "bottleneck," where information enters a sensory buffer, and the relevant information is selected on the basis of its physical characteristics. Information that is not selected decays rapidly and is not processed further (Broadbent, 1958). Other models of selective attention, such as Treisman's (1964) attenuation model, suggest that all information is subject to at least some semantic analysis. Thus information on an unattended channel can enter consciousness if it exceeds a threshold in relation to its meaning. If information is selected at this later stage, it can explain phenomena such as the "cocktail party effect" where attention is drawn to an unattended conversation when a semantically salient word is uttered.

In relation to visual spatial attention, a number of metaphors have been developed to explain the selective nature of attention. One prominent model refers to an attentional "spotlight," which brings items of interest within its beam, enhancing the processing of information within the beam and bringing them into consciousness (Posner, Snyder, & Davidson, 1980).

A modification of this model proposes a "zoom lens," where the size of spotlight of attention is adjusted to encompass stimuli of interest. This zoom feature causes a more diluted spread of attention for wider spotlights and more concentrated attention when a tight focus is required (Barriopedro & Botella, 1998). Interestingly, Hüttermann, Memmert, and Simons (2014) demonstrated that the shape of the attentional spotlight varied according to sporting expertise. For soccer players, who need to attend to balls along the horizontal meridian, the attentional spotlight was elongated in the horizontal dimension. In contrast, for volleyball where the ball moves along the vertical dimension, the players exhibited an attentional spotlight that was elongated along the vertical dimension. Finally, a gradient model has been suggested where attentional resources are concentrated around the focus of attention and then decrease in a continuous gradient away from that point (LaBerge & Brown, 1989). The slope of the gradient is also thought to depend on the nature of the task and can be broader for a task that requires a greater spread of attention (Hughes & Zimba, 1987).

For psychologists, and in particular sports psychologists, one of the most interesting and important things about selective spatial attention is how it affects the mistakes we make. A good example of this sort of mistake is inattentional blindness. A classic example of this phenomenon is provided by Simons and Chabris (1999). They asked participants to watch a video of a group of individuals passing a basketball between them and count the number of passes made. Unbeknownst to participants, a person dressed in a gorilla walked through the scene at some point in the game. Despite being in plain sight, most participants failed to report the presence of the gorilla. It therefore appears that their spatial attention was restricted to the area immediately surrounding the ball, causing the gorilla to pass through unnoticed.

Failure to attend to potentially important stimuli during sporting activity has the potential to affect performance and potentially change the outcome of games. This chapter will discuss limitations in selective spatial attention with special reference to how these processes are affected by changes in position across the visual field. In particular, it is well known that asymmetries exist in the way attention is distributed from left to right across the horizontal axis (Loftus & Nicholls, 2012). Similarly, attentional asymmetries are known to exist between the lower and upper hemispaces across the vertical axis (Thomas, Castine, Loetscher, & Nicholls, 2015).

Asymmetries in Clinical Populations

One of the most dramatic examples of how attentional asymmetries along the horizontal axis affect performance comes from the clinical syndrome of spatial neglect. In this syndrome, patients lose the ability to attend and respond to stimuli placed to the left of their midline

(Mattingley et al., 2004). The symptoms of spatial neglect are readily observed using tasks such as line bisection. Instead of placing a transector near the middle of a horizontal line, neglect patients placed the transector far to the right of the true middle (Bisiach & Vallar, 1988; Heilman, Jeong, & Finney, 2004; Heilman & Valenstein, 1979; Toth & Kirk, 2002). Spatial neglect also affects many everyday activities, causing patients to dress the right side of the body, to eat from the right side of their plate, and to collide with objects located on their left (Azouvi et al., 1996; Punt, Kitadono, Hulleman, Humphreys, & Riddoch, 2008, 2011). While spatial neglect is associated with damage to a broad range of sites within the attentional networks of the brain, it is most often associated with damage centered on the parietal region of the right hemisphere (Molenberghs, Sale, & Mattingley, 2012).

Attentional asymmetries for stimuli placed along the horizontal axis also depend on the distance the stimulus is placed from the observer. For some patients, leftward neglect is observed for objects placed in near space, but not far space (Halligan & Marshall, 1991). In contrast, other patients show leftward inattention for objects in far, but not near space (Vuilleumier, Valenza, Mayer, Reverdin, & Landis, 1998). This dissociation most likely reflects the operation of different neural circuits specialized for processing near and far space. In support of this proposition, Committeri et al. (2007) demonstrated a dissociation between extrapersonal and peripersonal space in a group of right hemisphere stroke patients. Patients with an intact ventral circuit, including the right frontal and superior temporal regions, had normal attentional processes within extrapersonal (far) space. Conversely, intact attention in peripersonal (near) space was associated with a dorsal circuit that coded proprioceptive and somatosensory inputs, including the right inferior parietal regions (see also Butlera, Eskes, & Vandorpe, 2003).

Patients with spatial neglect can also show signs of altitudinal neglect along the vertical axis. Butter, Evans, Kirsch, and Kewman (1989) reported a case for a woman with bilateral trauma to the dorsal sections of the occipital lobes extending into the cuneal and precuneal sections. When asked to bisect rods, using either vision or touch, she placed the bisector further upwards compared to controls. Because this asymmetry was not related to a primary sensory deficit, Butter et al. (1989) concluded that the disorder reflected an inability to orient attention toward the lower hemispace. Subsequent research by Làdavas, Carletti, and Gori (1994) used central and peripheral cues to manipulate attention in a group of patients with spatial neglect. Besides the expected inability to attend the hemispace contralateral to the lesion, Làdavas et al. (1994) also observed that the left/right asymmetry was more pronounced in the lower hemifield. Once again, this result suggests a problem with orienting attention toward the lower hemispace in neglect patients.

Horizontal Symmetries in the General Population

While patients who have suffered some form of brain injury can exhibit profound asymmetries in selective spatial attention, more subtle asymmetries are also evident in the general population. In relation to the horizontal axis, asymmetries in attention exist, whereby more attention is paid to the features of a stimulus that falls in the left hemispace compared to those features that fall to the right (McCourt, 2001). This bias in attention is clearly evident for tasks such as line bisection. When asked to transect a horizontal line, participants reliably place the transector slightly to the left of true middle (van Vugt, Fransen, Creten, & Paquier, 2000). This asymmetry in attention is not limited to motor tasks and also occurs for purely perceptual tasks. For example, when asked to decide to judge the relative lengths of the left and right segments of a line, participants reliably judge the element on the left side as longer (Nicholls et al., 2014). The leftward overattention extends beyond the visual modality and also occurs for the haptic exploration of rods (Bowers & Heilman, 1980).

The leftward attentional bias that occurs in the general population is often referred to as "pseudoneglect" (Bowers & Heilman, 1980). This term is apt given that pseudoneglect shares so many features in common with neglect. For example, both neglect and pseudoneglect are affected in a similar manner by increases in stimulus length (McCourt & Jewell, 1999), height (McCourt & Jewell, 1999), and shape (McCourt & Garlinghouse, 2000). There also seems to be a strong overlap in the neural circuits that affect both behaviors. Using fMRI, Çiçek, Deouell, and Knight (2009) examined brain activation as participants carried out manual and landmark versions of the line bisection task. Manual line bisection tasks require participants to mark the center of a line using devices such as a pencil and therefore emphasize the motor aspects of the task. In contrast, landmark tasks require participants to estimate whether a prebisected line has been bisected accurately and therefore emphasize the perceptual aspects of the task. For both tasks, there was right lateralized intraparietal sulcus and lateral peristriate cortex activity. These regions closely overlap with areas implicated in the manifestation of clinical neglect (Molenberghs et al., 2012).

A number of models have been put forward to explain the link between known asymmetries in the neural mechanisms that control attention and the attentional asymmetries themselves. Kinsbourne (1970) has proposed an "opponent" model where the level of activation within each hemisphere determines the level of attention payed to the contralateral hemispace (also known as the activation orientation model). Alternatively, Heilman and Valenstein's (1979) "hemispatial" model proposed that the right hemisphere is able to attend to both hemispaces, whereas the left hemisphere is only able to attend to the contralateral hemispace. A model proposed by Duecker and Sack (2015) has attempted to combine both models. Using data from transcranial magnetic stimulation, they showed that mechanisms within the posterior parietal cortex generate a contralateral bias of attention (opponent model) and this combines with an asymmetry in the frontal eye fields, which allows the right hemisphere to attend to both hemispaces (hemifield model).

It is also likely that cultural practices affect left/right attentional asymmetries. For example, habitual scanning of the eyes from left-to-right may cause an overestimation of the leftward features of an object (and vice versa for right-to-left scanning). In support of this proposition, Chokron and Imbert (1993) found that readers of French (left-to right) bisected lines to the left of true center, whereas readers of Hebrew (right-to-left) bisected lines to the right of center. Rinaldi, Di Luca, Henik, and Girelli (2014) administered star cancellation and line bisection tasks to a group of monolingual readers of Italian and Hebrew and bilingual readers of Hebrew. They found that cultural practices had a significant effect on left/right attentional asymmetries. The effect of reading direction, however, appeared to be interactive (modifying the underlying asymmetry generated by hemispheric specialization). Similarly, Smith, Szelest, Friedrich, and Elias (2014) have demonstrated that right-to-left reading reduces leftward attentional biases but does not reverse it.

Like spatial neglect, pseudoneglect is also affected by the distance between the observer and the stimulus. When a stimulus is placed within reach (peripersonal space), the general leftward bias associated with pseudoneglect is observed (Nicholls et al., 2014). When the stimulus is placed outside of reach (extrapersonal space), the leftward bias associated with line bisection can be annulled (Bjoertomt, Cowey, & Walsh, 2002; McCourt & Garlinghouse, 2000) or reversed toward a rightward bisection bias (Longo & Lourenco, 2006). Longo and Lourenco (2006) have demonstrated that "actionability" is the critical factor that determines the boundary between peripersonal and extrapersonal space. They presented lines at a range varying between 0.3 and 1.2 m. When the bisection was made using a laser pointer, leftward bisections were observed for near stimuli (actionable), which reversed to a rightward bisection bias for far stimuli (nonactionable). When all stimuli were made actionable by performing the bisection with a stick, leftward bisections were observed irrespective of viewing distance. This finding ties in nicely with primate research showing that tool-use allows distant objects to be processed by the "near" processing mechanisms of the brain (Iriki, Tanaka, & Iwamura, 1996).

Vertical Asymmetries in the General Population

Attentional biases are not limited to the horizontal plane in the general population but also occur in the vertical plane. For example, Drain and Reuter-Lorenz (1996) asked participants to view vertical lines and judge the position of a transector. They found that bisections were consistently misplaced upwards from the line's true midpoint. Upward biases for line bisection tasks have been reported by a number of others (Bradshaw, Nettleton, Nathan, & Wilson, 1986; McCourt & Olafson, 1997; van Vugt et al., 2000). An upward bias has also been reported for the grayscales task (Nicholls, Mattingley, Berberovic, Smith, & Bradshaw, 2004). In this task, participants are asked to make a relative luminance judgment between two vertically oriented bars, which changed from black at the top to white at the bottom (and vice versa for the other bar). Nicholls et al. (2004) found that participants biased their responses toward the stimulus with the salient feature on its upper side.

The upward bias in attention could be the result of perceptual or attentional factors. Drain and Reuter-Lorenz (1996) investigated this issue using a line bisection task. To control for perceptual factors, the bisection point was always placed in the vertical center of the screen. Spatial cues presented to the upper and lower end of the stimuli were used to manipulate attention.

Drain and Reuter-Lorenz found that the bias was affected by the spatial cues and therefore concluded that the upward bias was attentional in origin. They went on to suggest that the attentional asymmetry was related to relative activation of the dorsal and ventral visual pathways. In a comprehensive review of upper and lower visual field asymmetries, Previc (1990) suggested that the upper visual field has a stronger input into the ventral visual stream, which passes through the temporal lobe. In contrast, the lower visual field has a stronger connection with the dorsal visual stream, which passes through the parietal lobe. Given that the ventral pathway (the "what" pathway) is specialized for object processing, Drain and Reuter-Lorenz (1996) proposed that the line bisection task, because it is object-based, causes an upward attentional bias because it activated the ventral stream. It can be seen that the role of activation in vertical attentional biases proposed by Drain and Reuter-Lorenz (1996) is analogous to the hemispheric activation model proposed by Kinsbourne (1970).

The Relationship Between Horizontal and Vertical Attentional Biases

Attentional biases in the horizontal and vertical dimensions share many features in common. For example, the magnitude of attentional biases increases for longer stimuli in both the horizontal (McCourt & Jewell, 1999) and vertical dimensions. Similarly, attentional biases can be affected by the presentation of spatial cues for both horizontal (Nicholls & Roberts, 2002) and vertical (Drain & Reuter-Lorenz, 1996) stimuli. The nature of the cognitive/neural mechanisms that give rise to the attentional biases is also analogous. In both cases, differences in the amount of relative activation between the left/right hemispheres (Kinsbourne, 1970) or ventral/dorsal (Drain & Reuter-Lorenz, 1996) streams are thought to give rise to a bias of attention toward one side of space.

The relationship between horizontal and vertical attentional biases has been explored by Nicholls et al. (2004). In their task, the grayscales stimuli were presented in four orientations: horizontal, vertical, and 45 degree oblique forward (/) and backward (\). For the horizontal and vertical conditions, the expected leftward and upward attentional biases were observed. Interestingly, for the oblique forward condition, the biases counteracted one another (see Fig. 10.1). In this case, equal amount of attention is paid to the upper/right and lower/left quadrants of space. In contrast, for the oblique backward condition, the effects were additive. Thus the segment of the stimulus that fell in the upper/left quadrant received an especially large amount of attention compared to the segment that fell in the lower right segment.

Despite the fact the leftward horizontal and upward attentional biases combine to produce an extra strong bias toward the upper/left quadrant, the biases themselves appear to be independent. Nicholls et al. (2004) examined the correlation between an individual's attentional bias along the horizontal axis with their bias along the vertical axis. No evidence of an association was found between the axes, suggesting independent cognitive mechanisms. Churches, Loetscher, Thomas, and Nicholls (submitted) asked participants to mark the center of a variety of rectangles. As might be expected, participants perceived the center to be slightly to the

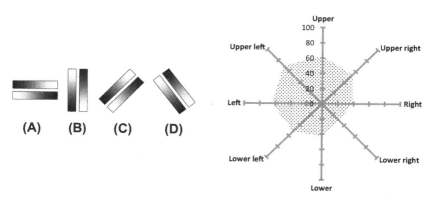

FIGURE 10.1 Participants viewed the stimuli in (A) horizontal, (B) vertical, (C) oblique forward, and (D) oblique backward conditions. The radar chart shows the amount of attentional bias along each of the four axes. Response asymmetry is measured in terms of response bias. For example, a score of 60 toward the upper direction indicates that participants selected the stimulus with the salient feature in the upper half of space 60% of the time. As can be seen, there is a shift of attention toward the upper/left quadrant.

left and up from the true center. Despite measuring horizontal and vertical biases within the same stimulus at the same moment, no correlation was observed between the biases along the two axes. There therefore seems to be strong evidence that the biases, despite sharing some features in common, arise for disparate cognitive/neural mechanisms.

Attentional Asymmetries and Everyday Behavior

Asymmetries in the way attention is spread along the horizontal and vertical axes has the potential to affect our everyday behaviors. One such behavior relates to the ability to walk between two obstacles. Turnbull and McGeorge (1998) investigated this issue by asking students to recall if they had collided with anything recently while walking. They reported a trend for participants to recall more collisions on the right, and this bias was significantly related to their asymmetry for line bisection. To investigate whether the self-report data collected by Turnbull and McGeorge could be found under laboratory conditions, Nicholls, Loftus, Meyer, and Mattingley (2007) asked participants to walk through a doorway that was only marginally wider than the participant. By observing the number of collisions and the side on which they occurred, Nicholls et al. (2007) found that there were significantly more collisions on the participant's right side. To investigate whether unilateral hemispheric activation played a role in the asymmetry, hemispheric activity was manipulated by asking participants to use their left, right, or both hands to fire a toy gun at a target as they passed through the doorway. Consistent with Kinsbourne's (1970) model of hemispheric activation, activation of the left hand (right hemisphere) increased rightward collisions whereas activation of the right hand (left hemisphere) caused leftward collisions. Nicholls, Loftus, Orr, and Barre (2008) followed up on the original study by Nicholls et al. (2007). Although no effect of unilateral activation was found, more rightward collisions were observed. Perhaps more importantly, an association was observed between collisions and line bisection, once again relating asymmetries in collisions to pseudoneglect. While a predominance of rightward collisions are frequently reported, it should be noted that this pattern of asymmetry is not always observed for navigation tasks (Fujikake, Higuchi, Imanaka, & Maloney, 2011; Hatin, Tottenham, & Oriet, 2012).

Besides ambulatory tasks, navigation asymmetries also exist for the operation of vehicles. Nicholls, Hadgraft, et al. (2010) asked participants to maneuver an electric wheelchair through a narrow aperture. The number of collisions with the left or right sides of the aperture was recorded. A significant bias toward collisions with the right side was recorded for the electric wheelchair. In a follow-up experiment, the task was changed so that the doorway was significantly wider than the wheelchair. In the case, although no rightward collisions were observed, a significant deviation to the right of true center was observed. Like the effect of line length for pseudoneglect (McCourt & Jewell, 1999), the asymmetry increased for wider apertures. The rightward bias also occurred when the wheelchair was operated via remote control and when an electric scooter was used instead of a wheelchair. The rightward deviation for operating vehicles therefore appears to be a highly robust phenomenon.

ATTENTIONAL ASYMMETRIES AND SPORT

If asymmetries in attention can affect everyday activities, such as navigation, can they also affect sporting performance? A number of studies have examined this question.

Golf

Few activities in sports are more likely to provoke the anxiety of participants than putting in golf (Mullen & Hardy, 2000). In an effort to understand what is necessary to accurately and reliably place the ball in the cup, researchers in sports psychology have studied a range of psychological states shown by golfers. In addition to anxiety, researchers have studied decision-making, imagery, goal setting, and emotional control (Smeeton, Williams, Hodges, & Ward, 2005). However, considering that the task of putting is a spatial one, it would appear that one psychological skill is paramount: accurate spatial attention.

The relationship between spatial attention and putting success was studied by Roberts and Turnbull (2010). The authors asked 30 inexperienced golfers to putt a golf ball into a hole placed 2.26 m away. This is well outside the personal space in which leftward pseudoneglect occurs. Rather it is at a distance where a rightward bias in attention would be anticipated (McCourt & Garlinghouse, 2000). The authors recorded the number of putts that were placed into the hole and, if they missed, the degree of deviation to the left and right of the hole. The authors also asked participants to complete a manual line bisection task using a bisection tool within their personal space.

In line with expectations, the results showed that, on the putting task, more putts passed to the right of the cup than to the left. Likewise, on the line bisection task, participants placed the subjective midpoint significantly to the left of the true midpoint. Interestingly, however, there was also a relationship between performance on the two tasks. Participants who bisected the lines to the left in the manual bisection task displayed a reduced rightward bias in the putting task. Moreover, participants with the greatest leftward bias on the manual task holed the greatest number of putts.

The degree of leftward bias shown in manual bisection tasks is correlated with the degree of activation in the right hemisphere of the brain, particularly the right temporoparietal junction, which is also involved in spatial memory (Benwell, Harvey, & Thut, 2014). Thus the finding that participants who produced the greatest leftward bias on the line bisection task were also the most skillful putters indicates that people with a greater activation of the right hemisphere during the task produced the most accurate putting performance.

Australian Rules Football

Australian rules football is a game played in Australia since 1859 (Lewis, 2006). It is a flowing game, similar to soccer, in which the ball is always in contention. However, there is one feature of Australian rules football which is unique to the sport and that makes it particularly interesting for research into perceptual asymmetries in sport. The goals in Australian rules football are marked by posts spaced 6.4 m apart. Then, at a further distance of 6.4 m from each goalpost, two additional posts are placed (called behind posts). Kicking the ball between the goalposts yields six points, but if the goal is missed to the right or left (but still passes within the gap between goalpost and behind post), one point is awarded. This scoring system gives a unique opportunity to use real world data to study the way perceptual biases relate to performance in sport.

Nicholls, Loetscher and Rademacher (2010) collected data from the Australian Football League, the preeminent Australian rules football competition, for the five football seasons between 2005 and 2009. In that time, 14,827 points were scored by kicks which passed between the behind post and the goalpost on either side of the goal. Like in other codes of football, goals are typically scored in Australian rules football when the goal is outside the kicker's personal space. Hence, the attention of the kickers, and their resulting kicks, should be biased to the right of the goal. And indeed, the data showed a significant bias for points to be scored by kicks which missed the goal on the right-hand side.

This was followed up by Nicholls, Loetscher, et al. (2010) with a series of experimental studies in the laboratory to further delineate the mechanisms contributing to the observed effect. In their first study, participants were asked to kick a ball at a single target post placed at a distance of 4 m. The mean deviation from the target was 23.9 mm. But this bias showed no significant deviation to the left or right. In the second study, two target posts were used to better resemble the characteristics of a goal. To kick toward the middle of the goal, the kicker must bisect the horizontal space between goalposts. The distance from the kicker to the goal was again 4 m, and the distance between the posts was varied between 500, 900, and 1500 mm. Consistent with the archival data from the Australian Football

League, there was a significant bias in the deviations from the true center of the goal toward the right. This bias was also modulated by the width of the goal itself. The rightward bias was present for the 900 and 1500 mm wide goals but not for the 500 mm wide goal. This is consistent with the literature, which shows that the perceptual biases are reduced or even reversed for short horizontal lines (Jewell & McCourt, 2000).

The finding that the two-goalpost condition produced a significant rightward bias while the single-goal condition did not strongly suggests that the rightward deviations in the two-goal condition are the result of misdirecting the midpoint of the goal rather than a mechanical bias induced while kicking the ball. However, to further show that this effect was related to attentional asymmetries, Nicholls, Loetscher, et al. (2010) conducted an experiment which removed the motor component of the task. In this final experiment, participants again stood 4 m from the two goalposts that were spaced at the same intervals used previously. Instead of kicking a ball, the participants were asked to use a 4-m long stick to mark the center of the goal space. The results showed a smaller mean deviation of 6.3 mm. Nevertheless, consistent with the results from the two-goal kicking condition, there was a significant bias in this deviation to the right of the true center. Again, this rightward deviation was greatest for the widest goal to the point that it was absent for the smallest goal width.

Soccer

One well-documented characteristic of soccer since it was codified in 1848 at Parker's Piece in Cambridge, UK, is the propensity of games to end in a draw (Cox, Vamplew, & Russell, 2002). For instance, in the group stage of World Cups between 1998 and 2010, about 30% of matches are drawn (Anderson & Sally, 2013). However, sporting contests need a winner, and soccer administrators have developed additional means of determining an outcome for teams who have scored the same number of goals at the end of the regulation playing time. Of the different measures available, the one employed as a final match-ending step in Fédération Internationale de Football Association (FIFA)-organized tournaments is the penalty shootout.

In a penalty shootout, each team takes turns attempting to kick a goal from the penalty spot, with only the opposing team's goalkeeper allowed to defend the goal. This task represents a dramatic change in tempo from the typically fast, flowing, and team-based environment of a soccer match. And, with the likelihood of a game being resolved this way, the penalty shootout has attracted much attention from sports psychologists looking to find a reliable method for improving a team's performance from the penalty spot. This research has included the documented increase in stress which is brought about by the penalty shootout in players (Jordet & Elferink-Gemser, 2011) and even in fans (Carroll, Ebrahim, Tilling, MacLeod, & Smith, 2002).

The arrangement of the players during a penalty kick is governed by Law 14 of the Laws of the Game (FIFA, 2012). The penalty spot is 11 m from the goal, and a professional striker kicks a penalty ball at around 112 km/h (Masters, van der Kamp, & Jackson, 2007). The laws also state that the goalkeeper must stand behind the goal line until the striker has kicked the ball, which means that the goalkeeper has around 700 ms to dive in the direction of the ball after its kicked (Anderson & Sally, 2013). These laws put the goalkeeper at a distinct disadvantage. Hence, one fruitful line of research has asked if there is anything the goalkeeper can do within the confines of these limitations to influence the side of the goal toward which the striker kicks. If this influence could be exerted, then the goalkeeper could prepare to jump before the ball is kicked rather than reacting to it after it is kicked. In particular, it is possible that by deliberately standing off center on the goal line, the goalkeeper could influence the striker to kick toward that side of the goal with a greater undefended area.

Masters et al. (2007) reviewed 200 penalty kicks from FIFA-organized events to see whether goalkeepers position themselves off center and whether this indeed does influence the location which the striker aims for. They reported that indeed goalkeepers stood off center for 96% of penalty kicks. The average deviation from the center was 99.5 mm. The soccer goal is 7.32 m wide and 2.44 m high, which means that these goalkeepers were creating an average difference of 2.9% in areas to their left and right with significantly more kicks aimed at the side of the goal with a greater undefended area. However, despite having established this influence on kicking direction, the goalkeepers did not make use of it. Masters et al. (2007) found that there was no relationship between the position of the goalkeeper on the goal line and the side to which he jumped. That is, goal keepers were able to exert some influence on the side to which the striker kicked but they did not seem to be aware of the bias they created.

This begged the question: if the goalkeeper was unaware of the bias being created, was the striker also unaware? To answer this, Masters et al. (2007) conducted a series of experiments in the laboratory to determine if the striker was kicking to the more undefended side of the goal because he accurately perceived that the goalkeeper was positioned off center and consciously decided to kick toward the less defended area. In the first experiment, participants were shown a computer-generated rectangle that was scaled to be 3% of an actual soccer goal. Another rectangle, which was scaled to be 3% the size of the German goalkeeper Oliver Kahn, was placed at 14 different deviations from the actual center. These created differences in the area to the left and right of the goalkeeper of between 0.5%

and 20%. Even at the most difficult level of 0.5%, participants could correctly report the side of the goal with the greater exposed area. However, at this same level of difficulty, the participants reported that their confidence in their judgment was not above chance. This suggests that strikers are able to detect which side of the goal is more undefended, but that their decision to kick to this side is not made after conscious consideration.

This experiment was followed up by two more realistic replications by Masters et al. (2007). When a 44% scaled goal and photo-realistic depiction of Oliver Kahn were used with a new sample of participants, the same pattern of results was found. In their final experiment, Masters et al. presented participants with the 44% scaled goal and goalkeeper but asked participants to kick a ball into the goal only when they thought Oliver Kahn was in the actual center. However, the goalkeeper always deviated from the center by 1.6–20%. At deviations of less than 3%, participants kicked the ball more than 90% of the time, suggesting that they did not perceive the goalkeeper as being off center. In addition, participants were more likely to direct their kicks on these stimuli to the less defended side.

It is worth noting that the three experimental studies conducted by Masters et al. (2007) used participants who were not professional soccer players. With this in mind, it is worth investigating whether the bias to kick toward the more undefended area can also be found experimentally in professional soccer players, which would confirm the evidence from the observational study reported by Masters et al. (2007). To this end, Weigelt, Memmert, and Schack (2012) conducted a study using similar stimuli and tested both amateur soccer players as well as professionals. The results showed that the bias by strikers to kick toward the less defended part of the goal was present across both groups but was stronger in the amateur group. This suggests that it is a bias which can be overcome with expertise training.

The ability of people to accurately notice differences as small as those reported in the goal-kicking studies of Masters et al. (2007) and Weigelt et al. (2012) is consistent with the ability of participants to report the longer end of a line in studies using prebisected lines (Jewell & McCourt, 2000). However, because in all these studies the goalkeeper was presented at a deviation from the center, the results are limited in their ability to determine if there was an overall bias in kicking to the right of center as was reported for Australian rules football by Nicholls, Loetscher et al. (2010).

To investigate this aspect of the findings in more detail, Weigelt and Memmert (2012) conducted a follow-up experiment that included trials in which the goalkeeper was placed in the actual center of the goals. The results indicated that when the goalkeeper was placed in the middle of the goal, participants kicked the ball into the right side of the net a significant 58.7% of the time, which is consistent with the finding of a rightward bias for goal kicking in Nicholls, Loetscher, et al. (2010).

Baseball

The research reviewed above on biases in kicking toward soccer and Australian rules football goals showed a bias to attend to the right side of a horizontal target in far space. This is consistent with the extensive literature detailing the same bias in laboratory studies reviewed earlier in this chapter (e.g., Jewell & McCourt, 2000). Also reviewed earlier in this chapter is the extensive laboratory literature demonstrating a bias to attend toward the upper part of a vertically oriented line (e.g., Nicholls et al., 2004). However, the studies of football codes reviewed above did not address this. Part of the reason for this is that in many sports, the technology does not exist to allow for the reliable collection of information on biases in these two dimensions. However, one sport which does systematically collect this information is baseball.

Ted Williams, perhaps the greatest baseball hitter of all time, is often quoted as having said that "I think without question the hardest single thing to do in sport is to hit a baseball" (Vecsey, 2008, p. 5). Indeed, hitters in baseball face the daunting task of making contact with a ball that can be thrown by the best pitchers at over 150 km/h and which can deviate by 508 mm as it crosses the 18 m from the pitcher's hand to the home plate (Mills, 2014). The only prior information about where the ball will be is an imaginary rectangle in the air above the home plate which runs from the midpoint between the top of the batter's shoulders and the top of the uniform pants to the hollow beneath the kneecap and crosses the width of the home plate. If the ball passes through this rectangle without being hit by the batter, the pitch is called as a strike against the batsman. If it passes outside of this rectangle, then it is called a ball against the pitcher.

That pitchers may favor one part of the strike zone over another does not necessarily suggest a perceptual bias. Pitchers may show this bias because they believe pitches placed in one part of the strike zone are harder to hit. Likewise, the bias shown by a hitter in making contact with pitches in certain locations may have a purely mechanical explanation. Instead, what is interesting to perceptual psychologists are the biases shown by the third person involved in each pitch: the umpire.

Since the playoffs at the end of the 2007 Major League Baseball season, the location of every pitch in Major League Baseball has been recorded by the PITCHf/x system. This gives us the opportunity to check the data available from the PITCHf/x cameras, which have captured the location of the ball as it passes through the strike zone to see if the umpires are biased in their decision to call a strike or a ball following each pitch.

These data have allowed researchers to conduct several interesting analyses, including the analysis of the vertical dimension in how umpires call the strike zone. Mills (2014) analyzed the data from the PITCHf/x cameras between 2008 and 2014 and showed that the middle of the called strike zone has been lowered each year. In 2008, the middle of the average called strike zone was 1.6 inches above the actual middle of the strike zone, but in 2014 it is only 0.1 inches above. This means that in 2008, umpires placed the midpoint of the imaginary rectangle well above the actual midpoint. But in 2014, they have got it pretty close to the actual midpoint. What changed in this time was that umpires were able to get feedback from the PITCHf/x cameras and started to call low pitches which passed through the actual strike zone as strikes instead of balls.

Another bias identified by Rosales and Spratt (2015) is that umpires are more likely to make an error in calling a pitch when it is on the inside edge of the strike zone for both left- and right-handed batsmen. This increase in errors for pitches which pass close to the batsman is such that pitches which pass through the actual strike zone on the side of the batsman are more likely to be called balls when they should have been called strikes. This manifests as a distortion of the called strike zone such that the mid-point of the called strike zone is further away from the batsman than the actual midpoint of the strike zone. This bias is in keeping with the finding from studies in a laboratory setting, which show that participants place the midpoint of lines away from other participants in the experiment (Szpak et al., 2015). That is, we all have a bias to withdraw our attention from other people.

Despite these biases, Rosales and Spratt (2015) showed that Major League Baseball umpires are incredibly good at their job. The average accuracy for calling pitches as a ball or a strike in the 2014 season was 92.42%. This level of accuracy is even more remarkable considering that umpires worked an average of 25 games that season and averaged 146 decisions per game.

Archery

The finding by Weigelt et al. (2012), that professional soccer players show a reduction in the biases for goal kicking compared to amateur players raises the more general question of how expertise affects spatial biases in sport. Prolonged training and expertise in spatial tasks, including playing music (Lega, Cattaneo, Merabet, Vecchi, & Cucchi, 2014) and driving taxis (Maguire et al., 2000), have been shown to affect the neural bases of space perception. Thus, it is plausible that prolonged training and the development of expertise in a sport may also affect the way space is processed in the brains of athletes.

This topic was addressed by Coudereau, Gueguen, Pratte, and Sampaio (2006) by investigating space perception in a sample of visually impaired athletes who regularly practiced a sport in which spatial accuracy is integral: archery. These athletes competed under the International Blind Sport Association B1 category, which includes people with no visual perception in the left or right eye and an inability to recognize shapes or silhouettes at any distance or in any direction. Their training in archery involved the use of sound clues to gauge the accuracy of each arrow. Due to the participants' inability to see, Coudereau et al. used a tactile bisection task similar to that developed by Çiçek et al. (2009). This involved the participants running their index fingers along the full extent of wooden dowels and indicating where they believed the center to be. Previous research using tactile line bisection tasks has shown that sighted participants typically bisect the dowel rods to the left of the objective midpoint, corresponding with the misbisection of the lines in standard visual bisection tasks (Brooks, Della Sala, & Darling, 2014).

Coudereau et al. (2006) measured the performance of 20 blind participants, 10 of whom where competitive archers and 10 of whom did not practice any high precision sport. The results showed that the nonarchers were in fact more accurate in identifying the middle of the dowel than the competitive archers. This effect, however, was explained by the difference in the nature of the deviations between the groups. The nonarcher group did not differ significantly from the midpoint. However, the archery group was not only less accurate, they were significantly biased toward the left in their estimation of the center.

Coudereau et al. (2006) note that the spatial biases shown by the visually impaired archers in their study resembled the bias shown by sighted people. That is, both professional visually impaired archers and sighted people are biased in placing the subjective midpoint to the left of the objective center on tactile line bisection tasks. This led the authors to hypothesize that the regular practice of a high precision spatial skill by the visually impaired archers had increased the functional localization of spatial processing in the right hemisphere in the same way as this ability is localized in sighted people (for review see Hugdahl, 2011).

SUMMARY

There are subtle, but consistent asymmetries in the way attentional resources are distributed along the horizontal and vertical dimensions. The asymmetries affect a number of everyday behaviors, including sport. This chapter has reviewed evidence showing that a number of sports miss to the right. It seems unlikely that this bias is the result of a simple mechanical or motor asymmetry and instead seems to be the result of an attentional asymmetry. It would be fascinating to determine whether similar asymmetries exist in other sports which require spatial judgments, such as shooting, rugby, hockey, and gridiron football.

References

Anderson, C., & Sally, D. (2013). *The numbers Game: Why everything you know about football is wrong*. London: Penguin.

Azouvi, P., Marchal, F., Samuel, C., Morin, L., Renard, C., Louis-Dreyfus, A., … Bergego, C. (1996). Functional consequences and awareness of unilateral neglect: study of an evaluation scale. *Neuropsychological Rehabilitation, 6*(2), 133–150.

Barriopedro, M. I., & Botella, J. (1998). New evidence for the zoom lens model using the RSVP technique. *Perception & Psychophysics, 60*(8), 1406–1414.

Benwell, C. S. Y., Harvey, M., & Thut, G. (2014). On the neural origin of pseudoneglect: EEG-correlates of shifts in line bisection performance with manipulation of line length. *Neuroimage, 86*(100), 370–380.

Bisiach, E., & Vallar, G. (1988). Hemineglect in humans. In F. Boller, J. Grafman, G. Rizzolatti, & H. Goodglass (Eds.). *Handbook of neuropsychology: Vol. 1*. (pp. 195–222). New York, NY: Elsevier Science.

Bjoertomt, O., Cowey, A., & Walsh, V. (2002). Spatial neglect in near and far space investigated by repetitive transcranial magnetic stimulation. *Brain, 125*, 2012–2022.

Bowers, D., & Heilman, K. M. (1980). Pseudoneglect: effects of hemispace on a tactile line bisection task. *Neuropsychologia, 18*(4–5), 491–498.

Bradshaw, J. L., Nettleton, N. C., Nathan, G., & Wilson, L. (1986). Tactual-kinesthetic matching of horizontal extents by the long-term blind: absence or reversal of normal left-side underestimation. *Neuropsychologia, 24*(2), 261–264.

Broadbent, D. (1958). *Perception and communication*. London: Pergamon Press.

Brooks, J. L., Della Sala, S., & Darling, S. (2014). Representational pseudoneglect: a review. *Neuropsychology Review, 24*(2), 148–165.

Butlera, B. C., Eskes, G. A., & Vandorpe, R. A. (2003). Gradients of detection in neglect: comparison of peripersonal and extrapersonal space. *Neuropsychologia, 42*, 346–358.

Butter, C. M., Evans, J., Kirsch, N., & Kewman, D. (1989). Altitudinal neglect following traumatic brain injury: a case report. *Cortex, 25*(1), 135–146.

Carroll, D., Ebrahim, S., Tilling, K., MacLeod, J., & Smith, G. D. (2002). Admissions for myocardial infarction and World Cup football: database survey. *British Medical Journal, 325*(7378), 1439–1442.

Chokron, S., & Imbert, M. (1993). Influence of reading habits on line bisection. *Cognitive Brain Research, 1*, 219–222.

Churches, O., Loetscher, T., Thomas, N. A., & Nicholls, M. E. R. (in press, accepted November 2015). Perceptual biases in the horizontal and vertical dimensions are driven by separate cognitive mechanisms. *Quarterly Journal of Experimental Psychology*.

Çiçek, M., Deouell, L. Y., & Knight, R. T. (2009). Brain activity during landmark and line bisection tasks. *Frontiers in Human Neuroscience, 3*, 7.

Committeri, G., Pitzalis, S., Galati, G., Patria, F., Pelle, G., Sabatini, U., … Pizzamiglio, L. (2007). Neural bases of personal and extrapersonal neglect in humans. *Brain, 130*, 431–441.

Coudereau, J. P., Gueguen, N., Pratte, M., & Sampaio, E. (2006). Tactile precision in right-handed archery experts with visual disabilities: a pseudoneglect effect? *Laterality: Asymmetries of Body, Brain and Cognition, 11*(2), 170–180.

Cox, R., Vamplew, W., & Russell, D. (Eds.). (2002). *Encyclopedia of British Football*. London: Routledge.

Drain, M., & Reuter-Lorenz, P. A. (1996). Vertical orienting control: evidence for attentional bias and "neglect" in the intact brain. *Journal of Experimental Psychology: General, 125*(2), 139–158.

Duecker, F., & Sack, A. T. (2015). The hybrid model of attentional control: new insights into hemispheric asymmetries inferred from TMS research. *Neuropsychologia, 74*, 21–29.

FIFA. (2012). *The laws of the game*. From http://www.fifa.com/mm/document/affederation/generic/81/42/36/lawsofthegame_2012_e.pdf.

Fujikake, H., Higuchi, T., Imanaka, K., & Maloney, L. (2011). Directional bias in the body while walking through a doorway: its association with attentional and motor factors. *Experimental Brain Research*, *210*(2), 195–206.

Halligan, P. W., & Marshall, J. C. (1991). Left neglect for near, but not far space in man. *Nature*, *350*, 498–500.

Hatin, B., Tottenham, L. S., & Oriet, C. (2012). The relationship between collisions and pseudoneglect: is it right? *Cortex*, *48*(8), 997–1008.

Heilman, K. M., Jeong, Y., & Finney, G. R. (2004). Spatial cognition. *Neurology*, *63*(11), 1994–1996.

Heilman, K. M., & Valenstein, E. (1979). Mechanisms underlying hemispatial neglect. *Annals of Neurology*, *5*(2), 166–170.

Hugdahl, K. (2011). Hemispheric asymmetry: contributions from brain imaging. *Wiley Interdisciplinary Reviews: Cognitive Science*, *2*(5), 461–478.

Hughes, H. C., & Zimba, L. D. (1987). Natural boundaries for the spatial spread of directed visual attention. *Neuropsychologia*, *25*(1A), 5–18.

Hüttermann, S., Memmert, D., & Simons, D. J. (2014). The size and shape of the attentional "spotlight" varies with differences in sports expertise. *Journal of Experimental Psychology: Applied*, *20*(2), 147–157.

Iriki, A., Tanaka, M., & Iwamura, Y. (1996). Coding of modified body schema during tool use by macaque postcentral neurons. *Neuroreport*, *7*, 2325–2330.

Jewell, G., & McCourt, M. E. (2000). Pseudoneglect: a review and meta-analysis of performance factors in line bisection tasks. *Neuropsychologia*, *38*(1), 93–110.

Jordet, G., & Elferink-Gemser, M. T. (2011). Stress, coping, and emotions on the world stage: the experience of participating in a major soccer tournament penalty shootout. *Journal of Applied Sport Psychology*, *24*(1), 73–91.

Kinsbourne, M. (1970). The cerebral basis of lateral asymmetries in attention. *Acta Psychologica*, *33*, 193–201.

LaBerge, D., & Brown, V. (1989). Theory of attentional operations in shape identification. *Psychological Review*, *96*(1), 101–124.

Làdavas, E., Carletti, M., & Gori, G. (1994). Automatic and voluntary orienting of attention in patients with visual neglect: horizontal and vertical dimensions. *Neuropsychologia*, *32*(10), 1195–1208.

Lega, C., Cattaneo, Z., Merabet, L. B., Vecchi, T., & Cucchi, S. (2014). The effect of musical expertise on the representation of space. *Frontiers in Human Neuroscience*, *8*, 250.

Lewis, W. (2006). *Events that shaped Australia*. Frenchs Forest, NSW: New Holland Publishers.

Loftus, A. M., & Nicholls, M. E. R. (2012). Testing the activation-orientation account of spatial attentional asymmetries using transcranial direct current stimulation. *Neuropsychologia*, *50*, 2573–2576.

Longo, M. R., & Lourenco, S. F. (2006). On the nature of near space: effects of tool use and the transition to far space. *Neuropsychologia*, *44*, 977–981.

Maguire, E. A., Gadian, D. G., Johnsrude, I. S., Good, C. D., Ashburner, J., Frackowiak, R. S. J., & Frith, C. D. (2000). Navigation-related structural change in the hippocampi of taxi drivers. *Proceedings of the National Academy of Sciences*, *97*(8), 4398–4403.

Masters, R. S. W., van der Kamp, J., & Jackson, R. C. (2007). Imperceptibly off-center goal-keepers influence penalty-kick direction in soccer. *Psychological Science*, *18*(3), 222–223.

Mattingley, J. B., Berberovic, N., Corben, L., Slavin, M. J., Nicholls, M. E. R., & Bradshaw, J. L. (2004). The greyscales task: a perceptual measure of attentional bias following right hemisphere damage. *Neuropsychologia*, *42*, 387–394.

McCourt, M. E. (2001). Performance consistency of normal observers in forced-choice tachistoscopic visual line bisection. *Neuropsychologia*, *39*(10), 1065–1076.

McCourt, M. E., & Garlinghouse, M. (2000). Asymmetries of visuospatial attention are modulated by viewing distance and visual field elevation: pseudoneglect in peripersonal and extrapersonal space. *Cortex*, *36*(5), 715–731.

McCourt, M. E., & Jewell, G. (1999). Visuospatial attention in line bisection: stimulus modulation of pseudoneglect. *Neuropsychologia, 37*(7), 843–855.

McCourt, M. E., & Olafson, C. (1997). Cognitive and perceptual influences on visual line bisection: psychophysical and chronometric analyses of pseudoneglect. *Neuropsychologia, 37*(3), 369–380.

Mills, B. M. (2014). Expert workers, performance standards, and on-the-job training: evaluating major league baseball umpires. *Social Science Research Network.* http://ssrn.com/abstract=2478447.

Molenberghs, P., Sale, M. V., & Mattingley, J. B. (2012). Is there a critical lesion site for unilateral spatial neglect? A meta-analysis using activation likelihood estimation. *Frontiers in Human Neuroscience, 6,* 78.

Mullen, R., & Hardy, L. (2000). State anxiety and motor performance: testing the conscious processing hypothesis. *Journal of Sports Sciences, 18*(10), 785–799.

Nicholls, M. E. R., Hadgraft, N. T., Chapman, H. L., Loftus, A. M., Robertson, J., & Bradshaw, J. L. (2010). A hit and miss investigation of asymmetries in wheelchair navigation. *Attention, Perception & Psychophysics, 72,* 1576–1590.

Nicholls, M. E. R., Loetscher, T., & Rademacher, M. (2010). Miss to the right: the effect of attentional asymmetries on goal-kicking. *PLoS One, 5*(8).

Nicholls, M. E. R., Loftus, A., Meyer, K., & Mattingley, J. B. (2007). Things that go bump in the right: the effect of unimanual activity on rightward collisions. *Neuropsychologia, 45,* 1122–1126.

Nicholls, M. E. R., Loftus, A. M., Orr, C. A., & Barre, N. (2008). Rightward collisions and their association with pseudoneglect. *Brain and Cognition, 68,* 166–170.

Nicholls, M. E. R., Mattingley, J. B., Berberovic, N., Smith, A., & Bradshaw, J. L. (2004). An investigation of the relationship between free-viewing perceptual asymmetries for vertical and horizontal stimuli. *Cognitive Brain Research, 19*(3), 289–301.

Nicholls, M. E. R., & Roberts, G. R. (2002). Can free-viewing perceptual asymmetries be explained by scanning, pre-motor or attentional biases? *Cortex, 38*(2), 113–136.

Nicholls, M. E. R., Roden, S., Thomas, N. A., Loetscher, T., Spence, C. J., & Forte, J. D. (2014). Close to me: asymmetrical environments do not affect spatial attention. *Ergonomics, 57,* 876–885.

Posner, M. I., Snyder, C. R. R., & Davidson, B. J. (1980). Attention and the detection of signals. *Journal of Experimental Psychology: General, 109*(2), 160–174.

Previc, F. H. (1990). Functional specialization in the lower and upper visual fields in humans: its ecological origins and neuropsychological implications. *Behavioural and Brain Sciences, 13,* 519–575.

Punt, T. D., Kitadono, K., Hulleman, J., Humphreys, G. W., & Riddoch, M. J. (2008). From both sides now: crossover effects influence navigation in patients with unilateral neglect. *Journal of Neurology, Neurosurgery, and Psychiatry, 79*(4), 464–466.

Punt, T. D., Kitadono, K., Hulleman, J., Humphreys, G. W., & Riddoch, M. J. (2011). Modulating wheelchair navigation in patients with spatial neglect. *Neuropsychological Rehabilitation, 21*(3), 367–382.

Rinaldi, L., Di Luca, S., & Girelli, L. (2014). Reading direction shifts visuospatial attention: an interactive account of attentional biases. *Acta Psychologia, 151,* 98–105.

Roberts, R., & Turnbull, O. H. (2010). Putts that get missed on the right: investigating lateralized attentional biases and the nature of putting errors in golf. *Journal of Sports Sciences, 28*(4), 369–374.

Rosales, J., & Spratt, S. (2015). Who is responsible for a called strike? Paper presented at the MIT Sloan sport Analytics Conference, Boston, USA.

Simons, D. J., & Chabris, C. F. (1999). Gorillas in our midst: sustained inattentional blindness for dynamic events. *Perception, 28,* 1059–1074.

Smeeton, N. J., Williams, A. M., Hodges, N. J., & Ward, P. (2005). The relative effectiveness of various instructional approaches in developing anticipation skill. *Journal of Experimental Psychology: Applied, 11,* 98–110.

Smith, A. K., Szelest, I., Friedrich, T. E., & Elias, L. J. (2014). Native reading direction influences lateral biases in the perception of shape from shading. *Laterality: Asymmetries of Body, Brain and Cognition, 20*(4), 418–433.

Szpak, A., Loetscher, T., Churches, O., Thomas, N. A., Spence, C. J., & Nicholls, M. E. (2015). Keeping your distance: attentional withdrawal in individuals who show physiological signs of social discomfort. *Neuropsychologia, 70,* 462–467.

Thomas, N. A., Castine, B. R., Loetscher, T., & Nicholls, M. E. R. (2015). Upper visual field distractors preferentially bias attention to the left. *Cortex, 64,* 179–193.

Toth, C., & Kirk, A. (2002). Representational bias does not affect bisection of lines with a pictorially or semantically defined top by patients with left hemispatial neglect. *Brain and Cognition, 50*(2), 167–177.

Treisman, A. (1964). Selective attention in man. *British Medical Bulletin, 20,* 12–16.

Turnbull, O. H., & McGeorge, P. (1998). Lateral bumping: a normal-subject analog to the behaviour of patients with hemispatial neglect? *Brain and Cognition, 37,* 31–33.

Vecsey, G. (2008). *Baseball: A history of America's favorite game.* New York: Modern Library.

van Vugt, P., Fransen, I., Creten, W., & Paquier, P. (2000). Line bisection performances of 650 normal children. *Neuropsychologia, 38*(6), 886–895.

Vuilleumier, P., Valenza, N., Mayer, E., Reverdin, A., & Landis, T. (1998). Near and far visual space in unilateral neglect. *Annals of Neurology, 43,* 406–410.

Weigelt, M., & Memmert, D. (2012). Goal-side selection in soccer penalty kicking when viewing natural scenes. *Frontiers in Psychology, 3,* 312.

Weigelt, M., Memmert, D., & Schack, T. (2012). Kick it like Ballack: the effects of goalkeeping gestures on goal-side selection in experienced soccer players and soccer novices. *Journal of Cognitive Psychology, 24*(8), 942–956.

PERFORMANCE IN SPORTS

11

Laterality in Individualized Sports

Thomas Heinen, Christina Bermeitinger
University of Hildesheim, Hildesheim, Germany

Christoph von Laßberg
University of Tübingen, Tübingen, Germany

INTRODUCTION

Lateralized behavior occurs in sports that are not obvious, such as in gymnastics or figure skating. However, empirical evidence on the relationship between laterality factors and athletic experience in individualized sports seems to be inconclusive (Loffing, Sölter, & Hagemann, 2014). Most studies find only very small or no relationships between athletic experience and laterality factors, such as handedness (e.g., Demura et al., 2006). In addition, there seems to be a slightly higher amount of left-handers in individualized sports reflecting fighting elements, whereas the distribution of right-handers and left-handers in other individualized sports seems to reflect the distribution of right-handers and left-handers in the general population (Abrams & Panaggio, 2012; Faurie & Raymond, 2013). The difference between right-handers and left-handers in sports reflecting fighting elements is usually explained by a functional advantage of left-handers over right-handers during fighting situations and/or selection in professional sports (Abrams & Panaggio, 2012; Raymond, Pontier, Dufour, & Møller, 1996; see Chapter 12: Performance Differences Between Left- and Right-Sided Athletes in One-on-One Interactive Sports of this book). In individualized sports such as gymnastics or athletics, there is no advantage of left-handers over right-handers per se, because in principle all skills can be performed diametrically with both sides of the body.

Human laterality, however, is not limited to aspects such as handedness or eyedness, but it also involves athlete's preference to perform rotations about the vertical axis of the body in one or the other direction (Sands, 2000; Stochl & Croudace, 2013). Rotational preference has received less attention than other aspects of laterality in general and in individualized sports in particular. However, in individualized sports, such as gymnastics or figure skating, most skills incorporate rotations about one or more body axes, and thus rotational preference seems to be an important aspect of laterality in individualized sports (Arkaev & Suchilin, 2004; King, 2005; Miller, 2008). Therefore the question arises: what constitutes athlete's rotational preference in individualized sports? To address this question, we will at first define the concept of rotation in sports, with a particular focus on rotations about the vertical axis. Afterward, theoretical and empirical aspects concerning rotational preference will be reviewed before we discuss laterality factors, as well as perceptual-cognitive aspects that may contribute to rotational preference. Finally, implications for practice in individualized sports will be given, and conclusions on rotational preference in individualized sports will be drawn.

ROTATIONAL MOVEMENTS

Rotation in individualized sports can be defined as a circular motion of the human about a rotational axis when engaged in sport-specific activity (cf., Yeadon, 2000). For instance, when performing a somersault, the gymnast rotates about his/her frontal horizontal axis (somersault axis), and when performing a pirouette, the gymnast rotates about his/ her vertical axis (twist axis). A cartwheel is performed about the sagittal horizontal axis (cartwheel axis, see Behnke, 2001; Fig. 11.1). Rotations about any axis orthogonal to the sagittal plane are clearly defined in the competition rules with regard to direction *and* amount of rotation (i.e., forward and backward rotation; single, double, triple somersault; FIG, 2013). These definitions account for the structural asymmetry of the human body in relation to the frontal plane, and they constitute an important starting point for methodical progressions in individualized sports (Arkaev & Suchilin, 2004).

Rotations about the athletes' vertical axis are only defined with regard to the amount of rotations but not with regard to the direction of rotation. For example, a *single twist* comprises a rotation about the vertical axis of 360 degrees, and a *triple twist* comprises a rotation about the vertical axis of 1.080 degrees. There are, in general, no rules constraining one or the other rotation direction in gymnastics and other individualized sports, and thus a twisting somersault in gymnastics or platform diving can for instance be

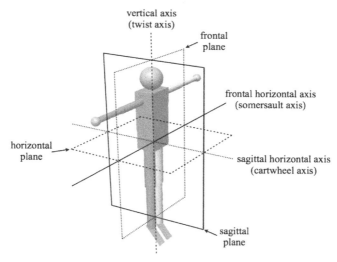

vertical axis
(twist axis)

frontal
plane

frontal horizontal axis
(somersault axis)

horizontal
plane

sagittal horizontal axis
(cartwheel axis)

sagittal
plane

FIGURE 11.1   Illustration of the cardinal planes and axes of movement. *Note:* The sagittal horizontal axis is orthogonal to the frontal plane (*dotted line*). The frontal horizontal axis is orthogonal to the sagittal plane (*solid line*) and the vertical axis is orthogonal to the horizontal plane (*dashed line*).

performed with a *clockwise* (CW) or *counterclockwise* (CCW) rotation about the vertical axis. The same is true for a toe loop in figure skating or a tour jeté in ballet dance.

Rotation direction about the vertical axis in individualized sports is usually defined as follows: A "clockwise rotation direction" corresponds to a rotation of the athletes' body about the vertical axis in a clockwise direction when observing the athlete from above in upright stance (see Fig. 11.2). A clockwise rotation about the vertical axis in upright stance corresponds to an initial *forward motion of the left shoulder* and *backward motion of the right shoulder* in relation of the alignment of the athlete's body. Therefore, identifying the shoulder that moves *backward* in a particular rotation about the vertical axis is a feasible task for the observer, thereby indicating the rotation direction of the gymnast. For example, if the *right* shoulder moves backward during a handstand with a full turn, this indicates a clockwise rotation about the vertical axis (Fig. 11.2). If the *left* shoulder moves backward during a pirouette in upright stance, this indicates a counterclockwise rotation.

On an individual level, untrained people or children usually exhibit a bias for rotating either clockwise or counterclockwise about their vertical axis when performing spontaneous rotations (Day & Day, 1997; Stochl & Croudace, 2013). The same is often true for athletes when performing sport-specific skills (Golomer, Rosey, Dizac, Mertz, & Fagard, 2009; Loffing et al., 2014; Sands, 2000; Starosta, 1986). Gymnasts for

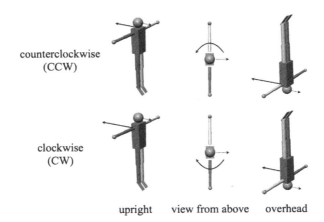

counterclockwise (CCW)

clockwise (CW)

upright   view from above   overhead

FIGURE 11.2   Illustration of counterclockwise (CCW) and clockwise (CW) rotation direction about the vertical axis in an upright position and when in an overhead position. A counterclockwise rotation corresponds to an initial backward motion of the left shoulder, while a clockwise rotation corresponds to an initial backward motion of the right shoulder. *Note:* The *dotted arrow* indicates viewing direction.

instance usually decide at a very young age whether to rotate clockwise or counterclockwise about their vertical axis in a particular skill, and they usually maintain this preference during their career (Arkaev & Suchilin, 2004; Brown, Tolsma, & Kamen, 1983; Sands, 2000). On a group or population level, such an individual tendency could be masked by a general counterclockwise bias for rotations about the vertical axis (Mohr, Brugger, Bracha, Landis, & Viaud-Delmon, 2004; Toussaint, Do, & Fagard, 2008). However, lateral preferences or rotational preferences in sport tasks also seem to vary depending on the demands of the task to be performed (Loffing et al., 2014).

Taken together, rotational movements are an inherent component of individualized sports, and athletes usually exhibit a particular bias for one or the other rotation direction when performing rotational movements about the vertical axis (Sands, 2000). This bias is one strong example of a directional tendency in humans, which is usually referred to as rotational preference, turning preference, or turning bias (Toussaint et al., 2008). In the following, we will refer to the concept of *rotational preference*, which can be defined as the tendency of athletes to favor one direction of rotation over the other in a sport-specific skill (Heinen, Vinken, & Velentzas, 2010; Stochl & Croudace, 2013). One could speculate that there exists a variety of factors constituting rotational preference in individualized sports (Stochl & Croudace, 2013). In the next step, we will at first review theoretical and empirical aspects concerning rotational preference in general and with regard to individualized sports in particular.

ROTATIONAL PREFERENCE

Generally speaking, hominids, such as humans or chimpanzees, show a tendency to preferably rotate in one direction about their vertical axis during motor activities (Nishida & Inaba, 2009; Schaeffer, 1928; Toussaint et al., 2008). Explanations for the tendency to favor one direction when rotating about the vertical axis comprise at least hypotheses about *hemispherical asymmetries in the dopamine system* or influences from other hormone systems (Bracha, Seitz, Otemaa, & Glick, 1987; Glick & Ross, 1981; Gordon, Busdiecker, & Bracha, 1992; Mead & Hampson, 1997; Mohr et al., 2004; Mohr, Landis, Bracha, Fathi, & Brugger, 2003), hypotheses about *asymmetries in the vestibular system* (Howard & Templeton, 1966; Previc & Saucedo, 1992), as well as hypotheses about *biomechanical and sensorimotor asymmetries* between the right and left side of the body (Boyadjian, Marin, & Danion, 1999; Lund, 1930; Reiss & Reiss, 1997; Souman, Frissen, Sreenivasa, & Ernst, 2009).

The *dopamine hypothesis* suggests that dopamine modulates visuospatial functioning and thus rotational preference (Bradshaw & Bradshaw, 1987; Le Moal & Simon, 1991; Mohr, Landis, Bracha, & Brugger, 2003). Higher dopamine levels were for instance found in rats' striatum contralateral to the preferred rotation direction in a T-maze (Glick & Ross, 1981). In addition, patients with hemi-Parkinsonism more often exhibit spontaneous rotations toward the hemisphere with lower dopamine levels (Bracha, Shults, et al., 1987).

Tops, Wijers, Koch, and Korf (2006) questioned the modulating role of cortisol in frontal dopaminergic activity and thus in rotational preference. The authors asked right-handed participants to either ingest a capsule of 35 mg hydrocortisone or a placebo. After 2 h, the participants were blindfolded and asked to perform two full turns about their vertical axis in clockwise and counterclockwise directions. Under higher cortisol levels, participants exhibited an increased clockwise turning bias. The authors argued that this bias might stem from a decrease in right hemisphere activity, thus supporting the dopamine hypothesis. However, the authors did neither assess participants' rotational behavior when vision was available nor across tasks with different (rotational) demands. Mohr et al. (2004) had participants perform three movement tasks while assessing turning behavior: (1) spontaneous turning behavior during 20 h within three consecutive days, (2) walking blindfolded and with ears plugged along a 20 m corridor, and (3) stepping blindfolded and with ears plugged on a spot for 60 s. Results revealed a small, yet significant preference for counterclockwise turning in long-term spontaneous behavior. However, rotational preference was not related across tasks. The authors did neither measure nor manipulate dopamine levels, so one cannot be sure if and how dopamine levels modulated turning behavior. The authors argue that differences in hemispheric dopamine levels may not explain human turning behavior alone, but rather aspects such as visuospatial control or task demands are likely to modulate human turning behavior.

The *vestibular asymmetry hypothesis* states that asymmetry in the labyrinth system could originate from the position of the fetus during the fetal phase of prenatal development and thus lead to a particular rotational preference (Previc & Saucedo, 1992). The information stimulating the vestibular system of the fetus due to accelerations and decelerations of the mother's body is likely to differ between the right and the left side, since the fetus usually does not lie in a symmetric position in the mother's womb. This difference could lead to a prevalence of one vestibular organ over the other, where unilateral dominance of the left-otolithic system could for instance promote a right-sided motoric dominance (Previc, 1991).

Fitzpatrick, Marsden, Lord, and Day (2002) had blindfolded participants laying down supine on a rotating platform. The platform rotated either to the left or the right or was held still. Galvanic vestibular stimulation was induced either to the left mastoid, the right mastoid, or not. To this end, small electrodes were attached over each mastoid process, and a small electrical stimulus ranging from 1.0 to 2.0 mA was delivered (depending on participants' perceived body rotation sensation). The participants reported feelings of a stronger rotation when the galvanic vestibular stimulation was congruent with the rotation of the platform, thereby highlighting the role of the sensitivity of the vestibular system in the perception of rotation. Participants were rotated about a vertical axis when lying in a supine position but not about the vertical axis when lying in an upright position. Thus the experiment demonstrated the role of asymmetrical vestibular information in rotational movements, but it is still questionable if the results can be generalized to rotational preference about the vertical axis. Fitzpatrick, Wardman, and Taylor (1999) used galvanic vestibular stimulation to experimentally induce asymmetrical information of the vestibular system. The authors asked healthy adults to move in a straight line to a target 4 m ahead in different experimental conditions (e.g., blindfolded with and without galvanic vestibular stimulation). Results revealed that participants exhibited no significant difficulties to walk to the target without visual cues. However, galvanic vestibular stimulation caused participants to veer in the direction of the anodal electrode when walking blindfolded. Participants were not affected by galvanic vestibular stimulation when they had their eyes open, thereby highlighting the compensating effect of visual information. The question, however, would be if the effects of the vestibular stimulation were potentially mediated by a participant's rotational preference.

The *biomechanical or sensorimotor asymmetry hypothesis* states that rotational preference in motor tasks is a function of different properties of the left and right limbs, such as differences in leg length and strength. It is furthermore thought that rotational preference covaries with laterality factors such as handedness or footedness (Boyadjian et al., 1999; Reiss & Reiss, 1997; Taylor, Strike, & Dabnichki, 2006). Given that if one leg is longer or stronger than the other one, this should lead to a small but systematic bias. This bias is compensated when visual information is available, but it should in particular make an impact on blindfolded stepping or walking.

Boyadjian et al. (1999) asked students of sports sciences to move 15 m as straight as possible in three experimental tasks, while being blindfolded: (1) walking, (2) riding a wheelchair, and (3) being pushed in a wheelchair while verbally instructing the pushing person. Results revealed that participants veered in all tasks, while about half of the subjects rotated in a different direction during wheelchair riding as compared to walking. The authors argue that veering in blindfolded walking results from the imbalance between two legs. However, participants were selected on the basis of their stability in exhibiting the same turning bias from trial to trial in blindfolded walking but not on the basis of any other measure of limb asymmetry (i.e., differences related to strength, length, flexibility, or functional status). Souman et al. (2009) asked participants to walk as straight as possible in different environments (i.e., Sahara desert, airstrip) under normal conditions and when blindfolded. The authors found that people tend to walk in circles when blindfolded if there is no other information for spatial orientation. The authors, however, did not find a relationship between turning bias and factors such as leg strength. Even a manipulation of leg length did not have a systematic effect on turning bias. The authors argue that veering from a straight path may result from accumulated noise in the sensorimotor system rather than from biomechanical differences between both legs.

Taken together the explanation of rotational preference in humans seems to be multifactorial and may stem from different hypotheses (Lenoir, van Overschelde, de Rycke, & Musch, 2006). Nevertheless, results from existing studies are for instance not straightforward in terms of verifying the biomechanical hypothesis, and one could speculate if hemispheric differences in dopamine concentration sufficiently explain rotational preference in athletes (Mohr et al., 2004; Souman et al., 2009). Additionally, lateralized vestibular information is not limited to its influence on the vestibular sense per se, but rather seems to be part of a multisensory system leading to the experience of the body as a coherent moving system (Latash, 2008; Previc, 1991). Some authors therefore simply argue: "[…] turning preference in humans is the result of a complex interaction between intrinsic preferences and externally imposed task constraints" (Lenoir et al., 2006, p. 179). Intrinsic preferences could play a stronger role in motor acquisition processes, which are an inherent component of individualized sports (Serrien, Ivry, & Swinnen, 2006). We will therefore refer to the relationships between lateral (intrinsic) factors and rotational preference in the next section.

LATERALITY FACTORS CONTRIBUTING TO ROTATIONAL PREFERENCE

It is generally accepted that lateralization of motor functions originates from prenatal and postnatal developments (e.g., Golomer et al., 2009; Previc, 1991). It is thus likely that a person exhibits at least some structural asymmetries together with particular side preferences for learning and performing skills the first time he/she engages in a particular sport. Imagine for instance a novice gymnast who takes part in his/her first class. The gymnast is exposed to a learning environment that may further bias or compensate for these asymmetries and preferences (see also Chapter 10: Near Misses and the Effect of Attentional Asymmetries on Sporting Performance of this book). One could easily think of a coach that also exhibits a particular side preference in demonstrations or when applying manual guidance and what this could mean for a developing gymnast with his/her individual asymmetries or preferences.

Given the aspects mentioned so far, one would expect particular differences in side preferences between individuals that may be related to factors such as lateral preferences, type of sport, demands, and complexity of the tasks to be performed or expertise level (Kimmerle, 2010; Loffing et al., 2014). It is furthermore argued that rotational preference should not be considered as an independent dimension of lateral preferences but rather in relationship to other aspects of laterality, such as handedness or footedness (Lenoir et al., 2006). Accordingly, measures of handedness, eyedness, and footedness should correlate positively with measures that reflect rotational preference.

Bradshaw and Bradshaw (1987) questioned the relationship between handedness and rotational preference. The authors assessed participants' rotational preference in a turning task and a linear walking task. Participants were blindfolded and wore earmuffs during both tasks. Results revealed that right-handed participants more often showed a clockwise turning bias and left-handers showed a counterclockwise bias in the turning task. The authors argue that the results are compatible with the dopamine asymmetries hypothesis.

Previc and Saucedo (1992) analyzed the relationship between turning behavior in a rotational task and handedness, eyedness, and footedness. The authors assessed participants' handedness, footedness, and eyedness by means of a questionnaire. In addition, participants were asked to perform a slight variation of the Fukuda stepping test while being blindfolded and wearing earmuffs (Fukuda, 1959; Toussaint et al., 2008). Results revealed significant correlations between eyedness and stepping test scores as well as between footedness and stepping test scores. No significant correlation was found between handedness and stepping test scores. The authors conclude that the relationship between motoric dominance and rotational preference may at least partially originate from vestibular asymmetries in normal, healthy humans (Previc, 1991).

Scharine and McBeath (2002) questioned the relationship between cultural influences (i.e., different traffic rules in America and England), measures of laterality, and rotational preference. The authors had participants from England and from the United States walk through a T-maze while assessing rotational preference at the T-junction. Results revealed that handedness predicted turning preference, i.e., right-handed people tended to turn to the right. English participants were less likely to turn to the right than were US participants. However, turning direction was unrelated to other laterality factors, such as eye dominance. The authors conclude that rotational preference may stem from genetic as well as cultural influences.

Stochl and Croudace (2013) aimed to identify predictors of preferred rotation direction in humans. The authors surveyed for instance handedness, footedness, rotational preference in global and local movements, as well as the perception of a rotating figure (spinning dancer illusion, see next Section) in men and women from different countries. Results revealed that handedness and footedness could predict preferred rotation direction in global (i.e., jumping and spinning) and local (i.e., drawing a circle) movements. In addition, sex was a predictor of the direction of global rotational movements. Most surprisingly, the perception of a rotating figure (spinning dancer illusion) was related to rotational preference. The authors thus argue that rotational preference and perceiving the spinning figure may be controlled by a shared underlying mechanism, thereby highlighting the potential influence of perceptual-cognitive aspects to rotational preference.

Lenoir et al. (2006) questioned the influence of task constraints on rotational preference. The authors assessed hand preference, foot preference, and turning behavior in humans during running and walking with different task demands (i.e., perform a turn on a whistle signal). Results revealed that neither hand preference nor foot preference had an effect on rotational preference (turning bias). Most surprisingly, the authors could show that a participant's natural rotational preference can be overruled by task constraints, such as an asymmetrical placement of the feet when asked to turn and run from a stationary position.

There seems to be concluding evidence that laterality measures are at least partially related to rotational preference. Whether such relationships are found may depend strongly on the task chosen to assess rotational preference. The direction in which people turn may not only be related to lateral preferences per se, but also to constraints imposed by the task demands. Additionally, it can be assumed that relationships between rotational preference and other lateral preferences in individualized sport could even more strongly depend on influences from learning and practicing in that particular sport. For example, when learning hammer throwing, coaches often instruct right-handed athletes to turn counterclockwise and left-handed athletes to turn in a clockwise direction (Bartonietz, 2008). It seems furthermore plausible that novice athletes in sports such as dance or gymnastics base their choice of the supporting leg during rotational movements upon their foot preference (Golomer & Mbongo, 2004; Heinen et al., 2010). However, in individualized sports such as gymnastics or free-style dance, there are in general no rules constraining one or the other rotation direction. A twisting somersault in gymnastics can for instance be performed with a clockwise or counterclockwise rotation about the vertical axis (FIG, 2013). The same is true for a toe loop in figure skating or a tour jeté in ballet dance. Influences that stem from learning processes could thus easily overrule relationships between rotational preference and laterality factors.

Brown et al. (1983) assessed for instance eye and hand dominance of nonathletes and college-level gymnasts. In addition, rotational preference was analyzed in four rather simple gymnastics skills. The authors found a small negative, yet significant relationship between hand dominance and rotation direction in the so-called swivel-hips maneuver on the trampoline for the gymnasts. In addition, another small positive relationship was found between eye dominance and rotation direction in a seat-drop with full twist on a trampoline for nonathletes. The authors argue that although significant relationships were found, the relationships do not seem to be of practical value.

Heinen et al. (2010) as well as Heinen, Jeraj, Vinken, and Velentzas (2012) explored relationships between rotational preference in several gymnastics skills and measures of laterality. Heinen et al. (2010) found a significant relationship between eyedness and rotational preference in upright stance, as well as a significant relationship between footedness and rotational preference in the roundoff. For instance, gymnasts who exhibited a clockwise rotational preference in upright stance were more right consistent in eyedness and footedness as compared to gymnasts who exhibited a counterclockwise turning rotational preference in upright stance. There were no significant relationships between handedness and rotational preference in any of the assessed gymnastics skills. Additionally, Heinen et al. (2012) found a significant relationship between lateral preference and rotational preference for nonexperts, but not for near-expert and expert gymnasts. The authors argue that aspects of laterality could be one constituting factor in the decision of the rotation direction in a particular skill. However, this may not be true for gymnasts on all expertise levels because other aspects may be more important in deciding to rotate in one direction or the other.

Golomer et al. (2009) addressed the question if classical dance training influences the side of the supporting leg and turning bias. The authors analyzed prepubertal untrained girls and trained female dance students' handedness, eyedness, footedness, and whole body spontaneous turns with either eyes open or closed. Turn direction did not differ with eyes open or closed. Untrained girls exhibited a slight leftward turning bias, whereas dance students showed a clear rightward turning bias. Footedness, eyedness, or handedness were not related to turn direction in untrained girls or dance students. The authors conclude that training may overrule natural rotational preference. The authors furthermore speculate that dance experts use some kind of spatial turn representation, thereby highlighting the potential influence of perceptual-cognitive information on rotational preference.

Taken together, rotational preference should not be considered as an independent dimension of lateral preferences (Lenoir et al., 2006). Accordingly, it can be thought that rotational preference and other aspects of lateral preference may at least partially relate to each other (Stochl & Croudace, 2013). However, complementary to genetic and cultural factors, influences that may stem from a particular training environment may bias or compensate for lateral preferences as well as rotational preferences (Brown et al., 1983). It could be speculated that perceptual-cognitive aspects more strongly account for athletes' rotational preference in individualized sports (Golomer et al., 2009; Stochl & Croudace, 2013). In the next section, we will therefore discuss perceptual-cognitive aspects that may be related to rotational preference in individualized sports.

RELATIONSHIP BETWEEN PERCEPTUAL-COGNITIVE SKILLS AND ROTATIONAL PREFERENCE

Athletes in individualized sports such as gymnastics or figure skating exhibit a particular rotational preference about their vertical axis (Heinen et al., 2012). This preference (clockwise or counterclockwise) seems to differ between skills (Sands, 2000). For instance, during her floor routine in the apparatus finals at the 2008 Olympic Games in Beijing, Shawn Johnson rotated in a clockwise direction about her vertical axis in a backward double tucked somersault with two twists (first lane) and in a backward straight somersault with three twists (second lane). She rotated also in a clockwise direction about her vertical axis in a forward straight somersault with one and a half twists (third lane), but, quite surprisingly, in a counterclockwise direction in a preceding forward straight somersault with one twist. In her roundoff, she rotated also in a counterclockwise direction about her vertical axis. Thus gymnasts' rotational behavior affirmed a common training observation in gymnastics; that is to say, gymnasts are likely to rotate in different directions about their vertical axis in different skills.

In this context, Sands (2000) analyzed female gymnasts' twist directions in different gymnastics skills. The study revealed no clear tendency for either a clockwise or a counterclockwise preference in twist direction of forward and backward somersaults. Furthermore, the author observed that if gymnasts placed their left hand down first in the roundoff (indicating a clockwise rotation about the vertical axis), they twisted in a counterclockwise direction in a backward somersault and a pirouette in about 80% of the time. Gymnasts placing their right hand down first during a roundoff (counterclockwise rotation about the vertical axis) will twist in a clockwise direction in a backward somersault and a pirouette about 75% of the time. The most surprising result was that gymnasts preferred different rotation directions in different skills, with the most obvious difference between the roundoff (a typical skill in which rotation about the vertical axis starts when the head is placed upside down) and the pirouette (a typical skill in which rotation about the vertical axis starts when the head is placed in an upright position).

Given that gymnasts should exhibit *one* rotational preference about their vertical axis, the question arises why rotational preference differs between skills? Experiencing the body as a coherent (moving) system is based on (integrated) information from a variety of sensory modalities (Latash, 2008). In individualized sports, this may especially be true when it comes to the perception and execution of rotations, since they are one inherent component in sports such as gymnastics or figure skating (Arkaev & Suchilin, 2004). Empirical evidence suggests that rotational preference is associated with aspects, such as visuospatial performance and representation (Golomer et al., 2009; Gordon et al., 1992) or specific motor experience (Heinen & Jeraj, 2013). Therefore, it is likely to assume that, in addition to laterality factors, there are also influences from perception and cognition on rotational preference in individualized sports.

Fig. 11.3 shows for instance a gymnast performing a roundoff and a straight jump with a full turn. Performing a roundoff with a clockwise rotation direction goes along with the optical impression that the environment flows to the right when bringing the arms to the floor (Fig. 11.3A). The same optical expression occurs when performing a straight jump with a full turn in a counterclockwise rotation direction (Fig. 11.3B). In both cases the gymnast would perceive an invariant optical impression during the initial, yet essential phase of the skill; that is to say the environment flows to the right from the perspective of the gymnast.

The idea of *perceptual invariance* may therefore not only be restricted to an invariance in vestibular information when performing skills such as the roundoff and a somersault with twists (Heinen et al., 2012), but also to an invariance in visual information (i.e., optic flow information; Davids, Button, & Bennett, 2008). This may at least in part explain why gymnasts' rotational preference about the vertical axis can be different between different skills. Nevertheless, different informational sources interact during

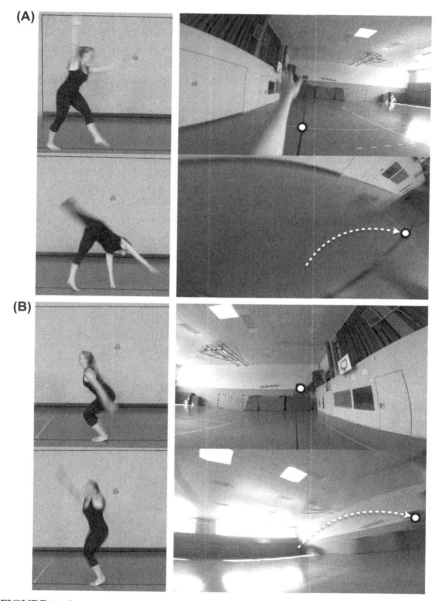

FIGURE 11.3   Illustration of a female gymnast performing the initial phase of a roundoff (A) and a straight jump with a full turn (B) together with the corresponding shift of the optical field from an egocentric perspective. The *dashed line with the arrow* highlights the movement of the white dot during the initial phase of both skills. *Note:* The gymnast exhibits a clockwise rotation about her vertical axis in the roundoff and a counterclockwise rotation in the straight jump.

goal-directed activity while visual information may be used as a reference (Mergner, Schweigart, Müller, Hlavacka, & Becker, 2000). The utilization of particular information becomes optimized with practice and experience (Vuillerme et al., 2001). Thus the informational source that guides athletes' actions may differ between different individuals, tasks, and sports (Raab, de Oliveira, & Heinen, 2009).

It is additionally thought that the observation of the actions of other people may activate a corresponding motor representation in the observer (Grèzes, Armony, Rowe, & Passingham, 2003). Athletic experience thus seems to modulate action-related perceptual-cognitive processing (Calvo-Merino, Glaser, Grèzes, Passingham, & Haggard, 2005; Grèzes et al., 2003; Ozel, Larue, & Molinaro, 2002). In addition, specific motor experience (i.e., rotational preference) is thought to relate to athletes' performance in perceptual-cognitive tasks incorporating rotations (Contakos & Carlton, 2007, 2008; Stochl & Croudace, 2013).

The reader may for instance be familiar with the "spinning dancer illusion" or "silhouette illusion" by Nobuyuki Kayahara (Fig. 11.4). It is an animation of a pirouetting female dancer that lacks visual depth cues.

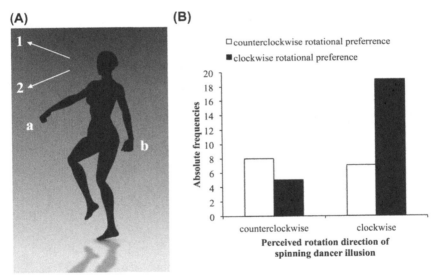

FIGURE 11.4 (A) Bistable picture of a dancing figure, similar to that used in the "silhouette illusion" or "spinning dancer illusion" by Nobuyuki Kayahara. *Note:* The reader may either perceive the figure facing and moving to the upper left "1" or lower left direction "2." When perceiving the figure facing to the upper left direction, "a" represents the dancing figure's left hand and "b" represents the dancing figure's right hand. The original animation of Nobuyuki Kayahara's "silhouette illusion" (spinning dancer) can be found here: http://procreo.jp/labo/labo13.html. (B) Absolute frequencies of gymnasts with different rotational preferences perceiving the spinning dancer as rotating either in a counterclockwise or clockwise direction.

Observers more often perceive the figure as spinning clockwise, while others perceive the figure spinning in a counterclockwise direction about its vertical axis (Troje & McAdam, 2010).

We asked $N = 39$ gymnasts to indicate their preferred rotation direction in upright stance. In addition, gymnasts were asked to observe the spinning dancer illusion and indicate the perceived rotation direction of the animation. Results revealed that more gymnasts ($N = 26$) perceived the spinning dancer rotating in a clockwise direction (Fig. 11.4). This difference is in line with previously published data and may be attributed to a viewing-from-above bias (Troje & McAdam, 2010). Furthermore, there was a systematic relationship between the perceived rotation direction of the spinning dancer illusion and gymnasts' rotational preference in upright stance ($\chi^2 = 4.30$; $p = 0.036$). Gymnasts who preferred turning in a clockwise direction on the office chair also perceived the spinning dancer more often as turning in a clockwise direction and vice versa (see also Stochl & Croudace, 2013). It can be concluded that rotational preference and perceiving rotations may at least partially relate to each other.

Differences in the perception and cognition of rotations could be related to different processes or perspectives (Kessler & Thomson, 2010). Perceiving the environment flowing around oneself could rely on an egocentric perspective, while perceiving the spinning dancer illusion could for instance rely on an allocentric perspective (Gibbs, 2006). Jola and Mast (2005) compared participants' mental rotation performance in two different mental rotation tasks. The authors asked nondancers and professional dancers to perform a mental object rotation task and a mental body rotation task in the same rotation conditions. Results revealed impaired performance for expert dancers in the mental object rotation task. The authors argue that expert dancers are likely to apply a different strategy to solve the task as compared to the nondancers (i.e., rotating oneself to align with the object stimuli in the task). However, the authors did neither find a difference in dancers' and nondancers' mental rotation performance in mental body rotation tasks, speculating that dancers may be more experienced in performing rotations about their vertical axis instead of the sagittal axis used to rotate the mental rotation stimuli.

Steggemann, Engbert, and Weigelt (2011) additionally compared mental rotation performance in experts with a particular expertise in performing rotational movements to that of nonexperts. Participants were asked to perform an object-based (spatial) mental rotation task and a perspective-transformation mental rotation task. Results revealed that motor experts showed superior mental rotation performance in the task involving a perspective transformation. The authors argued that specific motor expertise not only modulates the perception of action but also facilitates higher cognitive processes, such as those reflected in mental rotation tasks.

Heinen and Jeraj (2013) assessed mental rotation performance of male gymnasts who exhibited either a clockwise or a counterclockwise rotational preference about their vertical axis. Gymnasts were asked to perform a psychometric mental rotation test with either rotational-preference congruent stimuli or rotational-preference incongruent stimuli. Results revealed that mental rotation performance was better for rotational-preference congruent stimuli as compared to incongruent stimuli. The authors concluded that sensory-motor experience in a particular sport (i.e., rotational preference) may facilitate perceptual-cognitive processing of experience-congruent stimuli.

Taken together, rotational preference in individualized sports at least partially relates to athletes' perceptual-cognitive processing. Athlete's perceptual-cognitive processing may either be seen as a cause for a particular rotational preference (i.e., perceptual invariance in complex rotations) or as an effect that occurs due to a particular rotational preference (i.e., facilitated mental rotation performance). Given the discussed aspects so far, we argue that rotational preference in individualized sports is a complex phenomenon that may be best understood in the context of other laterality characteristics, as well as athletes' perceptual-cognitive processing. Finally, the question arises if there are any implications for practice in individualized sports that can be derived from the aspects just discussed? We will therefore try to highlight several implications before conclusions on rotational preference in individualized sports will be drawn.

IMPLICATIONS FOR PRACTICE

It is generally accepted in the coaching literature in individualized sports such as gymnastics that an athlete should maintain his/her rotation direction in a particular skill or a particular group of skills (Arkaev & Suchilin, 2004). Thus gymnasts usually decide at a young age whether to rotate in a clockwise or counterclockwise direction in a particular skill and maintain this preference throughout their careers (Sands, 2000). However, rotational preference may differ between different skills. In daily practice, the decision about rotation direction is often determined from self-reports of young athletes, indicating the direction in which they *feel good* when performing a particular skill or by observing their spontaneous rotational behavior in simple skills. In some cases, information about aspects such as handedness or footedness is incorporated in this decision.

Choosing individual rotation direction in favor of lateral preferences may facilitate skill acquisition processes (Serrien et al., 2006). However, if the training environment enforces gymnasts to develop more complex skills later in their career, such as the Kasamatsu on vault, it is required that the gymnast rotates about the vertical axis in a well-defined manner.

If a gymnast is for instance not able to rotate in a counterclockwise direction in a roundoff and in a clockwise direction in a forward-twisting somersault or vice versa, he or she will not be able to perform a Kasamatsu on vault. Taking this into consideration may potentially overrule spontaneous rotational preferences or the unfolding of lateral preferences in particular skills.

Some authors call for unbiased and functionally balanced athletes that are laterally not limited as performers (e.g., Golomer & Fery, 2001; Karageanes, 2005; Kimmerle, 2010). While exploring and practicing both rotation directions in simple skills such as pirouettes and jump turns could potentially be beneficial in terms of learning and transfer (Issurin, 2013; Schöllhorn, Hegen, & Davids, 2012), this may, however, be questionable for complex skills. Imagine for instance a gymnast performing a double-straight somersault with two twists. The question arises if it would be advantageous to acquire this particular skill in a way that it can be performed with either a clockwise or a counterclockwise rotation direction during the twist or if this could potentially lead to orientation problems thereby hampering performance (Day & Thatcher, 2006)? There may be no definite answer to this question at the moment, and each athlete in individualized sports has to find his/her own way of dealing with different rotation directions when performing complex skills. However, addressing this question experimentally could be one fruitful approach to clarify the role of rotation preference in the acquisition of complex skills.

There may be no definite answer on how to determine rotational preference in sports such as gymnastics, figures skating, or platform diving. First, it may be most advisable to let athletes explore both rotation directions (in different skills), thus ensuring that performers have the opportunity to demonstrate a particular preference. Therefore, it may be helpful if coaches try to eliminate virtually all teaching or demonstration biases that could potentially be existent in the gym (Kimmerle, 2010). Second, information about athletes' lateral preferences (i.e., Toussaint et al., 2008), their performance on diverse rotation tasks (i.e., Fukuda, 1959), and their performance on perceptual-cognitive tasks (i.e., Stochl & Croudace, 2013) could be taken into account when determining or defining athletes' rotation direction. Third, sport-specific demands could be considered. As mentioned above, if a gymnast will have to learn a Kasamatsu on vault later in his career, he should exhibit a particular rotational preference in a roundoff and in a twisting somersault. If this is not the case, he will hardly learn the Kasamatsu (Heinen et al., 2012). The aspects discussed so far should not discourage but rather sensitize athletes and coaches that rotational preference in individual sports is a complex, yet important and potentially performance-facilitating aspect that should be given appropriate attention in daily training.

CONCLUSIONS

Lateralized behavior occurs in sports that are not obvious, such as in gymnastics or figure skating. Rotational movements are an inherent component of individualized sports. Human laterality is thus not limited to aspects such as handedness or eyedness, but it also involves an athlete's preference to perform rotations about the vertical axis of the body in one or the other direction (Sands, 2000; Stochl & Croudace, 2013). Explanations for the tendency to favor one direction over the other when rotating about the vertical axis comprise diverse hypotheses (e.g., asymmetries in the vestibular system; Toussaint et al., 2008). Given the empirical evidence so far, one could argue that there exists a variety of intrinsic and extrinsic factors constituting rotational preference in individualized sports (Lenoir et al., 2006). Rotational preference and other aspects of lateral preference may at least partially relate to each other (Stochl & Croudace, 2013). In addition, an athlete's perceptual-cognitive processing may either be seen as a cause for a particular rotational preference or as an effect that occurs due to a particular rotational preference. Finally, there may be no definite answer on how to determine rotational preference in sports such as gymnastics, figure skating, or platform diving, but the coach may be advised to take as much information as possible into account (i.e., lateral preferences, athletes' performance in perceptual-cognitive tasks, task demands) as well as letting athletes explore both rotation direction in different skills so that a clear-cut, yet performance-facilitating rotational preference is given a chance to emerge.

References

Abrams, D. M., & Panaggio, M. J. (2012). A model balancing cooperation and competition can explain our right-handed world and the dominance of left-handed athletes. *Journal of the Royal Society Interface, 9*, 2718–2722.

Arkaev, L. I., & Suchilin, N. G. (2004). *How to create champions. The theory and methodology of training top-class gymnasts.* Oxford: Meyer & Meyer Sport.

Bartonietz, K. (2008). Hammer throwing: problems and prospects. In V. M. Zatsiorsky (Ed.), *Biomechanics in sport: Performance enhancement and injury prevention* (pp. 458–486). Oxford, UK: Blackwell Science Ltd.

Behnke, R. S. (2001). *Kinetic anatomy.* Champaign, IL: Human Kinetics.

Boyadjian, A., Marin, L., & Danion, F. (1999). Veering in human locomotion: the role of the effectors. *Neuroscience Letters, 265*, 21–24.

Bracha, H. S., Seitz, D. J., Otemaa, J., & Glick, S. D. (1987). Rotational movement (circling) in normal humans: sex difference and relationship to hand, foot and eye preference. *Brain Research, 19*, 231–235.

Bracha, H. S., Shults, C., Glick, S. D., & Kleinman, J. E. (1987). Spontaneous asymmetric circling behavior in hemi-parkisonism: a human equivalent of the lesioned-circling rodent behavior. *Life Sciences, 40*, 1127–1130.

Bradshaw, J. L., & Bradshaw, J. A. (1987). Rotational and turning tendencies in humans: an analog of lateral biases in rats? *International Journal of Neuroscience, 39*, 229–232.

Brown, J., Tolsma, B., & Kamen, G. (1983). Relationships between hand and eye dominance and direction of experienced gymnasts and non-athletes. *Perceptual and Motor Skills, 57*, 470.

Calvo-Merino, B., Glaser, D. E., Grèzes, J., Passingham, R. E., & Haggard, P. (2005). Action observation and acquired motor skills: an fMRI study with expert dancers. *Cerebral Cortex, 15*, 1243–1249.

Contakos, J., & Carlton, L. G. (2007). Thinking upside-down: the perception of human body rotation. *Journal of Sport & Exercise Psychology, 29*, S64.

Contakos, J., & Carlton, L. G. (2008). Cognitive acrobatics: spatial perception-action coupling of human body rotation. *Journal of Sport & Exercise Psychology, 30*, S72–S73.

Davids, K., Button, C., & Bennett, S. (2008). *Dynamics of skill acquisition. A constraints-led approach*. Champaign, IL: Human Kinetics.

Day, H. D., & Day, K. C. (1997). Directional preferences in the rotational play behaviors of young children. *Developmental Psychobiology, 30*, 213–223.

Day, M., & Thatcher, J. (2006). The causes of and psychological responses to lost move syndrome in national level trampolinists. *Journal of Applied Sport Psychology, 18*, 151–166.

Demura, S., Tada, N., Matsuzawa, J., Mikami, H., Ohuchi, T., Shirane, H., … Uchiyama, M. (2006). The influence of gender, athletic events, and athletic experience on the subjective hand and the determination of the dominant hand based on the laterality quotient (LQ) and the validity of the LQ. *Journal of Physiological Anthropology, 25*, 321–329.

Faurie, C., & Raymond, M. (2013). The fighting hypothesis as an evolutionary explanation for human handedness polymorphism: where are we? *Annals of the New York Academy of Sciences, 1288*, 110–113.

Fédération Internationale de Gymnastique (FIG). (2013). *2013–2016 Code de pointage*. Lausanne: FIG.

Fitzpatrick, R. C., Marsden, J., Lord, S. R., & Day, B. L. (2002). Galvanic vestibular stimulation evokes sensations of body rotation. *NeuroReport, 13*, 2379–2383.

Fitzpatrick, R. C., Wardman, D. L., & Taylor, J. L. (1999). Effects of galvanic vestibular stimulation during human walking. *Journal of Physiology, 517*, 931–939.

Fukuda, T. (1959). The stepping test: two phases of the labyrinthe reflex. *Acta Oto-Laryngologica, 50*, 95–108.

Gibbs, R. W. (2006). *Embodiment and cognitive science*. New York: Cambridge University Press.

Glick, S. D., & Ross, D. A. (1981). Lateralization of function in the rat brain. Basis mechanisms may be operative in humans. *Trends in Neurosciences, 4*, 196–199.

Golomer, E., & Fery, Y.-A. (2001). Unilateral jump behavior in young professional female ballet dancers. *International Journal of Neuroscience, 110*, 1–7.

Golomer, E., & Mbongo, F. (2004). Does footedness or hemispheric visual asymmetry influence centre of pressure displacements? *Neuroscience Letters, 367*, 148–151.

Golomer, E., Rosey, F., Dizac, H., Mertz, C., & Fagard, J. (2009). The influence of classical dance training on preferred supporting leg and whole body turning bias. *Laterality: Asymmetries of Body, Brain and Cognition, 14*, 165–177.

Gordon, H. W., Busdiecker, E. C., & Bracha, S. H. (1992). The relationship between leftward turning bias and visuospatial ability in humans. *International Journal of Neuroscience, 65*, 29–36.

Grèzes, J., Armony, J. L., Rowe, J., & Passingham, R. E. (2003). Activations related to "mirror" and "canonical" neurones in the human brain: an fMRI study. *NeuroImage, 18*, 928–937.

Heinen, T., & Jeraj, D. (2013). The athletes' body shapes the athletes' mind – new perspectives of mental rotation performance in athletes. *Problems of Psychology in the 21st Century, 7*, 23–31.

Heinen, T., Jeraj, D., Vinken, P. M., & Velentzas, K. (2012). Rotational preference in gymnastics. *Journal of Human Kinetics, 33*, 33–43.

Heinen, T., Vinken, P. M., & Velentzas, K. (2010). Does laterality predict twist direction in gymnastics? *Science of Gymnastics Journal, 2*(1), 5–14.

Howard, I. P., & Templeton, W. B. (1966). *Human spatial orientation*. New York, NY: John Wiley & Sons Inc.

Issurin, V. B. (2013). Training transfer: scientific background and insights for practical application. *Sports Medicine, 34*, 675–694.

Jola, C., & Mast, F. W. (2005). Mental object rotation and egocentric body transformation: two dissociable processes? *Spatial Cognition and Computation, 5*, 217–237.

Karageanes, S. J. (2005). *Principles of manual sports medicine*. Philadelphia, PA: Lippincott Williams & Wilkins.

Kessler, K., & Thomson, L. A. (2010). The embodied nature of spatial perspective taking: embodied transformation versus sensorimotor interference. *Cognition, 114*, 72–88.

Kimmerle, M. (2010). Lateral bias, functional asymmetry, dance training and dance injuries. *Journal of Dance Medicine & Science, 14*, 58–66.

King, D. L. (2005). Performing triple and quadruple figure skating jumps: implications for training. *Canadian Journal of Applied Physiology, 30*, 743–753.

Latash, M. L. (2008). *Neurophysiological basis of movement*. Champaign, IL: Human Kinetics.

Le Moal, M., & Simon, H. (1991). Mesocorticolimbic dopaminergic network: functional and regulatory roles. *Physiological Reviews, 71*, 155–234.

Lenoir, M., van Overschelde, S., de Rycke, M., & Musch, E. (2006). Intrinsic and extrinsic factors of turning preference in humans. *Neuroscience Letters, 393*, 179–183.

Loffing, F., Sölter, F., & Hagemann, N. (2014). Left preference for sport tasks does not necessarily indicate left-handedness: sport-specific lateral preferences, relationship with handedness and implications for laterality research in behavioural sciences. *PLoS One, 9*(8), e105800.

Lund, F. H. (1930). Physical asymmetries and disorientation. *American Journal of Psychology, 42*, 51–62.

Mead, L. A., & Hampson, E. (1997). Turning bias in humans is influenced by phase of menstrual cycle. *Hormones and Behavior, 31*, 65–74.

Mergner, T., Schweigart, G., Müller, M., Hlavacka, F., & Becker, W. (2000). Visual contributions to human self-motion perception during horizontal body rotation. *Archives Italiennes des Biologie, 138*, 139–166.

Miller, D. I. (2008). Springboard and platform diving. In V. M. Zatsiorsky (Ed.), *Biomechanics in sport: Performance enhancement and injury prevention* (pp. 326–348). Oxford, UK: Blackwell Science Ltd.

Mohr, C., Brugger, P., Bracha, H. S., Landis, T., & Viaud-Delmon, I. (2004). Human side preferences in three different whole-body movement tasks. *Behavioural Brain Research, 151*, 321–326.

Mohr, C., Landis, T., Bracha, H. S., & Brugger, P. (2003). Opposite turning behavior in right-handers and non-right-handers suggests a link between handedness and cerebral dopamine asymmetries. *Behavioral Neuroscience, 117*, 1448–1452.

Mohr, C., Landis, T., Bracha, H. S., Fathi, M., & Brugger, P. (2003). Human locomotion: levodopa keeps you straight. *Neuroscience Letters, 339*, 115–118.

Nishida, T., & Inaba, A. (2009). Pirouettes: the rotational play of wild chimpanzees. *Primates, 50*, 333–341.

Ozel, S., Larue, J., & Molinaro, C. (2002). Relation between sport activity and mental rotation: comparison of three groups of subjects. *Perceptual and Motor Skills, 95*, 1141–1154.

Previc, F. H. (1991). A general theory concerning the prenatal origins of cerebral lateralization in humans. *Psychological Review, 98*, 299–334.

Previc, F. H., & Saucedo, J. C. (1992). The relationship between turning behavior and motoric dominance in humans. *Perceptual and Motor Skills, 75*, 935–944.

Raab, M., de Oliveira, R. F., & Heinen, T. (2009). How do people perceive and generate options? In M. Raab, H. Hekeren, & J. G. Johnson (Eds.), *Progress in brain research Mind and motion: The bidirectional link between thought and action: Vol. 174.* (pp. 49–59). Amsterdam, NL: Elsevier.

Raymond, M., Pontier, D., Dufour, A.-B., & Møller, A. P. (1996). Frequency-dependent maintenance of left handedness in humans. *Proceedings of the Royal Society B, 263,* 1627–1633.

Reiss, M., & Reiss, G. (1997). Asymmetry of the stepping test. *Perceptual and Motor Skills, 85,* 305–306.

Sands, W. A. (2000). Twist direction. *Technique, 20*(2), 5–7.

Schaeffer, A. A. (1928). Spiral movement in man. *Journal of Morphology, 45,* 293–398.

Scharine, A. A., & McBeath, M. K. (2002). Right-handers and Americans favor turning to the right. *Human Factors, 44,* 248–256.

Schöllhorn, W. I., Hegen, P., & Davids, K. (2012). The nonlinear nature of learning. A differential learning approach. *The Open Sports Sciences Journal, 5*(Suppl. 1–M11), 100–112.

Serrien, D. J., Ivry, R. B., & Swinnen, S. P. (2006). Dynamics of hemispheric specialization and integration in the context of motor control. *Nature Reviews Neuroscience, 7,* 160–167.

Souman, J. L., Frissen, I., Sreenivasa, M. N., & Ernst, M. O. (2009). Walking straight into circles. *Current Biology, 19,* 1538–1542.

Starosta, W. (1986). Genetic or social determination of the direction of turns during physical exercises. *Kineziologija, 18,* 33–40.

Steggemann, Y., Engbert, K., & Weigelt, M. (2011). Selective effects of motor expertise in mental body rotation tasks: comparing object-based and perspective transformations. *Brain and Cognition, 76,* 97–105.

Stochl, J., & Croudace, T. (2013). Predictors of human rotation. *Laterality: Asymmetries of Body, Brain and Cognition, 18,* 265–281.

Taylor, M. J. D., Strike, S. C., & Dabnichki, P. (2006). Turning bias and lateral dominance in a sample of able-bodied and amputee participants. *Laterality: Asymmetries of Body, Brain and Cognition, 12,* 50–63.

Tops, M., Wijers, A. A., Koch, T., & Korf, J. (2006). Modulation of rotational behavior in healthy volunteers by cortisol administration. *Biological Psychology, 71,* 240–243.

Toussaint, Y., Do, M.-C., & Fagard, J. (2008). What are the factors responsible for the deviation in stepping on the spot? *Neuroscience Letters, 435,* 60–64.

Troje, N. F., & McAdam, M. (2010). The viewing-from-above bias and the silhouette illusion. *i-Perception, 1,* 143–148.

Vuillerme, N., Danion, F., Marin, L., Boyadjian, A., Prieur, J. M., Weise, I., & Nougier, V. (2001). The effect of expertise in gymnastics on postural control. *Neuroscience Letters, 303,* 83–86.

Yeadon, M. R. (2000). Aerial movement. In V. M. Zatsiorsky (Ed.), *Biomechanics in sport. Performance enhancement and injury prevention* (pp. 273–283). Oxford: Blackwell Science.

12

Performance Differences Between Left- and Right-Sided Athletes in One-on-One Interactive Sports

Florian Loffing, Norbert Hagemann

University of Kassel, Kassel, Germany

Any one who has watched a cricket-match in which a left-handed batsman was taking part, knows what trouble he causes to his opponents; how the fielders have to change either their positions or their functions every time he faces the bowler; and how odd he appears at the wrong, that is, the unusual, side of the wicket.
Lundie (1896, p. 9)

INTRODUCTION

According to anecdotal reports, competing against left-sided opponents may be a tough challenge in sports such as tennis (Sampras, 1998), cricket (Lundie, 1896), or fencing (see Chapter 3: In Fencing, Are Left-Handers Trouble for Right-Handers? What Fencing Masters Said in the Past and What Scientists Say Today, by Harris, in this book). Indeed, research suggests that in some interactive sports, left-sidedness, where left-handedness is the most prominent example (but includes footedness or stance), may be associated with a performance advantage. Here we elaborate on performance differences between left- and right-sided athletes in sports and the possible underlying mechanisms (for related reviews see also Grouios, 2004; Grouios, Koidou, Tsorbatzoudis, & Alexandris, 2002; Loffing & Hagemann, 2012). To this end, first we will give an overview of the prevalence of left-sidedness in various sports. We will then briefly summarize different explanations for why left-sided athletes may have an advantage in sports and ask whether left-sidedness is associated with a greater probability of winning in sporting contests. Following a summary of findings on handedness effects in perceptual-cognitive skills, we will critically discuss the evidence cited in favor of the various explanatory approaches. Last but not least, we will reflect on research directions that appear to be promising in the goal of creating a more comprehensive understanding of laterality effects in one-on-one interactive sports.

Throughout this chapter, we will primarily refer to athletes' left- versus right-sidedness or left versus right preference instead of left- versus right-handedness unless it seems appropriate or necessary to do so. The main reasons for this are that (1) an athlete's lateral preference for a sport-specific task may not necessarily coincide with his or her general handedness, which holds for bilaterally controlled actions in particular, and (2) undifferentiated reference to handedness may lead to inaccuracy in methodology or conclusions about the mechanisms or processes possibly underlying laterality effects in performance (Loffing, Sölter, & Hagemann, 2014; Wood & Aggleton, 1989).

PREVALENCE OF LEFT-SIDEDNESS IN SPORTS

Examples of the literature that examine the prevalence of left preferences observed in different sports are summarized in Table 12.1 (see also Grouios, 2004; Grouios, Tsorbatzoudis, Alexandris, & Barkoukis, 2000; Loffing & Hagemann, 2012; Raymond, Pontier, Dufour, & Møller, 1996). Since variation in left-sidedness across or within sports was found to be particularly evident in men, the following discussion focuses on data from male competition (for data on female athletes, e.g., see Breznik, 2013; Grouios et al., 2000; Loffing, Hagemann, & Strauss, 2012; Raymond et al., 1996).

Type of Sports: Direct Interactive, Indirect Interactive, and Noninteractive

In relation to the incidence in the normal population, left-sided athletes have been found more frequently at the elite level of duel-like interactive individual sports (e.g., fencing, table tennis, boxing) or team sports where one-on-one interactions between opponents are essential components of a game (e.g., baseball, cricket). Such overrepresentation is interpreted as indirect evidence for an advantage (Grouios et al., 2000; Raymond et al., 1996; Wood & Aggleton, 1989), which seems to occur only in interactive but not in noninteractive sports such as darts, snooker, or bowling (Table 12.1).

TABLE 12.1 Left-Sidedness and Sporting Success in Male Interactive and Noninteractive Competition

Type	Sport	Author(s)	Sample	Laterality Measure	N	% Left	Success	Explanation by Author(s)
Direct interactive	Boxing	Gursoy (2009)	Semi-professional or amateur boxers from a boxing club in Turkey	Handedness preference questionnaire (Oldfield, 1971)	22	36.4	+ LH lost fewer fights than RH	Innate superiority (spatiomotor skills)
		Loffing and Hagemann (2015)	Top boxers listed in *The Ring* magazine (1924–2012)	Fighting stance	2403	18.6	+ Better lose-win ratio in left than right boxers − % losses by KO higher in left than right boxers	NFDS, alternatives not excluded
		Grouios et al. (2000)	Class-A (very good) athletes from northern Greece	Handedness preference questionnaire (Briggs & Nebes, 1975)	26	26.1		NFDS
		Raymond et al. (1996)	Danish amateurs	N/A	95	6.3		Not specifically explicated
			Danish champions	N/A	26	23.1		Not specifically explicated
	Fencing	Azémar et al. (1983)	Top 25 in world ranking in 1980	Use of weapon (foil)	25	48.0		Neuropsychological advantage of crossed laterality (left hand × right eye)
			Participants at world championships in 1981	Use of weapon (foil)	127	34.6		
				Use of weapon (epée)	130	23.8		
				Use of weapon (saber)	95	12.6		

Continued

TABLE 12.1 Left-Sidedness and Sporting Success in Male Interactive and Noninteractive Competition—cont'd

Type	Sport	Author(s)	Sample	Laterality Measure	N	% Left	Success	Explanation by Author(s)
	Judo	Tirp et al. (2014)	Judoka ranked 7th or worse in the German university championship 2011	Combat stance (left/right=left/right leg forward)	221	20.8		NFDS (strategic), alternatives not excluded
			Judoka ranked 1st–5th at Olympic Games (1996–2012), German championships (2005–11), and German university championships (2008–12)	Combat stance (left/right=left/right leg forward)	619	36.7		
	Mixed martial arts	Baker and Schorer (2013)	Fighters listed in an online data source	Fighting stance	1468	17.4	○ Chance of winning: L~R	
	Ultimate fighting	Pollet et al. (2013)	UFC broadcasts 118–148	Fighting stance	245	20.4	○ Chance of winning: L~R	NFDS in parts, alternatives not excluded
	Wrestling	Ziyagil et al. (2010)	Athletes at two world championships (women and men)	Handedness preference questionnaire (Oldfield, 1971)	440	10	+ Rounds won: LH > MH > RH	Innate superiority (neurologic)

	Reference	Sample	Measure	N	%	Findings	Explanation
Indirect interactive							
Badminton	Loffing (2015)	Top 100 in YEWR 2009–14	Racket use	183	12.6		NFDS (time constraints)
	Raymond et al. (1996)	Danish elite	Racket use	22	22.7		
Baseball	Grondin et al. (1999)	Players in Major League Baseball (1871–1992)	Throwing hand	7196	13.5	Hitting performance: + LH>RH (as defined by throwing hand) + Left batter (BL) > right batter (BR) + BL-LH>BL-RH	Motor control (hand dominance and hand specialization)
			Batting side	7196	30.3		
Cricket	Brooks et al. (2004)	Batsmen in 14 teams in the 2003 cricket World Cup	Batting side	177	23.7	+ Positive association between team success and % innings of LH batsmen + Bat duration and batting averages: LH>RH + Dismissal by bowler's wicket: LH<RH	NFDS

Continued

TABLE 12.1 Left-Sidedness and Sporting Success in Male Interactive and Noninteractive Competition—cont'd

Type	Sport	Author(s)	Sample	Laterality Measure	N	% Left	Success	Explanation by Author(s)
	Ice hockey	Puterman et al. (2010)	Field players in the National Hockey League (NHL) in 2006/07	Shooting side	856	64		
			NHL goalkeepers in 2006/07	Catching side	84	90.5		NFDS (perception, anticipation)
			NHL field players in 1917–2006	Shooting side	3269	N/A (~63%)	+ Goals scored: Right-shooters > left-shooters ○ Goals assisted: left-shooters > right-shooters	
			NHL goalkeepers in 1957–2006	Catching side	167	N/A (~90%)	+ Goals per shot: right-catcher < left-catcher	
	Squash	Loffing (2015)	Top 100 in YEWR 2005–14	Racket use	230	10		NFDS (time constraints)
	Table tennis	Loffing (2015)	Top 100 in YEWR 2005–14	Racket use	220	22.7		NFDS (time constraints)
	Tennis	Loffing, Hagemann, et al. (2012)	Top 500 (or higher) in YEWR (1973–2011)	Racket use	3746	9.6		NFDS
			Top 100 in YEWR (1973–2011)		843	13.4		
			Top 10 in YEWR (1973–2011)		116	13.8		
			No. 1 in YEWR (1973–2011)		16	18.8		

	Sport	Sample	Subgroup	Success	N	%	Reserved interpretation
Noninteractive	Darts			Throwing hand	100	3	Reserved interpretation against an innate superiority, but not excluded
	Golf	Aggleton and Wood (1990)					
		English, Welsh and Scottish players	Professionals	Playing side	250	0.8	
			Amateurs	Playing side	160	7.5	
				Self-classification of handedness	160	16.2	
	Snooker	Official world snooker rankings (1987)		Hand holding the Cue	125	8.8	
	Ten-pin bowling	Top players in the USA in 1987		Bowling hand	131	9.9	

Notes: YEWR, year-end world rankings; *NFDS*, negative frequency-dependent selection; *L(H)*, Left(-hander); *MH*, Mixed-hander; *R(H)*, Right(-hander).

In the studies on boxing (Loffing & Hagemann, 2015), mixed martial arts (Baker & Schorer, 2013), and ultimate fighting (Pollet et al., 2013), fighting stance was classified "left" or "right" if a fighter's right or left shoulder was in front. Fighting "left" corresponds to a "southpaw" stance, whereas a "right" stance is also called "orthodox."

In the "success" column, "+" and "−" symbols indicate evidence in favor of and against a left-sided athletes' advantage, respectively, and 'O' denotes findings neither for nor against an advantage. Note that, in ice hockey, right-sidedness appears rarer than left-sidedness (Puterman et al., 2010) and, therefore, for ice hockey "+" symbols suggest evidence of a relatively rarer right-sided athletes advantage.

Interactive sports can be further differentiated into direct versus indirect interactive sports (Grouios et al., 2000; Raymond et al., 1996). *Direct interactive* sports comprise those contests where athletes are close to each other, have physical contact, and may thus directly interfere with and manipulate their opponent's actions (e.g., by pushing, grasping, punching, or kicking). In *indirect interactive* sports, athletes may also be close together (e.g., table tennis) but here they cannot directly physically manipulate their opponent's actions. While we are not aware of any quantitative measures that would allow classification of different sports according to their spatiotemporal or visuomotor demands, direct interactive sports seem to be more cognitively challenging from the perspective of the need to anticipate and read an opponent's intention as well as the necessity to choose and adjust actions under greater time pressure than in indirect interactive sports. Visual inspection of data illustrated in Table 12.1 as well as research on "class-A" athletes from northern Greece (Grouios et al., 2000) suggest that left-sidedness is more prevalent in direct as opposed to indirect interactive sports. Moreover, recent work indicates that within the class of structurally related indirect interactive racket sports (i.e., badminton, squash, table tennis, and tennis), the proportion of left-handed players increases with a decrease in the time available for players between actions (Loffing, 2015). Thus data suggest that left-sided athletes are more prevalent in sports with greater time pressure.

The higher rate of left preferences at more elite levels of participation is not evident in all cases for interactive sports, however. In particular, this pattern is not the case for those sports that vary in disciplines, as in fencing (i.e., epée, foil, and saber), or which are divided into different weight divisions, as in boxing (Loffing & Hagemann, 2015; Raymond et al., 1996). In fencing, left-hander frequencies observed in world rankings or in the final rounds of world championships suggest a left-hander advantage in epée and foil but not in saber (Azémar, Ripoll, Simonet, & Stein, 1983). Albeit confirmation of evidence for more than just a few time points is required, disciplines may impose varying demands on fencers' motor control and thus either favor left- or right-handed athletes depending on whether proactive or retroactive action control is required (Boulinguez, 1999). Likewise, differences between disciplines regarding fight characteristics, the weapons used, or target areas may explain the varying relevance of handedness for high achievement in fencing. In boxing, Loffing and Hagemann (2015) recently reported that frequencies of "southpaw" fighters, who were listed in *The Ring* magazine's annual ratings from 1998 to 2012, varied considerably across the 17 weight divisions, ranging from

14% (heavyweight) to 42.3% (junior middleweight).[1] This variation is difficult to explain because there are no differences in equipment or fighting rules between weight categories.

Temporal Variation in Left Frequencies

Evidence of left-sided athletes' (non)overrepresentation has often been inferred from cross-sectional data (Aggleton & Wood, 1990; Baker & Schorer, 2013; Grouios et al., 2000; Raymond et al., 1996; Wood & Aggleton, 1989) or based on longitudinal data aggregated without considering time as a factor (Grondin, Guiard, Ivry, & Koren, 1999; Holtzen, 2000; McLean & Ciurczak, 1982). Both approaches may have certain limitations because left frequencies may be unstable over time and information on variations in the distribution of lateral preferences is lost when data are combined, especially across a long time period.

Analyses that included longitudinal data and considered time as a factor have been reported for professional baseball (1957–2005: Clotfelter, 2008; 1876–1985: Goldstein & Young, 1996), boxing (1924–2012: Loffing & Hagemann, 2015), tennis (1973–2011: Loffing, Hagemann, et al., 2012), and ice-hockey (1917–2006: Puterman, Schorer, & Baker, 2010). In baseball, Goldstein and Young (1996) considered Major League Baseball players' handedness for pitching and batting, differentiating data by the decade players first entered the sport. Analyses revealed a logarithmic increase of pitcher and batter left-handedness across decades, both stabilizing around 30% from decade eight onwards (i.e., 1946–85). Batter left-handedness, however, increased more rapidly compared to pitcher left-handedness, particularly between decades two (1886–95) and five (1916–25). According to the authors, the converging pattern in pitcher-batter coevolution, stabilization of left-hander frequencies, and the close match between pitcher and batter laterality observed in the final four decades on the one side and estimates of pitcher and batter population

---

[1] Boxing in a "southpaw" stance is characterized by having the right leg/shoulder in front nearer to the opponent (the opposite occurs in an "orthodox" stance). As a rule of thumb, a "southpaw" stance is recommended to boxers who have a stronger left than right hand since this stance allows for more forceful punches with the left hand as well as preparation of left punches via jabs with the relatively weaker right hand (and vice versa for orthodox boxers). Boxers adopting a southpaw or orthodox stance, however, are not necessarily left- or right-handed. Indeed, recent work suggests that the normal population's preference for boxing in a southpaw stance seems to be much higher (males: 21.23%; females: 34.83%) and not a good predictor of left-handedness (males: $r_{pb} = 0.417$; females: $r_{pb} = 0.276$; Loffing et al., 2014).

laterality on the other suggest an evolutionary stable strategy of handedness in professional baseball.

Analyses of left-hander frequencies across year-end world rankings in men's tennis suggest a linear decrease of left-handers in the top 10 over time and an inverse U-shaped pattern of left-handers in top 100 players (Loffing, Hagemann, et al., 2012). With regard to the top 100 players, there was a particularly high representation of left-handers in the 1990s. Furthermore, year-wise logarithmic fitting of left-hander frequencies observed in different ranking intervals of 50 players (i.e., top 50, 51–100, 101–150, etc.) over a period from 1973 to 2011 revealed that, in early years, the proportion of left-handers increased with better ranking intervals, whereas toward the end of the period, there was almost no relationship between the incidence of left-handers and ranking interval. Collectively, it seems that being left-handed used to be associated with high achievement in men's professional tennis, but this is no longer the case. The disappearance of the left-handed advantage could be due to an increase in players' professionalism, more sophisticated training regimes, and better opportunities to prepare against forthcoming opponents given the proliferation of technologies such as video recording and statistics describing game-play tendencies. In another sample of tennis players from amateur leagues in Germany, the authors found an increase in left-hander frequencies from low to high performance levels, suggesting that left-handed players may still enjoy a measurable advantage in nonprofessional tennis.

The need to consider more than just a few time points to reliably address the question of differences in laterality distribution has also been demonstrated in boxing (Loffing & Hagemann, 2015). The frequency of boxers adopting a "southpaw" stance varies considerably (i.e., 3.28–33.15%) and increased from 1924 to 2012. Relative to task-specific normal population estimates, an excess of southpaw boxers was only found in 7 of the 89 years. Since these boxing findings were obtained from archival data, it is difficult to apply clear interpretations regarding the mechanisms underlying the strong variation and increase in southpaw frequencies as well as their rare overrepresentation. However, results demonstrate that snapshots of lateral preferences in sports may run the risk of inappropriate conclusions or assumptions of lateral preferences for performance in interactive one-on-one sports (Loffing & Hagemann, 2015).

WHY WOULD LEFT-SIDED ATHLETES HAVE AN ADVANTAGE IN SPORTS?

The above findings of elevated rates of left-sidedness in interactive sports relative to normal population estimates indicate that left-sided athletes might have an advantage in these sports. But why? Two main hypotheses are discussed in the literature to explain this. Here, we will briefly address the key elements of each hypothesis (see also Grouios, 2004; Loffing & Hagemann, 2012; for related reviews). The two explanations are not mutually exclusive; however, throughout later sections we will suggest that empirical evidence available so far tends to favor one hypothesis over the other.

Innate Superiority

According to the innate superiority hypothesis, a variety of processes or predispositions (potentially) associated with left-*handedness* are thought to be beneficial to sports performance. Since the emphasis of the hypothesis is on left-handedness, we will refer to left-versus right-handedness in this section. However, we will see later that a focus only on left-handedness may be problematic given that it is not always clear whether athletes who prefer their left side for carrying out actions are actually left-handed in a more general sense.

Left-handers may benefit from right-hemisphere specialization (Holtzen, 2000; Petit et al., 2015). Specifically, actions carried out with left extremities (e.g., left hand) are under control of the right hemisphere, which is also functionally dominant for visuospatial (Toga & Thompson, 2003) and spatiotemporal skills (Boulinguez, Ferrois, & Graumer, 2003). In manual tasks requiring such skills, neural processes may be more efficient (e.g., lower delay or less loss of information) for left compared to right hand actions and thus favor left hand actions (Bisiacchi, Ripoll, Stein, Simonet, & Azémar, 1985; Dane & Erzurumluoglu, 2003). Right hand actions, in turn, are controlled by the left hemisphere, and task-relevant commands have to pass between hemispheres via the *corpus callosum*, possibly resulting in delayed visuo-spatio-temporal functioning. This delay could be detrimental to performance, particularly in time-constrained situations (e.g., Boulinguez et al., 2003; Iwabuchi & Kirk, 2009; Taddei, Viggiano, & Mecacci, 1991). Right-hemisphere specialization has also been suggested to facilitate left-hand movements in aiming tasks (Guiard, Diaz, & Beaubaton, 1983) such as in fencing (Boulinguez, 1999). Moreover, functional dominance of the right hemisphere is thought to be beneficial in tasks requiring object manipulation in close distance contests such as judo (Mikheev, Mohr, Afanasiev, Landis, & Thut, 2002) or wrestling (Ziyagil, Gursoy, Dane, & Yuksel, 2010).

A second component of the innate superiority hypothesis is the position that the relative lack of lateralization (McLean & Ciurczak, 1982) and higher proficiency in motor skills for the nonpreferred hand in left-handers compared to right-handers (Judge & Stirling, 2003) may provide left-handers with an advantage in bimanual coordination tasks (Gorynia & Egenter, 2000). A third component is that left-handers might additionally benefit from hormonal configurations that differ to those of right-handers, which are optimal to sporting performance (Geschwind & Behan, 1982; Geschwind & Galaburda, 1985a, 1985b, 1985c). One hormone candidate is testosterone, where higher concentration seems to be associated with more aggression and a greater propensity to engage in competitive fights (Archer, 2006). Testosterone level was reported to be higher in left- than right-handers (Faurie et al., 2011). However, concentrations were not related to variables such as individuals' fight performance, making it unclear from these data whether handedness differences in testosterone may actually induce performance differences between left- and right-handers.

In conclusion, propositions offered in support of a left-handers' innate superiority predict that left-handers have a performance advantage across a range of different contests that necessitate both accurate motor and visuospatial functioning (e.g., fencing, darts, snooker), that require fine bimanual coordination (e.g., golf, batting in baseball or cricket), and/or in competitions that favor individuals with high concentrations of hormones linked with more aggressive behavior (Loffing & Hagemann, 2012).

Negative Frequency-Dependent Selection

Frequency-dependent selection describes "a process in which the survival/fitness advantage of a type is dependent on its relative frequency" (Takahashi & Kawata, 2013, p. 499). Negative frequency-dependent selection (NFDS) is at work if a type's advantage increases as its relative frequency decreases. In contrast to the innate superiority hypothesis, the NFDS hypothesis takes a "nurture" perspective by focusing on the smaller proportions of left-sided athletes. Specifically, this hypothesis argues that relatively rarer left-sided athletes benefit from their opponents' low familiarity with competing left-sided athletes in particular sporting contexts (Raymond et al., 1996).

In humans, as far as we know, left preferences are considerably rarer than right preferences for almost any manual task irrespective of whether it is controlled unilaterally or bilaterally (e.g., Gilbert & Wysocki, 1992; Loffing et al., 2014; Peters, Reimers, & Manning, 2006).[2] Consequently, from an NFDS viewpoint, athletes who prefer their left side for carrying out sport-specific actions such as playing tennis, fencing, throwing a

---

[2] An exception is ice hockey, where left-sided shooting and left-sided catching seem to be more prominent than right-sided shooting and right-sided catching, respectively (Puterman et al., 2010).

ball, or batting in baseball or cricket may have an advantage simply due to their relative rarity.[3]

The NFDS hypothesis predicts that left-sided athletes should have an advantage only in duel-like interactive contests where athletes are face-to-face with their opponents and where they can more or less directly influence their opponents' actions (e.g., fencing, boxing, racket sports). In this regard, the left-sided athletes' relative rarity may provide them with a "strategic advantage" (e.g., Grouios, 2004) or a "tactical advantage" (e.g., Sterkowicz, Lech, & Blecharz, 2010) in competition (Loffing & Hagemann, 2012; Wood & Aggleton, 1989). In contests that are noninteractive (e.g., darts, snooker, gymnastics), the NFDS predicts that left-sided athletes should not have an advantage. The NFDS principle further predicts that the left-sided athletes' advantage should decrease when the number of lefties is more common in a specific sporting population and increase when they become rarer.

Innate Superiority or Negative Frequency-Dependent Selection?

In fact, both hypotheses are difficult to clearly distinguish based on their respective predictions as to the sports where left-sided athletes should have an advantage. Consequently, based on current evidence, none of them should be considered as either right or wrong (see Box 12.1). As a preliminary conclusion, however, we state that the findings of an excess of left-oriented athletes in interactive but not in noninteractive sports argue for a larger explanatory power of the NFDS hypothesis and a left-sided athletes' strategic or tactical advantage given the characteristics of interactive sports (Aggleton & Wood, 1990; Wood & Aggleton, 1989). The temporal variation in left frequencies in tennis (Loffing, Hagemann, et al., 2012) and stabilization of pitcher and batter handedness in Major League Baseball over time (Goldstein & Young, 1996) further indicate that frequency-dependent selection processes may be at work. On the other hand, the generality of the NFDS account is challenged—without providing clear support in favor of an innate superiority account, however—by considerable differences in left frequencies between divisions in boxing (Loffing & Hagemann, 2015) or disciplines in fencing (Azémar et al., 1983; Raymond et al., 1996).

[3] If we focus on handedness as an example, the NFDS account may suggest a "left-handers' opponents' disadvantage" more so than a "left-handers' advantage," which is effectively a left-handers' advantage. The term "left-handers' opponents' disadvantage" is bulky and complex, although it better represents the mechanisms assumed to underlie left-right performance asymmetries from the NFDS perspective. In contrast, the term "left-handers' advantage" may fit with the "innate superiority" explanation. However, we consider this more as a side note for further thought and, to keep it simple, we use the term "left-handers' advantage" or similar expressions such as "left-sided athletes' advantage" for both hypotheses.

BOX 12.1

LEFT-SIDEDNESS IN NONINTERACTIVE SPORTS

In noninteractive sports such as darts, snooker, golf, or gymnastics, the proportions of left-sided athletes do not exceed normal population estimates (e.g., Aggleton & Wood, 1990; Raymond et al., 1996). At first sight, the clear dissociation of sports where left-siders are over-represented (i.e., interactive) or not (i.e., noninteractive) fits well with the NFDS hypothesis and appears difficult to reconcile with an innate superiority account (Loffing & Hagemann, 2012). For example, better spatiomotor skills assumed in left-handers as opposed to right-handers should provide the former with an advantage in sports that put high demands on such skills as in darts or snooker. Likewise, similar to hitting in baseball, where lack of lateralization and better bimanual coordination in players who throw and bat left-handed was cited as one possible reason for their high batting performance (McLean & Ciurczak, 1982; for a critical discussion of that interpretation, see Wood & Aggleton, 1989), bimanual coordination is also an important skill in golf where no excess of left-sided play was found in either professionals or amateurs (see Table 12.1).

On closer inspection, however, Aggleton and Wood (1990) noted an interesting finding that seems to have almost gone unnoticed in past discussions of a left-sider's advantage and that may tentatively argue in favor of the innate superiority argument. Specifically, in their amateur sample the proportion of players who reported themselves as being left-handed was quite high (16.3%; 13.8% mixed-handed). If we ignore for the moment that self-assessment of handedness may be subject to bias (see Chapter 4: Measurement of Laterality and Its Relevance for Sports by Utesch, Mentzel, Strauss, & Büsch, in this book), there actually seemed to be a higher rate of left-handedness among golfers. Moreover, after splitting amateur golfers into two groups according to their handicap (poor: handicap >10; good: handicap ≤10), Aggleton and Wood (1990) found that the proportion of self-classified left- and mixed-handers was considerably higher in the group of good compared to the group of poor players, while the proportion of golfers playing left-sided was almost identical in both groups. Albeit confirmation of these findings is warranted and alternative explanations related to equipment and coaching need to be controlled for (Aggleton & Wood, 1990; Eastwood, 1972), data may be indicative of left-handers being, at least slightly, neurologically predisposed to tasks requiring bimanual coordination (Gorynia & Egenter, 2000).

LEFT-SIDEDNESS AND SPORTING SUCCESS

Apart from an overrepresentation of left-sided athletes in interactive sports, are "lefties" also more successful than their right-sided counterparts in these sports? Research addressing this question is quite rare compared to studies investigating the incidence of left-sided athletes in elite sports, and findings are far from conclusive (see Table 12.1 for an overview).

Direct Interactive Sports

Comparison of variables representing sporting success between left- and right-sided athletes have been reported for boxing (Gursoy, 2009; Loffing & Hagemann, 2015), judo (Sterkowicz et al., 2010; Tirp, Baker, Weigelt, & Schorer, 2014), wrestling (Ziyagil et al., 2010), and mixed martial arts (Baker & Schorer, 2013; Pollet & Riegmann, 2014; Pollet, Stulp, & Groothuis, 2013). In two cross-sectional studies, Gursoy (2009) and Ziyagil et al. (2010) determined athletes' handedness via handedness questionnaires and found indicators of better performance in left- than right-handed boxers and wrestlers, respectively (see Table 12.1). In a longitudinal study, Loffing and Hagemann (2015) differentiated boxers according to their fighting stance and revealed that southpaws had better lose–win ratios compared to orthodox boxers. Findings from the above studies generally fit with the idea of a left-sided athlete's advantage (see also Sterkowicz et al., 2010; Tirp et al., 2014); however, it is not clear if laterality differences in performance records were due to an innate superiority or NFDS, because neither fighters' combat stance (Gursoy, 2009; Ziyagil et al., 2010) nor their handedness was taken into consideration (Loffing & Hagemann, 2015). No distinct performance differences between fighters adopting a left versus right stance were identified in mixed martial arts (Baker & Schorer, 2013; Pollet & Riegmann, 2014; Pollet et al., 2013).

Indirect Interactive Sports

Simulations based on world ranking data from 2005 to 2008 suggest that at Grand Slam tournaments, left-handed, lower-ranked players are more likely to win against right-handed, higher-ranked players (del Corral & Prieto-Rodríguez, 2010). Moreover, according to Breznik's (2013) analyses of tennis matches between opposite-handed players carried out between 1968 and 2011, left-handers won more matches than expected in both male and female competition. A qualification to this finding, however, is that this effect was evident only in Challenger and Future tournaments where upcoming, lower-ranked players participate, but not in more prestigious Grand Slams or other tournaments on the ATP (Association of Tennis Professionals)/WTA (Women's Tennis Association) tour.

Batting "left-handed" (i.e., right foot in front and swinging the bat on the left body side) seems to also provide an advantage in cricket (Brooks, Bussière, Jennions, & Hunt, 2004) and baseball (Grondin et al., 1999; McLean & Ciurczak, 1982). To illustrate in cricket, team success was found to be positively related to the proportion of innings pitched by left-handed batsmen, with the estimated net run rate peaking at 50.5% left-handed innings (Brooks et al., 2004). Furthermore, left-handed batsmen had longer bat duration, higher batting averages, and were less likely to be sent off by a bowler's wicket; however, their scoring rates were no faster than those of right-handers. Closer inspection of the data revealed that the left-handed batters' advantage varied depending on the strength of the opposing teams; it was higher against relatively weaker, rather than stronger, teams. From these findings, the authors tentatively infer that "left-handers have a strategic advantage that decreases as left-handers become more common in a competition (e.g., a domestic league or the world ODI circuit) because bowlers become more adept at bowling when left-handers are relatively common" (Brooks et al., 2004, p. S66, ODI, One-Day International). Empirical confirmation of this interesting suggestion, however, is still lacking.

Interestingly, in contrast to other manual tasks, in professional ice hockey the prevalence of left-shooting field players and left-catching goalkeepers is higher than right-shooting and right-catching, respectively (Puterman et al., 2010). Multiple linear regressions on performance measures obtained from regular season play in a longitudinal sample of National Hockey League players revealed that right-shooters scored more goals than left-shooters, whereas left-shooters assisted more goals than right-shooters. Further, right-catching goalkeepers had higher save percentages (i.e., fewer goals per shot) compared to left-catching goalkeepers (Table 12.1). Focusing on penalty shootouts, these findings were replicated in goalkeepers, whereas no scoring difference was found between left- and right-sided shooters. Collectively, part of the above performance differences could fit with the NFDS account; however, in the "opposite" direction as right-sidedness in shooting and catching was relatively rarer, thus possibly favoring right-shooters and right-catchers.

LATERALITY EFFECTS IN TASK-SPECIFIC PERCEPTUAL-COGNITIVE SKILLS

To counteract the spatiotemporal constraints encountered in interactive sports, athletes develop task-specific perceptual-cognitive skills that include early visual anticipation of their opponent's action intentions and optimal selection of actions from a set of options (Yarrow, Brown, & Krakauer, 2009). Given the left-sided athletes' relative rarity, athletes are primarily exposed to right-sided opponents during practice and competition.

This, in turn, may result in the predominant formation of skills specific to and optimal for competition against right-sided athletes through processes such as reinforcement learning (Sinervo & Calsbeek, 2006). Consequently, athletes may be expected to demonstrate inferior or suboptimal performance in perceptual-cognitive skills when confronted with left-sided opponents, possibly providing the latter with a strategic or tactical advantage (Loffing & Hagemann, 2012).

Indeed, findings from laboratory-based experiments suggest that athletes have more difficulties anticipating left- than right-handed opponents' action intentions in tennis (Hagemann, 2009), volleyball (Loffing, Hagemann, Schorer, & Baker, 2015; Loffing, Schorer, Hagemann, & Baker, 2012), or team-handball goalkeeping (Loffing, Sölter, Hagemann, & Strauss, 2015). To exemplify, Hagemann (2009) asked a total of 108 novice, intermediate, and expert tennis players (18 left-handers and 18 right-handers per group) to predict the outcome of left- and right-handed tennis strokes presented as videos on a notebook monitor. Prediction accuracy was lower against left- than right-handed strokes across groups, and this effect was more pronounced in experts compared to the other two skill groups. Moreover, the handedness effect occurred irrespective of the participants' handedness: both left- and right-handed participants made larger errors against left- than right-handed shots. Thus it seems that observers' low perceptual familiarity with left-handed actions primarily drives the handedness effect and that this effect is less influenced, if at all, by observers' manual preferences.

Asymmetry in perceptual familiarity with left- and right-handers' actions can explain handedness effects in visual anticipation as suggested by a perceptual training study with novices in team-handball goalkeeping (Schorer, Loffing, Hagemann, & Baker, 2012). Exclusive confrontation with left- or right-handed penalty-takers during training resulted in hand-specific improvements in the prediction of penalty-throw direction from pretest to posttest. Specifically, a left-handed training group improved against left-handed but not right-handed penalties, whereas the right-handed training group showed larger increment in accuracy against right-than left-handed penalties. A mixed training group was confronted with a balanced ratio of left- and right-handed penalties during training and showed similar improvements against left- and right-handed throws from pretest to posttest.

In addition to reading an opponent's play, athletes also need to decide on their next intended action, such as where to place the ball in an opponent's half in tennis. One tactic is to direct a ball toward an opponent's backhand side because for most players the backhand is a weaker shot compared to the forehand. In a computer-based experiment, Loffing, Hagemann, and Strauss (2010) found that expert, intermediate, and novice tennis players, irrespective of their own handedness, directed more balls to the backhand side of right- rather than left-handed video opponents. Thus participants did not "mirror" their tactics when faced with left- compared to right-handed opponents. Further analyses of ball trajectories recorded from professional tennis singles' matches corroborated this finding: a lower proportion of balls were directed to left- as opposed to right-handers' backhand side. Collectively, these findings fit with the assumption that tactical preferences acquired through predominant play against right-handers may not be "mirrored" one-to-one against left-handers. Theoretically, such automaticity in players' tactics could provide left-handers with a (tactical) advantage. Empirical evidence in support of this causal relationship, however, still needs to be provided.

SO FAR, SO GOOD? A CRITIQUE AND SUGGESTIONS FOR FURTHER EXPLANATORY APPROACHES

Findings reported by Wood and Aggleton (1989) illustrate two important methodological issues: (1) it is important to consider how athletes' handedness (or other laterality measures) is operationalized (see Table 12.1 for examples), and (2) an athlete's handedness (e.g., as assessed via self-report preference questionnaires or performance tasks) may not necessarily coincide with his or her handedness for carrying out sport-specific tasks (see also Loffing et al., 2014). These factors seem to be particularly relevant for sports where both hands are involved since the association between general handedness preference (e.g., determined by the Edinburgh Handedness Inventory; Oldfield, 1971) and lateral preference for the control of bilateral actions (e.g., golfing, batting in baseball, boxing, wrestling) is much lower compared to sport tasks that are controlled unilaterally (e.g., holding a racket in tennis or a weapon in fencing, throwing a ball) (Loffing et al., 2014; Wood & Aggleton, 1989). Consequently and as noted at the beginning of this chapter, undifferentiated usage of the term "handedness" may be inappropriate especially for bilateral tasks. Rather, more neutral expressions such as "lateral preference" seem in order to (a) ensure a more sophisticated discussion of laterality effects on sport performance, (b) prevent usage of inappropriate reference values to test for left overrepresentation (e.g., comparison of observed incidence of left preference for combat stance with estimates of left-handedness for throwing), and (c) limit premature conclusions with regard to possible handedness-dependent performance differences (Loffing et al., 2014). These limitations are important to bear in mind when reporting the occurrence of lateral preferences in sports as well as when interpreting data in favor of different explanatory accounts (e.g., innate superiority vs. negative frequency dependence).

Moreover, the availability of only one type of laterality measure (i.e., athletes' handedness determined by established tests vs. athletes' handedness for a sport-specific task, for example, obtained from visual inspection of pictures or videos) may limit interpretation of findings with regard to different hypotheses. Specifically, if we only know an athlete's functional handedness for sport-specific tasks, we may support or reject the NFDS account (e.g., Loffing, Hagemann, et al., 2012; Raymond et al., 1996), but it will be almost impossible to properly reject or confirm the innate superiority hypothesis given that we do not know about athletes' "overall" handedness (Puterman et al., 2010; see also Chapter 4: Measurement of Laterality and Its Relevance for Sports, by Utesch et al., in this book, for a discussion of laterality measures). Conversely, if only athletes' "overall" handedness is known but not their lateral preferences for a sport-specific task (e.g., Gursoy, 2009; Ziyagil et al., 2010), data might or might not fit with propositions of the innate superiority hypothesis; however, this time the NFDS hypothesis is difficult to verify or falsify. Thus we should be aware that either way, clear-cut conclusions are limited and that at least sometimes interpretation of data may be guided more by our beliefs about underlying mechanisms rather than by what the data really allow us to infer. This limitation may be solved through simultaneous consideration of different laterality measures. However, we acknowledge that it will be a tough challenge to comprehensively assess elite athletes' handedness via established laterality tests (but: see Wood & Aggleton, 1989, for handedness assessment in professional cricketers). Where possible, a solution could be to consider athletes' lateral preferences for different sport-specific tasks such as lateral preference for throwing and batting in baseball (Grondin et al., 1999; McLean & Ciurczak, 1982) or cricket (Brooks et al., 2004; Wood & Aggleton, 1989).

In addition to the above issues, other methodological concerns relate specifically to the innate superiority or the NFDS hypothesis. In the following sections, we will briefly touch on examples and outline additional explanatory approaches (for further discussion, e.g., see Faurie & Raymond, 2013; Groothuis, McManus, Schaafsma, & Geuze, 2013; Loffing & Hagemann, 2012).

Innate Superiority

Findings interpreted in support of the innate superiority were often derived from research or tasks that were not representative of the respective sports' underlying performance demands. For example, sporting athletes have often been faced with simplistic reaction time tasks that do not represent the natural demands in domains such as in team handball (Dane & Erzurumluoglu, 2003) or fencing (Bisiacchi et al., 1985). In these sports, an athlete's (decision for) action is likely based on selective processing of a wealth of sensory input and context-specific knowledge (Yarrow et al., 2009). In other words, differences in left- versus right-hander performances identified in elegant and experimentally controlled settings may turn out to be practically irrelevant in more realistic testing scenarios or in real-life performance on the field (Dicks, Davids, & Button, 2009; Williams & Ericsson, 2005).

A second objection to the methods used in the innate superiority research relates to the fact that athletes who perform a sport-specific task with the left hand (e.g., playing tennis) or left-sided (e.g., batting in cricket or baseball) may not necessarily be left-handed in more general terms (Loffing et al., 2014; Wood & Aggleton, 1989). The assumption that they are seems problematic, particularly when an overrepresentation or enhanced success rate of "left-handed" athletes is interpreted as evidence in favor of a neuroanatomically based advantage (e.g., Holtzen, 2000).

Negative Frequency-Dependent Selection

To strengthen the argument that a left-sided athlete's advantage is due to NFDS, it remains to be demonstrated that their advantage actually increases/decreases as they become rarer/more common (Groothuis et al., 2013). In Major League Baseball, Clotfelter (2008) did not detect this sort of a relationship for left-handed pitchers in longitudinal data (1957–2005). However, he found an indication of NFDS in right-handed pitchers who were more successful in the years they were less common. The author speculates that hitters might perform best when the population of pitchers is dominated by one hand (e.g., right-handedness), whereas pitchers' performance might be facilitated if the pitching population is more balanced. As an underlying mechanism, analogous to search-image formation in frequency-dependent predation (Punzalan, Rodd, & Hughes, 2005), Clotfelter (2008) suggests that, through repeated exposure to left- or right-handed pitchers, hitters may form cognitive representations of pitcher handedness. These representations may enable better batting performance in years of clear asymmetry in pitcher handedness (i.e., dominance of one pitcher handedness; here: right-handedness) compared to years of more balanced pitcher handedness. Findings of lower batting averages as well as left- and right-handed pitchers' higher earned run averages in years of more balanced pitcher handedness seems to provide some initial support for this assumption (Clotfelter, 2008).

Another issue that warrants further examination is whether laboratory findings of athletes' difficulties anticipating left-handed opponents' action intentions (Hagemann, 2009; Loffing, Hagemann, et al., 2015; Loffing, Schorer, et al., 2012) or of not mirroring tactics when confronted with left- as opposed to right-handers (Loffing et al., 2010) can be replicated in more realistic field settings. More work is also needed to understand if, and to what extent, handedness effects in perceptual-cognitive skills actually contribute to suboptimal performance against left-handers.

Suggestions for Additional Explanations

Apart from the possible explanations for the left-sided advantage cited above, further hypotheses for why left-sided athletes might enjoy an advantage in interactive one-on-one sports have occasionally been discussed (e.g., Grouios, 2004; Loffing & Hagemann, 2012).

First, left-sided athletes might be characterized by personality traits that facilitate high achievement in interactive sporting contests (Allen, Greenlees, & Jones, 2013). The search for differences in personality between left- and right-handers has a long tradition (e.g., see Grimshaw & Wilson, 2012; McManus, 2002), but convincing evidence in favor of performance-facilitating traits is rare. Tentative support comes from Coren (1994), who found that left-handers ($n = 43$) scored higher on measures of dominance than right-handers ($n = 887$). Likewise, Dane and Sekertekin (2005) reported that a group of 18 left-handed soccer players scored higher on measures of aggressiveness compared to 33 right-handed soccer players. Whether these or handedness differences in other measures can be confirmed and identified as practically relevant to explain laterality differences in sport performance, however, remains to be shown.

A second alternative hypothesis centers on the fact that in some interactive sports, left-sided athletes might simply benefit from a psychological advantage in that "the very popularity of the notion that there is a 'leftie advantage' may give the left-hander a slight psychological edge when facing a right-handed opponent" (Wood & Aggleton, 1989, p. 237). On the one hand, the belief in or early experience of having an advantage because of being left-sided may boost left-sided athletes' confidence and possibly help stabilize high-level performance (cf. findings on the "winner effect," Hsu, Earley, & Wolf, 2006). On the other hand, once a right-sided athlete knows that he or she will be facing a left-sided opponent, he or she might anticipate problems (Sampras, 1998), and this could increase the likelihood of their actual occurrence via a self-fulfilling prophecy. Albeit speculative for the moment, we expect that taking a closer look at the psychological processes underpinning competition between left- and right-sided athletes may add fruitful knowledge to understanding performance differences.

A final alternative hypothesis centers on the idea that a left-sided athlete's overrepresentation in interactive sports could be due to their greater attraction to these sports compared to right-sided people. In this regard, whether or not there is an elevated rate of left-sidedness in a sport might depend on early selection processes during childhood (Grouios, 2004). Conversely, another selection mechanism that may favor left-sided athletes may be that coaches or talent scouts prefer to choose left- over right-sided athletes in interactive sports either for specific individual promotion or for inclusion in a team such as in cricket (Brooks et al., 2004), baseball (Hirotsu & Wright, 2005), or team handball (Baker et al., 2013; Schorer, Cobley, Büsch, Bräutigam, & Baker, 2009). This preference could be due to coaches' or scouts' experience that performing left-sided might be beneficial in these sports and/or because of team-tactical considerations. For example, in team handball, left-handers should be positioned on the right wing and right backcourt because from there they have better shooting angles toward the opposing goal than right-handed players (Schorer et al., 2009). Whether and to what extent different kinds of selection processes promote enhanced frequencies of left-sided athletes in specific sports are interesting questions for further research.

CONCLUSION

Previous research has helped to narrow down the sports where left-sided athletes may have an advantage and possibly why (Loffing & Hagemann, 2012). Our review focused on sports where manual actions are central, but the discussion of performance differences between left- and right-sided athletes in one-on-one interactive sport situations also extends to footedness, for example, in soccer penalties (see Box 12.2). From the evidence reviewed here, we may conclude that a large part of the performance differences between left- and right-sided athletes in interactive sports may be explained by negative frequency-dependent selection mechanisms in combination with the respective sports' performance demands. Of course, this does not exclude the possibility that other processes or mechanisms inherent to left-handedness or more generally to left-hand control may facilitate performance.

For sport practitioners, one obvious consequence of the left-sided advantage is to include left- and right-sided athletes into training (e.g., Harris, 2010; Sampras, 1998; Schwed, 1975) and/or to provide athletes with the opportunity to specifically counteract low familiarity with rarer "lefties," for example, via video-based perceptual training (Schorer et al., 2012). However, real experiences with left-sided athletes appear to be most important to allow athletes to develop perceptual-motor strategies and successfully react on otherwise unfamiliar consequences of left-sided actions. These unfamiliar consequences include different ball flight angles or reversed spin in ball flight when returning serves in tennis (Loffing, Hagemann, & Strauss, 2009) or batting in cricket (Edwards & Beaton, 1996). If coaches or athletes systematically and increasingly adopt a strategy of increasing exposure to lefties in sports where left-sided athletes seem to have an advantage today, an interesting question is whether their

---

BOX 12.2

LEFT-FOOTER ADVANTAGE IN SOCCER PENALTIES?

Footedness is strongly related to handedness (e.g., Tran, Stieger, & Voracek, 2014). Consequently, right-footedness is also more common than left-footedness (Coren, 1993); however, the imbalance is not as dramatic compared to handedness. For example, about 20% of the normal population prefer their left foot for kicking a ball, which is similar to the proportion in professional soccer players (for details, see Chapter 14: Laterality Effects on Performance in Team Sports: Insights From Soccer and Basketball by Stöckel & Carey, in this book).

In soccer penalties, however, the frequency of left-footed kickers seems to be higher than expected. For example, in an analysis of 999 penalties taken in the first German soccer league (1. Bundesliga) between 1995 and 2007, Baumann, Friehe, and Wedow (2011; see also Dohmen, 2008) reported that 35% of these penalties were kicked with the left foot. Moreover, left-footed kickers (76.22%) had a higher probability of scoring than right-footers (72.15%). These findings indicate a possible left-footers' advantage in soccer penalties. The underlying perceptual-cognitive mechanisms for this advantage could be similar to those suggested for explaining a left-handers' advantage in interactive sports (Hagemann, 2009).

To preserve the chances of successfully saving a penalty, soccer goalkeepers try to anticipate a penalty-taker's shot direction and initiate defensive moves accordingly. For example, a goalie may anticipate based on knowledge of a shooter's kicking preferences and/or a penalty-taker's movement during his or her run-up and/or kicking motion before making contact with the ball (for a review, e.g., see Memmert, Hüttermann, Hagemann, Loffing, & Strauss, 2013). Laboratory experiments suggest that goalkeepers have more difficulties anticipating the outcomes of left-footed as opposed to right-footed soccer penalties (Loffing & Hagemann, 2014; McMorris & Colenso, 1996). Consequently, the above-cited elevated proportion of left-footed penalty-takers and seemingly higher success rates in these kickers might be attributed, at least in part, to differences in goalkeepers' perceptual-cognitive skills against left- versus right-footed penalty-takers. Alternatively, left-footed kickers might also be more skilled in kicking with their dominant foot compared to right-footers, as suggested by a study on Australian rules footballers (Cameron & Adams, 2003).

However, data in support of a left-footed penalty-takers' advantage are far from definite. Out of 459 penalties taken in the Italian ($n = 242$ kicks; 1997–2000) and the French first-division league ($n = 217$ kicks; 1997–99),

continued

BOX 12.2   *(cont'd)*

only 16.34% were kicked left-footed and the scoring rate was worse in left-footers (66.67%) than right-footers (76.56%) (Coloma, 2007). Hughes and Wells (2002) did not find evidence of a footedness difference in scoring success in a sample of 129 penalties taken in FIFA World Cup finals and finals of the European Champions League. Finally, in an analysis of 478 penalties taken at FIFA World Cup finals, Schorer, Rienhoff, Loffing, and Baker (2015) found that while left-footers (kicking 19.87% of all penalties) were as successful as right-footers in penalties during regular match-play (86.7% vs. 84.0%), left-footers' success rate was lower compared to right-footers for penalties during play-off matches (69.2% vs. 75.1%). Thus in high-pressure situations where an individual's failure may eliminate a team from a tournament or from winning the cup, left-footers appeared to choke more than right-footers. Collectively, in light of the obvious ambiguity in findings, more systematic investigation of the effect of footedness on kicking in soccer penalties seems warranted.

---

advantage will persist in the future. The NFDS hypothesis predicts that the advantage would decrease or even disappear (Loffing, Hagemann, et al., 2012), possibly more so in low than high time-pressure interactive sports (Loffing, 2015), whereas the innate superiority hypothesis would not predict any systematic changes over time.

Despite often confident interpretations of findings in either direction (i.e., innate superiority vs. negative frequency dependence), we hope to have made clear in this chapter that there is still much to be learned about the mechanisms and processes potentially provoking performance differences between left- and right-sided athletes. The points listed below extend or emphasize previously cited directions for further research. By doing so, we would like to invite and stimulate concerted efforts on these issues.

To allow for the complexity of the processes underlying skilled performance in sports, we suggest extending the research framework through inclusion of potentially performance-relevant psychological measures such as personality traits (Aggleton & Wood, 1990). Although it is a tough challenge, we also advocate more unambiguous evidence in favor of and against different explanatory approaches (Groothuis et al., 2013; Loffing & Hagemann, 2015). This may be realized, for example, through experiments including training interventions (e.g., Schorer et al., 2012) or through longitudinal analyses of comprehensive performance datasets (e.g., Clotfelter, 2008). Last but not least, while previous research focused on laterality effects in adult competition (for an exception, e.g., see Sterkowicz et al., 2010), we anticipate that directing our attention toward youth athletes will deepen our understanding of possibly mediating effects of laterality on the development of sporting expertise (see also Chapter 5: Laterality and its Role in Talent Identification and Athlete Development, by Schorer, Tirp, Steingröver, & Baker, in this book).

References

Aggleton, J. P., & Wood, C. J. (1990). Is there a left-handed advantage in 'allistic' sports? *International Journal of Sport Psychology, 21*, 46–57.

Allen, M. S., Greenlees, I., & Jones, M. (2013). Personality in sport: a comprehensive review. *International Review of Sport and Exercise Psychology, 6*, 184–208.

Archer, J. (2006). Testosterone and human aggression: an evaluation of the challenge hypothesis. *Neuroscience & Biobehavioral Reviews, 30*, 319–345.

Azémar, G., Ripoll, H., Simonet, P., & Stein, J. F. (1983). Étude neuro-psychologique du comportement des gauchers en escrime. *Cinésiologie, 22*, 7–18.

Baker, J., Kungl, A.-M., Pabst, J., Strauss, B., Büsch, D., & Schorer, J. (2013). Your fate is in your hands? Handedness, digit ratio (2D:4D), and selection to a national talent development system. *Laterality: Asymmetries of Body, Brain and Cognition, 18*, 710–718.

Baker, J., & Schorer, J. (2013). The southpaw advantage? - lateral preference in mixed martial arts. *PLoS One, 8*, e79793.

Baumann, F., Friehe, T., & Wedow, M. (2011). General ability and specialization: evidence from penalty kicks in soccer. *Journal of Sports Economics, 12*, 81–105.

Bisiacchi, P. S., Ripoll, H., Stein, J. F., Simonet, P., & Azémar, G. (1985). Left-handedness in fencers: an attentional advantage? *Perceptual and Motor Skills, 61*, 507–513.

Boulinguez, P. (1999). Les avantages liés à la latéralité manuelle en escrime sont-ils l'expression d'asymétries cérébrales fonctionnelles? *Schweizerische Zeitschrift für Sportmedizin und Sporttraumatologie, 47*, 63–67.

Boulinguez, P., Ferrois, M., & Graumer, G. (2003). Hemispheric asymmetry for trajectory perception. *Cognitive Brain Research, 16*, 219–225.

Breznik, K. (2013). On the gender effects of handedness in professional tennis. *Journal of Sports Science and Medicine, 12*, 346–353.

Briggs, G. G., & Nebes, R. D. (1975). Patterns of hand preference in a student population. *Cortex, 11*, 230–238.

Brooks, R., Bussière, L. F., Jennions, M. D., & Hunt, J. (2004). Sinister strategies succeed at the cricket World Cup. *Proceedings of the Royal Society of London. Series B: Biological Sciences, 271*, S64–S66.

Cameron, M., & Adams, R. (2003). Kicking footedness and movement discrimination by elite Australian rules footballers. *Journal of Science and Medicine in Sport, 6*, 266–274.

Clotfelter, E. D. (2008). Frequency-dependent performance and handedness in professional baseball players. *Journal of Comparative Psychology, 122*, 68–72.

Coloma, G. (2007). Penalty kicks in soccer: an alternative methodology for testing mixed-strategy equilibria. *Journal of Sports Economics, 8*, 530–545.

Coren, S. (1993). The lateral preference inventory for measurement of handedness, footedness, eyedness, and earedness: norms for young adults. *Bulletin of the Psychonomic Society, 31*, 1–3.

Coren, S. (1994). Personality differences between left- and right-handers: an overlooked minority group? *Journal of Research in Personality, 28*, 214–229.

del Corral, J., & Prieto-Rodríguez, J. (2010). Are differences in ranks good predictors for Grand Slam tennis matches? *International Journal of Forecasting, 26,* 551–563.

Dane, S., & Erzurumluoglu, A. (2003). Sex and handedness differences in eye-hand visual reaction times in handball players. *International Journal of Neuroscience, 113,* 923–929.

Dane, S., & Sekertekin, M. A. (2005). Differences in handedness and scores of aggressiveness and interpersonal relations of soccer players. *Perceptual and Motor Skills, 100,* 743–746.

Dicks, M., Davids, K., & Button, C. (2009). Representative task designs for the study of perception and action in sport. *International Journal of Sport Psychology, 40,* 506–524.

Dohmen, T. J. (2008). Do professionals choke under pressure? *Journal of Economic Behavior & Organization, 65,* 636–653.

Eastwood, P. (1972). Studies in games playing: laterality in a games context. In H. T. A. Whiting (Ed.), *Readings in sports psychology* (pp. 228–237). London: Lepus.

Edwards, S., & Beaton, A. (1996). Howzat?! Why is there an over-representation of left-handed bowlers in professional cricket in the UK? *Laterality: Asymmetries of Body, Brain and Cognition, 1,* 45–50.

Faurie, C., Llaurens, V., Alvergne, A., Goldberg, M., Zins, M., & Raymond, M. (2011). Left-handedness and male-male competition: Insights from fighting and hormonal data. *Evolutionary Psychology, 9,* 354–370.

Faurie, C., & Raymond, M. (2013). The fighting hypothesis as an evolutionary explanation for the handedness polymorphism in humans: where are we? *Annals of the New York Academy of Sciences, 1288,* 110–113.

Geschwind, N., & Behan, P. (1982). Left-handedness: association with immune disease, migraine, and developmental learning disorder. *Proceedings of the National Academy of Sciences of the United States of America, 79,* 5097–5100.

Geschwind, N., & Galaburda, A. M. (1985a). Cerebral lateralization. Biological mechanisms, associations, and pathology: I. A hypothesis and a program for research. *Archives of Neurology, 42,* 428–459.

Geschwind, N., & Galaburda, A. M. (1985b). Cerebral lateralization. Biological mechanisms, associations, and pathology: II. A hypothesis and a program for research. *Archives of Neurology, 42,* 521–552.

Geschwind, N., & Galaburda, A. M. (1985c). Cerebral lateralization. Biological mechanisms, associations, and pathology: III. A hypothesis and a program for research. *Archives of Neurology, 42,* 634–654.

Gilbert, A. N., & Wysocki, C. J. (1992). Hand preference and age in the United States. *Neuropsychologia, 30,* 601–608.

Goldstein, S. R., & Young, C. A. (1996). "Evolutionary" stable strategy of handedness in major league baseball. *Journal of Comparative Psychology, 110,* 164–169.

Gorynia, I., & Egenter, D. (2000). Intermanual coordination in relation to handedness, familial sinistrality and lateral preferences. *Cortex, 36,* 1–18.

Grimshaw, G. M., & Wilson, M. S. (2012). A sinister plot? Facts, beliefs, and stereotypes about the left-handed personality. *Laterality: Asymmetries of Body, Brain and Cognition, 18,* 135–151.

Grondin, S., Guiard, Y., Ivry, R. B., & Koren, S. (1999). Manual laterality and hitting performance in major league baseball. *Journal of Experimental Psychology: Human Perception & Performance, 25,* 747–754.

Groothuis, T. G. G., McManus, I. C., Schaafsma, S. M., & Geuze, R. H. (2013). The fighting hypothesis in combat: how well does the fighting hypothesis explain human left-handed minorities? *Annals of the New York Academy of Sciences, 1288,* 100–109.

Grouios, G. (2004). Motoric dominance and sporting excellence: training versus heredity. *Perceptual and Motor Skills, 98,* 53–66.

Grouios, G., Koidou, I., Tsorbatzoudis, H., & Alexandris, K. (2002). Handedness in sport. *Journal of Human Movement Studies, 43,* 347–361.

Grouios, G., Tsorbatzoudis, H., Alexandris, K., & Barkoukis, V. (2000). Do left-handed competitors have an innate superiority in sports? *Perceptual and Motor Skills*, *90*, 1273–1282.

Guiard, Y., Diaz, G., & Beaubaton, D. (1983). Left-hand advantage in right-handers for spatial constant error: preliminary evidence in a unimanual ballistic aimed movement. *Neuropsychologia*, *21*, 111–115.

Gursoy, R. (2009). Effects of left- or right-hand preference on the success of boxers in Turkey. *British Journal of Sports Medicine*, *43*, 142–144.

Hagemann, N. (2009). The advantage of being left-handed in interactive sports. *Attention, Perception, & Psychophysics*, *71*, 1641–1648.

Harris, L. J. (2010). In fencing, what gives left-handers the edge? Views from the present and the distant past. *Laterality: Asymmetries of Body, Brain and Cognition*, *15*, 15–55.

Hirotsu, N., & Wright, M. (2005). Modelling a baseball game to optimise pitcher substitution strategies incorporating handedness of players. *IMA Journal of Management Mathematics*, *16*, 179–194.

Holtzen, D. W. (2000). Handedness and professional tennis. *International Journal of Neuroscience*, *105*, 101–119.

Hsu, Y., Earley, R. L., & Wolf, L. L. (2006). Modulation of aggressive behaviour by fighting experience: mechanisms and contest outcomes. *Biological Reviews*, *81*, 33–74.

Hughes, M. D., & Wells, J. (2002). Analysis of penalties taken in shoot-outs. *International Journal of Performance Analysis in Sport*, *2*, 55–72.

Iwabuchi, S. J., & Kirk, I. J. (2009). A typical interhemispheric communication in left-handed individuals. *Neuroreport*, *20*, 166–169.

Judge, J., & Stirling, J. (2003). Fine motor skill performance in left- and right-handers: evidence of an advantage for left-handers. *Laterality: Asymmetries of Body, Brain and Cognition*, *8*, 297–306.

Loffing, F. (2015). *Left-hander frequency in professional racket sports is related to underlying time constraints* (Manuscript submitted for publication).

Loffing, F., & Hagemann, N. (2012). Side bias in human performance: a review on the left-handers' advantage in sports. In T. Dutta, M. Mandal, & S. Kumar (Eds.), *Bias in human behaviour* (pp. 163–182). Hauppauge, NY: Nova Science.

Loffing, F., & Hagemann, N. (2014). Zum Einfluss des Anlaufwinkels und der Füßigkeit des Schützen auf die Antizipation von Elfmeterschüssen. [On the effect of a shooter's approach angle and kicking foot on the anticipation of penalty-kicks]. *Zeitschrift für Sportpsychologie*, *21*, 63–73.

Loffing, F., & Hagemann, N. (2015). Pushing through evolution? Incidence and fight records of left-oriented fighters in professional boxing history. *Laterality: Asymmetries of Body, Brain and Cognition*, *20*, 270–286.

Loffing, F., Hagemann, N., Schorer, J., & Baker, J. (2015). Skilled players' and novices' difficulty anticipating left- vs. right-handed opponents' action intentions varies across different points in time. *Human Movement Science*, *40*, 410–421.

Loffing, F., Hagemann, N., & Strauss, B. (2009). The serve in professional men's tennis: effects of players' handedness. *International Journal of Performance Analysis in Sport*, *9*, 255–274.

Loffing, F., Hagemann, N., & Strauss, B. (2010). Automated processes in tennis: do left-handed players benefit from the tactical preferences of their opponents? *Journal of Sports Sciences*, *28*, 435–443.

Loffing, F., Hagemann, N., & Strauss, B. (2012). Left-handedness in professional and amateur tennis. *PLoS One*, *7*, e49325.

Loffing, F., Schorer, J., Hagemann, N., & Baker, J. (2012). On the advantage of being left-handed in volleyball: further evidence of the specificity of skilled visual perception. *Attention, Perception, & Psychophysics*, *74*, 446–453.

Loffing, F., Sölter, F., & Hagemann, N. (2014). Left preference for sport tasks does not necessarily indicate left-handedness: sport-specific lateral preferences, relationship with handedness and implications for laterality research in behavioural sciences. *PLoS One*, *9*, e105800.

Loffing, F., Sölter, F., Hagemann, N., & Strauss, B. (2015). Accuracy of outcome anticipation, but not gaze behavior, differs against left- and right-handed penalties in team-handball goalkeeping. *Frontiers in Psychology*, *6*.

Lundie, R. A. (1896). Left-handedness. *Chamber's Journal of Popular Literature, Science and Arts*, *73*, 9–12.

McLean, J. M., & Ciurczak, F. M. (1982). Bimanual dexterity in major league baseball players: a statistical study. *The New England Journal of Medicine*, *307*, 1278–1279.

McManus, I. C. (2002). *Right hand, left hand: The origins of asymmetry in brains, bodies, atoms and culture*. London: Weidenfeld & Nicolson.

McMorris, T., & Colenso, S. (1996). Anticipation of professional soccer goalkeepers when facing right- and left-footed penalty kicks. *Perceptual and Motor Skills*, *82*, 931–934.

Memmert, D., Hüttermann, S., Hagemann, N., Loffing, F., & Strauss, B. (2013). Dueling in the penalty box: evidence-based recommendations on how shooters and goalkeepers can win penalty shootouts in soccer. *International Review of Sport and Exercise Psychology*, *6*, 209–229.

Mikheev, M., Mohr, C., Afanasiev, S., Landis, T., & Thut, G. (2002). Motor control and cerebral hemispheric specialization in highly qualified judo wrestlers. *Neuropsychologia*, *40*, 1209–1219.

Oldfield, R. C. (1971). The assessment and analysis of handedness: the Edinburgh inventory. *Neuropsychologia*, *9*, 97–113.

Peters, M., Reimers, S., & Manning, J. T. (2006). Hand preference for writing and associations with selected demographic and behavioral variables in 255,100 subjects: the BBC internet study. *Brain and Cognition*, *62*, 177–189.

Petit, L., Zago, L., Mellet, E., Jobard, G., Crivello, F., Joliot, M., ... Tzourio-Mazoyer, N. (2015). Strong rightward lateralization of the dorsal attentional network in left-handers with right sighting-eye: an evolutionary advantage. *Human Brain Mapping*, *36*, 1151–1164.

Pollet, T. V., & Riegmann, B. R. (2014). Opponent left-handedness does not affect fight outcomes for ultimate fighting championship hall of famers. *Frontiers in Psychology*, *5*, 375.

Pollet, T. V., Stulp, G., & Groothuis, T. G. G. (2013). Born to win? Testing the fighting hypothesis in realistic fights: left-handedness in the ultimate fighting championship. *Animal Behaviour*, *86*, 839–843.

Punzalan, D., Rodd, F. H., & Hughes, K. A. (2005). Perceptual processes and the maintenance of polymorphism through frequency-dependent predation. *Evolutionary Ecology*, *19*, 303–320.

Puterman, J., Schorer, J., & Baker, J. (2010). Laterality differences in elite ice hockey: an investigation of shooting and catching orientations. *Journal of Sports Sciences*, *28*, 1581–1593.

Raymond, M., Pontier, D., Dufour, A. B., & Møller, A. P. (1996). Frequency-dependent maintenance of left handedness in humans. *Proceedings of the Royal Society of London. Series B: Biological Sciences*, *263*, 1627–1633.

Sampras, P. (1998). Don't let southpaws scare you: after losing some tough matches to left-handers, we learned how to handle them. *Tennis*, *34*, 142–145.

Schorer, J., Cobley, S., Büsch, D., Bräutigam, H., & Baker, J. (2009). Influences of competition level, gender, player nationality, career stage and playing position on relative age effects. *Scandinavian Journal of Medicine & Science in Sports*, *19*, 720–730.

Schorer, J., Loffing, F., Hagemann, N., & Baker, J. (2012). Human handedness in interactive situations: negative perceptual frequency effects can be reversed!. *Journal of Sports Sciences*, *30*, 507–513.

Schorer, J., Rienhoff, R., Loffing, F., & Baker, J. (2015). Left kickers choke during play-offs in soccer penalties. *Talent Development & Excellence*, *7*, 91-94.

Schwed, P. (1975). *Sinister tennis. How to play against and with left-handers.* New York: Doubleday.

Sinervo, B., & Calsbeek, R. (2006). The developmental, physiological, neural, and genetical causes and consequences of frequency-dependent selection in the wild. *Annual Review of Ecology, Evolution, and Systematics, 37,* 581–610.

Sterkowicz, S., Lech, G., & Blecharz, J. (2010). Effects of laterality on the technical/tactical behavior in view of the results of judo fights. *Archives of Budo, 6,* 173–177.

Taddei, F., Viggiano, M. P., & Mecacci, L. (1991). Pattern reversal visual evoked potentials in fencers. *International Journal of Psychophysiology, 11,* 257–260.

Takahashi, Y., & Kawata, M. (2013). A comprehensive test for negative frequency-dependent selection. *Population Ecology, 55,* 499–509.

Tirp, J., Baker, J., Weigelt, M., & Schorer, J. (2014). Combat stance in judo – laterality differences between and within competition levels. *International Journal of Performance Analysis in Sport, 14,* 217–224.

Toga, A. W., & Thompson, P. M. (2003). Mapping brain asymmetry. *Nature Reviews Neuroscience, 4,* 37–48.

Tran, U. S., Stieger, S., & Voracek, M. (2014). Evidence for general right-, mixed-, and left-sidedness in self-reported handedness, footedness, eyedness, and earedness, and a primacy of footedness in a large-sample latent variable analysis. *Neuropsychologia, 62,* 220–232.

Williams, A. M., & Ericsson, K. A. (2005). Perceptual-cognitive expertise in sport: some considerations when applying the expert performance approach. *Human Movement Science, 24,* 283–307.

Wood, C. J., & Aggleton, J. P. (1989). Handedness in "fast ball" sports: do left-handers have an innate advantage? *British Journal of Psychology, 80,* 227–240.

Yarrow, K., Brown, P., & Krakauer, J. W. (2009). Inside the brain of an elite athlete: the neural processes that support high achievement in sports. *Nature Reviews Neuroscience, 10,* 585–596.

Ziyagil, M. A., Gursoy, R., Dane, S., & Yuksel, R. (2010). Left-handed wrestlers are more successful. *Perceptual and Motor Skills, 111,* 65–70.

13

Biomechanical Considerations of Laterality in Sport

Lucy Parrington

Swinburne University of Technology, Melbourne, VIC, Australia

Kevin Ball

Victoria University, Melbourne, VIC, Australia

INTRODUCTION

Proficient athletes appear to display effortless movement and fluid coordination patterns with mechanical equivalency between limbs. Whether the skill in question be cyclic in nature, such as running, or discrete motion, such as kicking a football, it is commonly believed that technical similarities between the dominant and nondominant limbs is beneficial to sporting performance. Symmetry between dominant and nondominant limbs in repetitive tasks is also believed to be beneficial in reducing the chances of limb compensation and repetitive-use injury.

Biomechanists have the ability to assess these factors. Biomechanics researchers are primarily concerned with the evaluation of right/left limb kinematics and coordination profiles and any underpinning kinetic mechanisms. Research may be conducted on a large sample of athletes in order to establish a guide of what general parts of the movement require focus during training. The applied biomechanist may also assess the technique of one or more athlete(s), in order to evaluate the movement characteristics necessary to evoke any changes required to either improve technique or reduce the chances of injury.

This chapter will explore the biomechanics of laterality, focusing on the effects of laterality on performance and injury. The proceeding chapter is divided into four main sections, including the biomechanical assessment of asymmetries, limb dominance in cyclic and repetitive movement

Laterality in Sports
http://dx.doi.org/10.1016/B978-0-12-801426-4.00013-4

patterns, and assessments of dominant and nondominant limb skills. The final section discusses methodological issues related to biomechanical approaches to assessing laterality.

BIOMECHANICAL ASSESSMENT OF ASYMMETRIES

How limb dominance and movement asymmetries affect performance or increase risk of injury across varying sports still requires clarification. Generally, bilateral differences between the right and left sides of the body are believed to cause a decrement to performance, or predispose athletes to injury. This makes the assessment of symmetry/asymmetry between the limbs an important process that should be conducted at the start of any training or program. Athletes should also be monitored regularly throughout the completion of training blocks or throughout their competitive season, such that modifications to training programs can be made when required in order to minimize the effects of asymmetries.

It may be possible for athletes to perform well despite movement discrepancies between left and right limbs; however, athletes and coaches may be concerned if asymmetries cause problems with mechanical efficiency, or if a lack of technical skill from one limb constrains the overall ability of the athlete. If an athlete has issues with mechanical efficiency, additional energy may be required in order to produce the movement, thereby causing a detriment to the potential performance of the athlete. Technical skill discrepancies between sides of the body in sports where rules allow either limb to be used (e.g., soccer, handball) are disadvantageous, because athletes are then reliant on the preferred or dominant limb. We will take a deeper look into preferred and nonpreferred limb use in kicking and throwing skills later in this chapter.

Asymmetries that put athletes at greater risk of injury may be of primary concern to team practitioners, especially where differences can be trained and improved. There is a wealth of research that indicates balance, muscular control, strength, and flexibility differences between limbs can predispose athletes to injury. Examples of this include balance (anterior reach asymmetry on Y-balance test associated with increased noncontact injury risk, Smith, Chimera, & Warren, 2014; anterior reach asymmetry on Star Excursion Balance Test associated with lower extremity injury, Plisky, Rauh, Kaminski, & Underwood, 2006) and strength asymmetries (ankle strength, Baumhauer, Alosa, Renström, Trevino, & Beynnon, 1995; eccentric hamstring strength, Fousekis, Tsepis, Poulmedis, Athanasopoulos, & Vagenas, 2010; hip flexor/knee extensor imbalances, Knapick, Bauman,

Jones, Harris, & Vaughan, 1991; hip muscle imbalance in females, Nadler et al., 2001; hamstring to quadriceps muscle ratio asymmetry, Söderman, Alfredson, Pietilä, & Werner, 2001).

A multidisciplinary approach involving biomechanics, skill acquisition, strength and conditioning, and physiotherapy is required to identify, correct, and monitor asymmetries in athletes in order to improve performance and reduce the chance of injury. Biomechanics researchers play a major role in the identification and evaluation of asymmetries. Now we will look at the methods by which asymmetries can be identified.

HOW DO WE IDENTIFY AND ASSESS ASYMMETRIES?

The identification and assessment of right–left asymmetries can be made using a number of different computational or observational methods. We will first look at the use of computational methods, starting with the commonly conducted method of strength assessment known as isokinetic dynamometry.

Strength Testing Using Isokinetic Dynamometry

An isokinetic dynamometer is a device used within sports and exercise science as well as clinical testing environments that is used to evaluate joint torque. Isokinetic dynamometers are able to test the strength (torque) and power of different muscle groups. The equipment can be modified in order to assess a number of different upper and lower body limb motions. The isokinetic dynamometer isolates the joint of interest, which allows targeted testing of particular muscle groups. In addition to this, settings can be changed to evaluate muscle performance across differing speeds and particular ranges of motion and can accommodate isometric, isokinetic, and isotonic (both eccentric and concentric) muscle action. The ability to precisely test joint torque over a number of different settings provides a thorough evaluation method to compare between right and left limbs and identify any injury risk or areas for improvement.

Kinetic Evaluation

Force plate analysis can be conducted on static balance tasks, gait, and jumping and landing tasks to help identify right–left movement asymmetries. The force plates used in biomechanics research (e.g., mainly strain gauge or piezoelectric) have the ability to measure three orthogonal ground reaction forces (Fx, Fy, and Fz), moment components (Mx, My, and Mz), and center of pressure. Thus this instrument can be used across a number of movement tasks, for example:

1. Gait analysis:
   Assessment of ground reaction forces between right and left foot steps is a well acknowledged method for the evaluation of right–left asymmetries in walking and running (Herzog, Nigg, Read, & Olsson, 1989).
2. Jumping and landing techniques:
   Testing vertical ground reaction forces in jumping has been identified as a valid and reliable tool for the assessment of bilateral strength asymmetry, demonstrating significant correlations with isokinetic strength testing (Impellizzeri, Rampinini, Maffiuletti, & Marcora, 2007). Similarly, testing the force profile of the right and left legs during landing can identify potential injury risks (Dufek & Bates, 1991), or predict reoccurring injury (e.g., postreconstructive ACL tear, Paterno et al., 2010).
3. Center of pressure profiles in balance tasks:
   Measuring the center of pressure to provide an estimate of the center of gravity and a representation of balance is generally well accepted in the evaluation of static balance tasks (Benda, Riley, & Krebs, 1994). Thus the evaluation of center of pressure on the right and the left leg using single-leg standing tasks can help to identify balance asymmetries.

Two-Dimensional or Three-Dimensional Kinematic Assessment

Kinematic assessment can also be used to identify bilateral differences in upper and lower extremity movement. Kinematic assessment involves using media such as video cameras, high-speed video, or three-dimensional motion analysis systems, with markers on the body to be tracked through the movement. Using this tracked data in either two-dimensional or three-dimensional space, joint and body segment positions, velocities, and accelerations can be calculated and compared between sides of the body. This type of analysis may be conducted on fundamental movements or sport-specific tasks to identify right–left differences and identify injury risks (Gundersen et al., 1989; Pappas & Carpes, 2012; Zifchock, Davis, Higginson, McCaw, & Royer, 2008).

Functional Assessment

Functional assessment is a popular way of identifying movement limitations or asymmetry that does not require advanced biomechanical hardware or software. These assessments may involve the rating of movement quality from the practitioner or using simple measurements. One type of functional assessment, which has gathered popularity since 2010, is the use

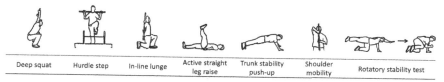

| Deep squat | Hurdle step | In-line lunge | Active straight leg raise | Trunk stability push-up | Shoulder mobility | Rotatory stability test |

FIGURE 13.1   Examples of the seven key movements tested during the FMS. *Adapted from Functional Movement Systems [FMS]. (March 02, 2015). Functional movement screening. Retrieved from:* http://www.functionalmovement.com.

of Functional Movement Screening (FMS™). This screening tool is used to identify movement limitations and limb asymmetries by examining a combination of strength, balance, flexibility, range of motion, and coordination during seven selected movement patterns (see Fig. 13.1). As the athlete completes each of the movements, the practitioner rates the athlete from zero to three. The sum of these scores is then used to identify the functional movement of the athlete. As with any rating tool, it is important that intra-rater reliability is high. The FMS has been identified as having high intra-rater reliability (ICC = 0.98). In addition, researchers have identified that athletes with lower FMS scores were more likely to incur injury in comparison with their higher-scoring counterparts (Kiesel, Plisky, & Voight, 2007).

ASYMMETRY AND LIMB DOMINANCE IN CYCLIC AND REPETITIVE MOVEMENT PATTERNS

The lateralization of motor functions is believed to occur as a result of heritable traits and developmental factors throughout the lifespan (Carter-Saltzman, 1980; Llaurens, Raymond, & Faurie, 2009). Focusing on developmental factors here, having a preference to use one side of the body can cause uneven flexibility, range of movement, strength development, and neural development occurring on the favored side. Thus laterality factors such as handedness or footedness and side dominance can lead to bilateral asymmetries. It is even quite common to see kinematic and kinetic asymmetries in repetitive and cyclic/alternating motor tasks such as running, cycling, and swimming. This is despite the fact that both limbs should be moving through similar ranges of motion, and thus adaptive changes are expected to occur evenly on either side of the body. In addition to this, repetitive training or habitual recreational activity that further favors one side of the body may also lead to, or exacerbate, asymmetries. For example, on reflection of the possible factors leading to asymmetries in swimming technique, Sanders and colleagues state:

> "Although the opportunity for muscular development on both sides should be equivalent given the symmetrical nature of swimming, the bilateral differences inherited from other activities may be reinforced rather than removed due to unwittingly favoring the stronger muscles" *Sanders, Thow, & Fairweather (2011, p. 4).*

Now we will look at the way in which asymmetries appear in different fundamental movements.

RUNNING

Running has been a popular form of physical activity for recreation, competition, or cross-training since the 1970s (Novacheck, 1998). Currently around 30 million people in the United States run at least once a week (Running USA, 2014). In addition to the number of people who run for recreation or competition, there are many people who partake in repeated bouts of running as a part of his or her selected sport (e.g., soccer, basketball, lacrosse).

Throughout the running gait cycle, there are alternate periods of deceleration and acceleration (Cavanagh, 1990; Novacheck, 1998). The equal ability to absorb and generate force throughout these periods by both the dominant and nondominant limb therefore becomes a topical point where asymmetry is concerned. Atypical mechanics, for example, such as an increase in the load per foot touchdown being absorbed, or an increase in propulsion by one side of the body, may be detrimental to the runner after prolonged training. Unfortunately the role that laterality is considered to play in running asymmetries has not been well-defined.

Fluctuating and Directional Asymmetries in Running

The level of symmetry/asymmetry and its association with bilateral dominance in running appears to be highly individual and dependent upon what is being measured. Research has identified that the dominant leg of runners has the ability to generate more force, though the influence this has on running mechanics remains in question. Both sprinters and distance runners have been found to exhibit bilateral strength asymmetries of approximately 8% (Vagenas & Hoshizaki, 1986, 1991). Distance runners were found to have statistically stronger knee flexion, extension, and total strength in the dominant leg. Yet, interestingly, the flexion to extension ratio was greater in the nondominant leg, indicating more balance between knee flexion strength and extension strength on the nondominant side.

The ability to generate more force from a strength-dominant leg was found to be beneficial in the sprint takeoff. Vagenas and Hoshizaki (1986) found greater takeoff velocity, and sprint times were achieved when the dominant leg was placed in front of the sprint-starting blocks. The determination of the strength dominant leg was determined through a single leg jump on a force platform. Pappas, Paradisis, and Vagenas (2015) determined the dominant leg of their participants through a similar functional strength task: a single leg triple jump. Their findings indicated that the dominant leg produced greater maximum ground reaction force during contact and a longer flight time in comparison with the nondominant leg during treadmill running. No significant asymmetries were found for leg stiffness parameters.

As well as measuring functional strength, Vagenas and Hoshizaki (1991) demonstrated that the dominant limb of distance runners allowed more eversion when the subtalar joint was passively tested for range of movement. Eversion range of motion and eversion to inversion range of motion ratio were found to be significantly greater in the dominant leg (for fluctuating asymmetry) and in the left leg (for directional asymmetry), while inversion range of motion was significantly greater in the nondominant leg.

Kinematic analyses have not provided definitive information relating to the influence of lower limb dominance on running parameters. For example, Brown, Zifchock, and Hillstrom (2014) found no significant differences between the dominant and nondominant leg in runners in either an unfatigued or fatigued state. On the other hand, Vagenas and Hoshizaki (1988, 1992) found a number of fluctuating and directional asymmetries in rearfoot motion (Fig. 13.2). Both studies indicated multifaceted lower limb

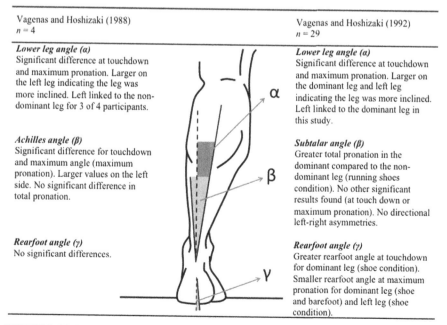

Vagenas and Hoshizaki (1988)
n = 4

Lower leg angle (α)
Significant difference at touchdown and maximum pronation. Larger on the left leg indicating the leg was more inclined. Left linked to the nondominant leg for 3 of 4 participants.

Achilles angle (β)
Significant difference for touchdown and maximum angle (maximum pronation). Larger values on the left side. No significant difference in total pronation.

Rearfoot angle (γ)
No significant differences.

Vagenas and Hoshizaki (1992)
n = 29

Lower leg angle (α)
Significant difference at touchdown and maximum pronation. Larger on the dominant leg and left leg indicating the leg was more inclined. Left linked to the dominant leg in this study.

Subtalar angle (β)
Greater total pronation in the dominant compared to the nondominant leg (running shoes condition). No other significant results found (at touch down or maximum pronation). No directional left-right asymmetries.

Rearfoot angle (γ)
Greater rearfoot angle at touchdown for dominant leg (shoe condition). Smaller rearfoot angle at maximum pronation for dominant leg (shoe and barefoot) and left leg (shoe condition).

FIGURE 13.2 Summary of selected rearfoot motion results of Vagenas and Hoshizaki (1988, 1992).

asymmetries, yet few results were reflected in both studies. Differences in findings in lateral dominance and running research may be an outcome of the methodological approaches used in the collection of data, participant samples, determination of dominant limb, parameters of interest, and mode of calculation for the assessment of asymmetry.

Considerations When Assessing Lateral Dominance and Asymmetries

As a number of researchers have reported mixed laterality in participants, with the level and direction of symmetry/asymmetry per parameter per participant varied (e.g., some kinematic measures greater on the left and others on the right), there may be potential issues with comparing right–left differences averaged across participants (Gunderson et al., 1989; Schieb, 1987; Vagenas & Hoshizaki, 1988). If comparisons between the dominant and nondominant leg are to be made, then the determination of the participant's dominant leg is an important factor for consideration. Unfortunately, there is a lack of consensus on the best method to approach this.

Pappas et al. (2015) noted a variety of criteria to determine leg dominance, including self-reports (perceived dominance, takeoff legs for jumping, kick leg preference) or functional tests (single leg jumps/hops on a force plate or for distance). It should be noted that a high level of agreement has been found between self-reported preferred kicking leg and perceived dominant leg, but that the perceived dominant leg may not actually reflect the stronger leg of participants (Vagenas & Hoshizaki, 1986). Finally, as bilateral differences in rearfoot kinematics during the contact phase have been indicated to vary as an outcome of the shoe and condition (Vagenas & Hoshizaki, 1988, 1992), this should be considered when assessing asymmetries from both an individual and group basis.

Asymmetry and Running Injuries

Some level of asymmetry in runners is believed to be normal, but whether asymmetry leads to injury or injury leads to asymmetry is a hard question to answer. Distance runners have the potential to clock up to 20,000 or more impacts per limb over just three training days per week. This means that small bilateral differences could potentially cause a negative effect after prolonged use.

The role that repeated impact loads and excessive eversion and pronation have with the contribution to overuse injuries has been debated within running-related literature (e.g., Cavanagh & Lafortune, 1980; Hreljac, 2004; Hreljac, Marshall, & Hume, 2000; James, Bates, & Osternig, 1978; Nielsen et al., 2014; Nigg, 2001; Zadpoor & Nikooyan, 2011). Yet, it is not clear whether the presence of asymmetry within these factors plays a causal role in overuse injuries. Similarly, there has been little to indicate that muscular imbalances or misalignments cause overuse injury (van Mechelen, 1992). It is plausible, however, that if asymmetries place one limb excessively outside the acceptable biological range, then the runner may be at risk of injury.

Studies have shown that runners with an injury history demonstrated patterns with greater vertical impact forces and loading rates (Hreljac et al., 2000). Furthermore, previously injured runners exhibited greater impact forces (Zifchock, Davis, & Hamill, 2006) and elevated peak tibial accelerations and range of hip internal rotation on the injured side (Zifchock et al., 2008). Yet the asymmetry levels for these parameters were found to be similar between injured and noninjured runners (Zifchock et al., 2006, 2008). Likewise, Bredeweg, Buist, and Kluitenberg (2013) demonstrated that asymmetries in impact peak, active peak, and loading rate were not significantly higher in previously injured runners.

On the other hand, Ciacci et al. found subelite sprinters who presented with previous hamstring strain injury to have greater knee flexion and less hip extension on the injured limb at the point of toe-off. The previously injured sprinters displayed symmetry indexes that exceeded clinical thresholds (15%, Ciacci, Di Michele, Fantozzi, & Merni, 2013), while in comparison, the symmetry indexes of uninjured sprinters were lower than the clinical threshold, demonstrating greater symmetry between the limbs.

CYCLING

Performance in cycling is determined by the ability to generate a high power output through the pedals. Both the right and left legs are expected to complete the same motion, yet despite the symmetrical requirements of the right and left sides of the body, cyclists have been found to frequently present with asymmetrical techniques. These bilateral differences appear to be dependent on the cycling configuration (e.g., cadence or resistance). Examples of pedaling asymmetries found in cycling studies include differences in force production (Daly & Cavanagh, 1976; Sanderson, 1990), crank torque (Carpes, Rossato, Faria, & Mota, 2007), and power output (Smak, Neptune, & Hull, 1999). Disparate findings have been found on asymmetries in cycling in relation to different workloads. While most studies (which we will cover in greater detail below) have demonstrated asymmetries between the left and right legs, they have failed to find consistent trends associated with increases or decreases in intensity. As a result, some authors believe that differences are dependent upon individual variability, experience, cadence, and workload, with bilateral changes associated with pedaling rate indicated to be subject-specific (e.g., Smak et al., 1999).

Limb Preference and Cycling Mechanics

In contrast to running research, many cycling studies have assessed bilateral comparisons using limb preference, determined by the preferred kick leg (e.g., Carpes, Rossato, Faria, & Mota, 2008; Smak et al., 1999) or by footedness questionnaire (e.g., Carpes Diefenthaeler, Bini, Stefanyshyn, Faria & Mota, 2010, 2011). The decision to assess asymmetries by this method may have stemmed from earlier findings, which demonstrated the effects of laterality on force propulsion during changes to pedal cadence using kick-leg preference but not strength dominance (Daly & Cavanagh, 1976).

Research suggests that the preferred leg is able to generate greater propulsive forces than the nonpreferred leg during cycling (e.g., peak crank torque, Carpes et al., 2007, 2008; greater average crank power, Smak et al., 1999). Interestingly, when Smak and colleagues observed asymmetries between preferred and nonpreferred sides, the results revealed a pattern whereby the preferred leg generated greater average crank power, while the nonpreferred side contributed more to average positive and negative power. It was suggested that the greater crank power in the preferred leg may be an outcome of a greater knee extensor moment that occurs during the power phase of the preferred leg. The authors also identified the greater hip extensor moment in the nonpreferred leg during the upstroke, which they suggested might hinder crank propulsion (of the preferred leg). If the preferred leg is not "hindering" the propulsion of the nonpreferred leg, this may help describe why the nonpreferred side contributed more to average positive and negative power.

Limb Preference and Muscle Activation

Carpes et al. (2010) conducted an interesting investigation into leg preference, efficiency, and muscle activation using unilateral cycling to assess legs in isolation. The study demonstrated similarity between preferred and nonpreferred legs for the magnitude of muscle activation, efficiency, and the oxygen uptake during unilateral pedaling. This finding occurred across both experienced and inexperienced cyclists, leading the authors to believe that any asymmetries in pedaling are not related to neuromuscular or muscle metabolism factors. Nonetheless, the authors acknowledge mechanical differences between unilateral and bipedal cycling. In unilateral cycling, there is no chance to catch out the possibility of one limb compensating for another.

Carpes et al. (2011) further investigated muscle activation in incremental and constant load bipedal cycling tests. In this study the authors found no difference in the magnitude of muscle activation between legs, but identified asymmetric patterns of variability in the electromyography signals that were influenced by exercise intensity in cyclists. Generally, across intensities, a higher coefficient of variation was exhibited in the nonpreferred limb.

The Effects of Intensity on Cycling Asymmetries

A number of authors have attempted to observe whether bilateral leg asymmetries change in accordance with increases in cycling intensity (Bertucci, Arfaoui, & Polidori, 2012; Carpes et al., 2007, 2008, 2010, 2011; Sanderson, 1990; Smak et al., 1999). In cycling, exercise intensity can be increased by increasing the power output (workload), which can be modified through changes to resistance or increased pedal cadence.

Whether pedal cadence plays a mediating role in the level of bilateral asymmetry appears to be dependent upon the parameter of interest and the total power output. For example, Sanderson (1990) demonstrated increased pedal cadence significantly increased work asymmetry (force specifically in the direction of pedaling) when working at a low workload (100 W). In comparison, Smak et al. (1999) found that increasing pedal cadence decreased percentage difference of average negative power between limbs. It should be noted, however, that the constant work rate used in Smak et al. (260 W) was higher than the two work rates used in Sanderson's research (100 and 235 W).

Cyclists in Sanderson's study exhibited lower work asymmetry at the higher workload; however, force asymmetry (the total linear impulse) generally remained constant across the conditions tested. Other research groups have indicated that peak crank torque asymmetry was less noticeable at the beginning and end points of a 40 km time-trial, which were characterized by higher intensity bouts (Carpes et al., 2007). It is unknown whether the increase in intensity here is due to an increase in pedal cadence or resistance.

More research conducted by Bertucci et al. (2012) on Masters-level cyclists appears to be in contrast with other previous findings. Bertucci et al. (2012) found asymmetries in peak torque between the right and left limbs for all power output conditions measured above 100 W (i.e., 150, 200 and 250 W).

The diverse findings here appear to support the idea that while bilateral asymmetries do occur frequently in cycling, the differences are dependent upon a number of factors such as individual differences, experience, and workload.

SWIMMING

Swimming performance is dependent upon the optimization of maximizing propulsion and minimizing resistive effects, while working within the physiological capabilities of the swimmer (Sanders, 2013). Bilateral

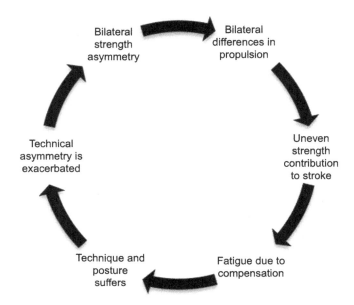

FIGURE 13.3 Example of bilateral asymmetries cycle: potential causes and effects. *Adapted from Sanders, R., McCabe, C., Alcock, A., Wright, L., Donald, N., Riach, I., & Fairweather, M. (2013). Case studies of asymmetries in swimming. In T. Shiang, W. Ho, P. Huang, & C. Tsai (Eds.), Proceedings of the 31st international conference on biomechanics in sports. Taipei, Taiwan. Retrieved from:* https://ojs.ub.uni-konstanz.de/cpa/article/download/5523/5017. *and Sanders, R.H. (2013). How do asymmetries affect swimming performance? Journal of Swimming Research, 21, 1–17. Retrieved from:* http://swimmingcoach.org/journal/manuscript-sanders-vol21.pdf.

differences in strength, flexibility, technique, and anthropometry can lead to issues relating to propulsion, resistance, or swimming efficiency, which result in performance decrements. Sanders and colleagues explain that these factors may be interconnected and thus should not be viewed in isolation (Fig. 13.3).

For example, right–left strength and flexibility asymmetries in either upper or lower limbs can cause uneven stroke contributions, which affects the propulsive ability of the swimmer. These asymmetries may manifest in problems with technique or posture, which can additionally increase resistive drag (Sanders, 2013). Here, we will focus predominantly on how side dominance and strength asymmetries can affect swimming performance.

Effects of Breathing Side Dominance

In front-crawl swimming, technical asymmetries can result from side dominance and the tendency to favor one side when breathing (Psycharakis & Sanders, 2008; Seifert, Chehensse, Tourny-Chollet, Lemaitre, & Chollet, 2008; Seifert, Chollet, & Allard, 2005). Seifert et al. (2005) found that a large number of participants (61%) exhibited a laterality profile where their dominant arm was on the preferred breathing side.

Breathing laterality has been strongly linked to force and coordination asymmetry (Seifert et al., 2008; Tourny-Chollet, Seifert, & Chollet, 2009) and power output (Potts, Charlton, & Smith, 2002). Seifert et al. (2008) found coordination asymmetries in unilateral breathing patterns to the preferred side, and greater asymmetry when swimmers were required to breathe only on their nonpreferred side. Furthermore, swimmers demonstrated greater shoulder roll according to the preferred breathing side (Psycharakis & Sanders, 2008).

The effect of side dominance and breathing asymmetry on performance has been found less in swimmers with bilateral, in comparison with unilateral, breathing patterns (Potts et al., 2002; Seifert et al., 2005). In order to avoid reinforcing any asymmetrical technique characteristics and any related imbalance, recommendations have been given to swimmers to train with symmetrical breathing patterns to reduce the tendency toward asymmetry arising from unilateral breathing techniques (Seifert et al., 2008).

Effects of Bilateral Strength Differences

Bilateral differences in strength may result in a different contribution to propulsion and affect the timing and coordination of the different stroke phases, which can decrease mechanical efficiency and overall performance. The duration of force application of the catch and pull in front-crawl swimming was found to be greater on the dominant side in comparison with the nondominant side in swimmers with force asymmetries (51.7% and 48.4%, respectively, Tourny-Chollet et al., 2009). This force asymmetry was related to the longer relative duration of medial rotator activity in these phases. Furthermore, bilateral asymmetry has been shown to occur more during the power phase (defined as from the catch to exit) in comparison with the recovery phase (Barden, Kell, & Kobsar, 2011). Barden and colleagues suggested that this finding was related to arm dominance. Interestingly, however, the hypothesis of Barden et al. that bilateral asymmetry would increase with swimming intensity, due to greater propulsive forces sought each stroke, was not supported. Instead, their research team found the inverse, where increased swimming intensity decreased the bilateral timing asymmetry of the phases.

Bilateral strength asymmetries may present issues relating to rotational balance, contribution to propulsion, and fatigue in swimmers. A stronger pull originating from one side of the body can result in unbalanced rotational torques, which affect the alignment and posture of the swimmer and in turn resistance. After observing asymmetries in power output using a simulated swim bench protocol, Potts and colleagues highlighted the following:

> "the potential performance gains expected from a relatively higher, but imbalanced muscular output, may be negated by the associated increase in resistive forces"
> *Potts et al., 2002, p. 978.*

In addition to unwanted resistive forces, bilateral strength differences may cause decreased mechanical efficiency in the stroke. That is, the alternation between strong and weak strokes in front-crawl or backstroke swimming or combined force during symmetrical swimming patterns would not be as strong as if both sides were making equal contributions (Sanders, 2013). Unequal stroke contributions due to strength asymmetry may further result in fatigue of the dominant strength or weaker limb, as the dominant limb is used to compensate for the weaker side, and the weaker side works harder to keep up (Sanders, 2013).

Sanders (2013) explains that the detriment caused by bilateral propulsion asymmetry will differ depending on the type of swimming stroke. In symmetrical strokes (e.g., breaststroke and butterfly), bilateral differences in the magnitude of the pull force can cause unwanted yawing rotations, which misalign the body and cause increased resistance (Sanders, 2013). In alternating strokes (e.g., front crawl and backstroke) the effect of any imbalance is dependent upon the distance between the midline of the body and the line of action of the hand during the pull. In backstroke, this distance is greater in comparison with front-crawl swimming, which means that there will be a greater bilateral torque difference as a result of strength imbalances in this swimming style. Introducing technical changes (i.e., changing the path of the hand) to help compensate for the difference may reinforce bilateral strength asymmetries and is not recommended (Sanders, 2013).

For more information the reader is directed to Sanders (2013) for a comprehensive discussion on how asymmetries can affect different phases of the stroke including propulsion, breathing, and recovery and entry.

COUNTERING THE EFFECTS OF BILATERAL ASYMMETRY

Asymmetries are believed to be detrimental, depending on the magnitude of the asymmetry, and therefore may potentially predispose athletes to injury. Because of the continuous and repetitive nature of cyclic movements, asymmetrical impact forces, joint torques, and muscle forces could lead to further bilateral changes in the biomechanics of the movement, which may in turn become detrimental to the athlete.

Biomechanical assessment can be conducted on athletes to evaluate asymmetries, which will allow targeted training interventions to offset any issues if necessary. Thus coaches and trainers should be aware of the need for athletes to maintain strength and flexibility throughout their training regime in order to maximize performance and minimize any chance of injury.

Whether assessing the kinematic or kinetic patterns of athletes, or assessing functional strength or flexibility, there are some considerations that need to be made. One important consideration is related to the determination of what level of asymmetry is classified as detrimental. For example, the clinical threshold used to assess asymmetry in Ciacci et al. (2013) was 15%. However, Karamanidis, Arampatzis, and Brüggmann (2003) demonstrated variability in symmetry indices, which were variable-dependent (e.g., <8% for linear/angular displacements vs. >15% for angular velocity).

Some researchers have quantified the level of asymmetry using different indices. Thus the mode of calculation can play an important role in assessment. Exell, Gittoes, Irwin, and Kerwin (2012) developed the idea of using composite kinetic and kinematic scores to help quantify asymmetry during sprinting. The composite asymmetry index accounted for intralimb variability, and the authors propose that these scores could be used in future investigations.

Given that asymmetries appear to be common across both uninjured and injured populations, another consideration is whether the identification of asymmetries through the assessment of running gait does not provide enough evidence for injury potential. For example, Ciacci et al. (2013) suggest that the kinematic assessment of sprinting could be used as a method for identifying hamstring strain risk because they had identified that hamstring strain was related to asymmetries in sprinting technique. But despite this relationship, the causal link between bilateral asymmetry and hamstring strain is yet to be determined.

Asymmetries across running, cycling, and swimming can be highly variable among subjects and may present in unique combinations. In addition to this, a number of factors, such as shoe condition and type of running shoe for runners or pedal rate for cyclists, indicated to potentially change the asymmetry profile, further highlighting the individuality of asymmetries. As a consequence, dealing with bilateral asymmetries may require an individual-based approach, rather than a blanket approach to address the needs of the athlete.

The first step in avoiding or reducing bilateral asymmetries should involve assessment during the movement or across a range of functionally related movements to accommodate for the individual. This process is important in order to identify where the asymmetry is occurring and a requirement in knowing what area (or areas) require improvement. It is important for coaches and other training staff to make an informed decision on whether to correct an asymmetry. Past researchers (e.g., Schieb, 1987) have cautioned that attempting to change ingrained patterns of movement may increase injury potential or decrease performance. Hamill, Gruber, and Derrick (2014), for example, indicated that attempting to change the foot strike pattern of one limb to match the other may not be an appropriate solution to avoid foot strike asymmetry in running. Furthermore, the authors indicated that changing between foot strike patterns can cause different joint stiffness actions required by the ankle and knee, suggesting that an attempt to change the pattern may not actually reduce injury potential, but rather change the injury potential.

Where problematic imbalances are present, task-specific programs can be developed aimed at addressing any movement issues. Sanders et al. (2013) provide examples of individualized targeted approaches used to correct asymmetries and improve swimming technique. These types of athlete-specific targeted intervention programs have been indicated to result in improved muscle balance, technique, and overall performance (Carson, 1999). Thus coaches should work with strength and conditioning staff and physiotherapists to implement programs with their athletes that concentrate on coordination, strength, and flexibility.

BIOMECHANICAL ASSESSMENTS OF PREFERRED AND NONPREFERRED LIMB SKILLS (DOMINANT AND NONDOMINANT LIMB SKILLS)

A number of team ball sports allow athletes to perform primary components of a skill using either the right or left limb. An example of some sports that fall into this category are football codes, such as Association, Australian, and Gaelic football, and the rugby codes, as well as throwing sports, including European handball, cricket, and water polo. In these sports, athletes may choose to pass the ball with either the preferred or nonpreferred side, depending on the requirements of the sequence of play. Performance dependence on one side of the body can therefore leave athletes stuck in particular game scenarios. This becomes particularly noticeable at the elite level, where proficiency to complete skills with either limb is regarded as a necessary ability in order to cope with game demands. Thus the ability to pass, shoot, or dribble competently with both limbs, according to the particular requirements of game play, is regarded as a desirable attribute, and bilateral equality between the limbs is suggested to provide an advantage over competitors who have a performance dominance on one side (Grouios, Kollias, Koidou, & Poderi, 2002; McLean & Tumilty, 1993; Parrington, Ball, & MacMahon, 2015; Sachlikidis & Salter, 2007).

In fact, ambidextrous players have been found to have a greater goal-scoring efficiency (soccer) in comparison with players who have left or right performance dominance (Starosta, 1988).

Many researchers agree that symmetry between the limbs is therefore important to address in the development of athletes. One suggested method to increase ambidexterity is to train the nonpreferred limb to mirror the preferred limb. This approach sees that performance on the nonpreferred (nondominant) limb will be improved if the movement pattern is more technically similar to the preferred limb (kicking, Ball, 2011; throwing, Sachlikidis & Salter, 2007; handballing, Parrington et al., 2015). In order to make practical suggestions and aid in the provision of coaching cues, biomechanists have focused on the identification of mechanical differences between the preferred and nonpreferred limbs. Conducting this type of analysis allows the chief components of the movement to be addressed in the less efficient movement pattern. One factor that needs to be further evaluated is whether or not equivalent performance can be achieved on either limb through different movement patterns. In this section, we will discuss the biomechanical differences that have been assessed in lower and upper body skills such as kicking and throwing.

KICKING

Many kicking sports require the use of both the preferred and nonpreferred legs. This need for laterality in the kicking task varies across the different football codes, ranging from frequent in Association and Australian football to advantageous in the rugby codes. In Association football, the most successful players in high-level competition have been shown to make shots with either leg (Starosta, 1988), and success rates with both the preferred and nonpreferred leg passes have shown similar levels of efficiency in internationals (Carey et al., 2001). In Australian football, with up to 45% of kicks performed with the nonpreferred leg (Ball, 2008), the ability to kick with either leg is an essential attribute for players. In the rugby codes, while the majority of kicks are taken with the preferred leg, nonpreferred leg kicks are emerging as a "surprise tactic" (Ball, 2011) or to enable kicking with the leg furthest from the defender to decrease the chance of it being blocked (e.g., Biscombe & Drewett, 1998).

Consistently among kicking research, the nonpreferred leg has produced poorer performance compared to the preferred leg in terms of distance, speed, or accuracy (e.g., Barfield, 1995; Dörge, Bull-Andersen, Sørensen, & Simonsen, 2002; Nunome, Ikegami, Kozakai, Apriantono, & Sano, 2006). Foot and ball speeds have been significantly lower in all studies (Table 13.1), suggesting the nonpreferred leg is swung through more

TABLE 13.1 Foot and Ball Speeds Comparing Preferred (P) and NonPreferred (NP) Leg Kicking

	Group	Task	Foot Speed (m/s)		Ball Speed (m/s)		Foot:Ball Speed Ratio	
			P	NP	P	NP	P	NP
PUNT KICK								
Smith, Ball, and MacMahon (2009)	Elite AF	Max	26.5	22.6	32.6	27.0	1.23	1.20
Ball (2011)	Elite AF	45m pass	19.4	17.0				
Farrow and Ball (2011)	Junior AF	Max	16	14	12	9	0.75	0.64
Ball (2013)	Elite AF	Max	22.1	19.4				
PLACE KICK								
Dörge et al. (2002)	Club S	Max	18.6	17.0	24.7	21.5	1.33	1.26
Nunome et al. (2006)	Elite S	Max	23.8	20.6	32.1	27.1	1.35	1.32

AF, Australian Football; S, Association Football.

slowly. Foot to ball speed ratios, an indication of the quality of impact between the foot and the ball, were also smaller for the nonpreferred leg, although in all studies this difference was not significant.

What Contributes to Decreased Performance on the Nonpreferred Side?

Coordination is an obvious possibility contributing to the differences between the preferred and nonpreferred leg kicks. The biomechanical mechanism to optimize end point speed is to sequence movement with proximal segments peaking in speed early in the movement and distal segments peaking late. This is in contrast to a simultaneous movement in which all muscles might be switched on at the same time, which optimizes force evident, for example, in a push up. Specific to kicking, this motion would be characterized by the trunk and pelvis rotating first, then the thigh and the hip, and finally the knee extending to maximize foot speed.

This sequencing has been found to be better in the preferred compared to the nonpreferred leg in Association football kicking. Dörge et al. (2002) performed a kinetic analysis of seven skilled soccer players performing maximal instep kicks with both legs. Examining how the upper leg affected the lower leg in the acceleration or downswing phase of the kick, they determined that the better performance of the preferred leg was due to a better intersegmental patterning between these two segments.

Coordination differences have also been found in the punt kick between the preferred and nonpreferred leg. Hancock and Ball (2008) collected three dimensional kick leg data for five elite AF players performing kicks with the preferred and nonpreferred legs. Using knee angle-knee angular velocity phase plane diagrams, differences between kick legs were found to be range of motion (ROM) and speed rather than timing- and coordination-based. However, Falloon, Ball, Taylor, and MacMahon (2010) and Ball (2011) expanded this evaluation to include the hip and pelvis, finding a different coordination pattern evident between the kick legs. The preferred leg exhibited greater knee and pelvis ROM and knee angular velocity at ball contact. Conversely the nonpreferred leg produced greater hip angle ROM and hip angular velocity at ball contact. This finding indicated the nonpreferred leg did not exhibit as efficient a proximal to distal (whip-like) motion, so momentum built up in the proximal segments was not transferred to the distal segments and foot. Interestingly, this pattern was also evident in junior kickers (9–11 years old), indicating this movement pattern is established very early (Farrow & Ball, 2011). Also of interest, a greater range of motion at the knee and less at the hip has been found for skilled players compared to novices (Chow, Davids, Button, & Koh, 2007), suggesting the nonpreferred leg exhibits a more "novice-like" pattern.

Strength is another obvious area that might influence the difference in performance between sides of the body. Much of the research attempting to link strength differences between preferred and nonpreferred sides of the body has been equivocal (e.g., Barfield, 1995; Capranica, Cama, Fanton, Tessitore, & Figura, 1992), but this is largely due to the different speeds that strength tests have been performed (Ball, 2011; Nunome et al., 2006). For example, knee extension angular velocities of 300 degree per second are often used to measure isokinetic strength. This compares to the 1500 degree per second the knee is extending at the point of ball contact in the kick. However, some indication of the influence of strength can be gathered through three-dimensional analysis evaluating joint kinetics (or forces at the joints). Nunome et al. (2006) examined six elite soccer players performing maximal kicks and calculated joint moments at the knee and hip. The knee extension moment was significantly greater for the preferred compared to the nonpreferred leg kicks, indicating strength differences contributed to performance while no coordination differences were evident. Nunome et al. (2006) suggested that given the players tested were all elite, coordination had developed to a high level already for both legs so the differences then became an issue of strength.

The punt kick represents an interesting issue for laterality. The punt kick begins with the ball in the hands. During execution, the ball is directed and released from the hand so it drops to the desired position for the foot to make impact. As such, the punt kick tests laterality of both upper body and lower body. The finer motor skill of directing, and in the case of kicking sports in which the ball is ovoid, and orienting the ball is controlled by the upper body, while the forceful interceptive action of the foot hitting the ball is controlled by the lower body. This is further tested when performers have differences in laterality preferences between the arms and legs. For example, Cameron Smith, the Australian Rugby League captain and kicker is left-footed but right-handed. Studies have found some players drop the ball with the contralateral hand (i.e., using the left hand to drop the ball for a right-footed kick) or releasing with both hands at the same time. These two techniques affect the posture of the kicker and in particular do not allow for a tension arc where the trunk twists about its long axis in preparation for downswing so reducing the speed of the foot that can be developed. Further, Ball (2011) noted that kick leg motion on the nonpreferred side during the kick might be affected by a less consistent ball release that can be expected when using the ipsilateral arm on the nonpreferred side to release the ball so control is maintained more at the hip with its greater degrees of freedom (compared to the knee) so that players might make adjustments to ensure they connect with the ball.

While differences have been shown in studies comparing preferred and nonpreferred leg kicking, not all individual performers have showed these differences. Ball (2011) reported that 2 of the 17 players tested in his study exhibited similar kicking performance and technique for both legs. This finding raises philosophical issues regarding the examination of laterality. Ball argued that if the target population was defined as elite performers, then the inclusion of these two was appropriate. However the research was partly aimed at identifying differences between preferred and nonpreferred leg kicks so that these might be trained. This population, then, would not include these two players as they would not require remedial work. Equally, understanding why these two players are capable of producing similar performance would be best answered by examining these players separately.

THROWING

Sports such as water polo, European handball, and cricket all afford situations where either the preferred hand or nonpreferred hand could be used to throw the ball. Here, the ability to throw equally well using either arm could be beneficial to performance. For example, being able to quickly throw the ball toward the wickets in cricket if picked up with the nonpreferred hand may save time in comparison with having to transfer the ball between hands. Another example could be the advantage gained over a goaltender in European handball, when attacking players have the ability to shoot for the goal using either the preferred or nonpreferred hand.

Performance Decrement Due to Preference/Dominance

When we first perform fundamental skills such as throwing, laterality/handedness effects might direct us to choose to use one limb in preference of the other. As we continue to practice, this limb can become more preferable to use because it is easier to complete the skill. In this instance, we become better at performing on the preferred side and reinforce the functional dominance of that side. As a result, performance as an outcome of accuracy and/or speed is not as good on the nonpreferred side. These findings have been demonstrated across a number of different populations including children aged 12 to 14 (Ning, Faro, Sue, & Hamilton, 1999), recreational athletes (Hore, Watts, Tweed, & Miller, 1996), elite junior athletes (Sachlikidis & Salter, 2007), and experienced athletes (van den Tillaar & Ettema, 2006, 2009). In addition to performance differences, a number of kinematic differences have been found relating to the overarm throw movement pattern on the nondominant/nonpreferred side. A list of the key findings from each of these studies is provided in Table 13.2.

In comparison with the movement pattern demonstrated on the preferred/dominant arm side, nonpreferred arm throws are often described as displaying less than optimal coordination (Sachlikidis & Salter, 2007),

TABLE 13.2 List of Studies and Results for Dominant Versus Nondominant Overarm Throwing

Authors	Evaluation	Key Findings (For the Nondominant Arm, in Comparison With the Dominant)
Sachlikidis and Salter (2007)	Biomechanical comparison of dominant and nondominant arm throws for speed and accuracy, in elite junior cricketers	• Slower ball speed (for both speed and accuracy emphasized throws) • Less accuracy • Lower maximum lead leg knee lift • No lead leg knee extension during arm acceleration phase • Less elbow flexion before extension • Less shoulder external rotation at the start of the arm acceleration phase • No delay between the initiation of pelvic and upper torso internal rotation • Suboptimal coordination pattern
Hore et al. (1996)	Kinematic comparison of dominant and nondominant overarm (isolated upper arm) throws for accuracy in recreational baseball/softball players	• Less accuracy • Height of ball impact on the target grid was related to hand trajectory length and hand orientation at ball release, but not hand trajectory height
van den Tillaar and Ettema (2006)	Kinematic comparison of dominant and nondominant arms in experienced handball players	• Slower ball speed • Less accuracy • Increased variability • Decreased shoulder internal rotation velocity • Decreased range of internal rotation of the shoulder
van den Tillaar and Ettema (2009)	Kinematic comparison of dominant and nondominant arms, specifically looking at speed accuracy trade-offs in experienced handball players	• Slower ball speed • Less accuracy • Increased variability • Decreased shoulder internal rotation velocity • Decreased range of internal rotation of the shoulder • Increased ball release height • Increased shoulder abduction • Increased trunk tilt sideways angle • Suboptimal timing of joint movements
Ning et al. (1999)	Kinematic comparison of dominant and nondominant arms for accuracy in school aged children (12–14 years)	• Slower ball velocity and acceleration • Less accuracy • Slower hand velocity and acceleration • Slower wrist velocity and acceleration • Slower elbow velocity and acceleration • Slower shoulder acceleration

or undeveloped movement patterns, similar to what is exhibited by novice performers (Williams, Haywood, & Painter, 1996).

Improving Performance on the Nondominant Side

The general consensus from throwing-related literature is that identifying the differences between dominant and nondominant (or preferred and nonpreferred) throwing is an important step in evaluation. By knowing what parts of the throw are lagging in the nondominant arm, we can more specifically target areas for improvement. Furthermore, if we train the nondominant to mirror the dominant arm, then this could improve the technique in the nondominant and thus improve ambidexterity and reduce limb dominance.

Based on a collaboration of the above literature, those wishing to improve ambidexterity on their nondominant side should improve the following:

1. Increase stride length
    a. Lift the lead leg knee higher
    b. Extend the lead leg during the arm acceleration phase
2. Increase range of motion at the elbow and shoulder of the throwing arm
    a. Increase elbow flexion before elbow extension
    b. Increase shoulder external rotation (at the start of the acceleration phase)
3. Generate greater hand velocity
    a. Increase rotation velocity at the shoulder, elbow, and wrist
4. Timing
    a. Shoulder external rotation should be delayed until after lead leg foot contact
    b. Forward rotation of the upper torso should occur after the forward rotation of the pelvis.

Notes on Other Upper-Limb Dominant Versus Nondominant Performance

Reduced performance and technical differences have been identified for other upper-body skills, such as Australian football "handball" passing (Parrington et al., 2015). Handballing is a passing maneuver in Australian football, which involves an underarm movement to strike the ball using the clenched fist of one hand, out of the other hand, which is holding the ball. The ability to perform efficiently with both the preferred and nonpreferred arm is an important skill attribute for elite players competing in the Australian Football League. Results from the study of preferred versus nonpreferred arm handballing have demonstrated similar findings to those of throwing, with decreased performance on the nonpreferred side. The nonpreferred handballs represented similar findings to those of throwing including slower linear and rotational trunk motion, slower shoulder flexion velocity, and slower hand speed in comparison with handballs performed on the preferred side. The authors recommended that Australian footballers should increase the number of repetitions made during practice using the nonpreferred side in order to increase performance.

IMPROVING THE AMBIDEXTERITY OF SKILLS

It is possible for sports people to improve their ambidexterity and therefore reduce reliance on one preferred limb. This can be beneficial for athletes whom, by reducing the preference for or dominance of one limb, add an extra dynamic to their skill set, as well as being valuable for those returning from injury. Targeted bilateral skill training can be used in order to improve the performance of the nondominant or nonpreferred limb (Hagerman, 2002; Teixeira, De Oliveira, Romano, & Correa, 2011; Teixeira, Silva, & Carvalho, 2003). These interventions require more frequent use of the nonpreferred limb, which can be less favorable for athletes during training and practice but should not affect the performance of the preferred limb. The use of therapeutic interventions may also be of use to decrease strength dependence on one side of the body, which has been shown in athletes recovering postsurgery (Impellizzeri, Rampinini, Maffiuletti, & Marcora, 2007).

COMMENT ON LATERALITY AND PERFORMANCE

Most of the research described throughout this chapter has used the outcome of the movement as the performance criterion and has used discrete point analysis to evaluate differences between limbs. To understand more about bilateral differences, however, an understanding of the coordination profiles and the muscle activation profiles may provide a greater understanding to why these differences in technique occur.

Bilateral differences appear to occur across athletic populations, which begs the question of whether achieving symmetry will improve performance or decrease injury potential. In the case of preferred versus nonpreferred limb skills, it is unknown whether or not both limbs can achieve the same performance, but yet be the outcome of a different movement pattern by each side; if this is the case, then attempting to mirror performance may not be as desirable as achieving an optimal coordination pattern for the nonpreferred side. While introducing training to improve symmetry in technique may seem desirable, it is important to consider the cost–benefit relationship. Where asymmetries in technique cause injury concerns, then seeking an intervention that may help to reduce or alleviate this asymmetry may be constructive. In some instances, however, attempting to change a well-ingrained technique on one side to match the other may not be beneficial and may hinder performance for a period of time, or increase the chances of injury. These factors should be taken into consideration before any intervention is implemented.

SUMMARY

In this chapter, we have explored the important connection between biomechanics and laterality in sport, with a particular focus on laterality effects on performance and injury. We have looked at the methods in which biomechanists and other practitioners assess bilateral symmetries/asymmetries, discussed dominance in cyclic movement patterns and repetitive movements, and looked into the assessment of preferred and nonpreferred skills.

Throughout this section, the overriding feature is that biomechanically we are concerned if issues related to laterality affect the performance of an athlete, or predispose the athlete to injury. While improving athletic performance is identified as an essential component of practice and training, assessing bilateral asymmetries is of particular concern when trainable changes can then be made in order to decrease the risk of injury.

It is integral for biomechanics researchers and practical consultants to work with other sports practitioners to address any laterality issues in athletes. From the perspective of improving technique, it is important for biomechanists to collaborate with motor learning and skill acquisition specialists, as well as coaches, in order to provide the best form of information and instruction to athletes. Targeted interventions may be beneficial to reduce moderate laterality effects; however, the method by which this is optimized requires further research and evaluation. Where targeted technique interventions or treatment is required in order to make changes to movement patterns to reduce bilateral asymmetries, biomechanists may be required to work with physiotherapists or rehabilitation specialists, strength and conditioning coaches, or athletic trainers in order to treat any underlying issues.

References

Ball, K. (2008). Biomechanical considerations of distance kicking in Australian rules football. *Sports Biomechanics, 7*, 10–23.

Ball, K. (2011). Kinematic comparison of the preferred and non-preferred foot punt kick. *Journal of Sports Sciences, 29,* 1545–1552.

Ball, K. (2013). Loading and performance of the support leg in kicking. *Journal of Science & Medicine in Sport, 16,* 455–459.

Barden, J. M., Kell, R. T., & Kobsar, D. (2011). The effect of critical speed and exercise intensity on stroke phase duration and bilateral asymmetry in 200-m front crawl swimming. *Journal of Sports Sciences, 29,* 517–526.

Barfield, W. R. (1995). Effects of selected kinematic and kinetic variables on instep kicking with dominant and non-dominant limbs. *Journal of Human Movement Studies, 29,* 251–272.

Baumhauer, J. F., Alosa, D. M., Renström, P. A., Trevino, S., & Beynnon, B. (1995). A prospective study of ankle injury risk factors. *The American Journal of Sports Medicine, 23,* 564–570.

Benda, B. J., Riley, P. O., & Krebs, D. E. (1994). Biomechanical relationship between center of gravity and center of pressure during standing. *IEEE Transactions on Rehabilitation Engineering, 2,* 3–10.

Bertucci, W. M., Arfaoui, A., & Polidori, G. (2012). Analysis of the pedaling biomechanics of master's cyclists: a preliminary study. *Journal of Science and Cycling, 1,* 42–46.

Biscombe, T., & Drewett, P. (1998). *Rugby: Steps to success.* Champaign, IL: Human Kinetics.

Bredeweg, S. W., Buist, I., & Kluitenberg, B. (2013). Differences in kinetic asymmetry between injured and non-injured novice runners: a prospective cohort study. *Gait & Posture, 38,* 847–852.

Brown, A. M., Zifchock, R. A., & Hillstrom, H. J. (2014). The effects of limb dominance and fatigue on running biomechanics. *Gait & Posture, 39,* 915–919.

Capranica, L., Cama, G., Fanton, F., Tessitore, A., & Figura, F. (1992). Force and power of preferred and non-preferred leg in young soccer players. *The Journal of Sports Medicine and Physical Fitness, 32,* 358–363.

Carey, D., Smith, G., Smith, D. T., Shepherd, J. W., Skriver, J., Ord, L., & Rutland, A. (2001). Footedness in world soccer: an analysis of France '98. *Journal of Sports Sciences, 19,* 855–864.

Carpes, F. P., Diefenthaeler, F., Bini, R. R., Stefanyshyn, D., Faria, I. E., & Mota, C. B. (2010). Does leg preference affect muscle activation and efficiency? *Journal of Electromyography and Kinesiology, 20,* 1230–1236.

Carpes, F. P., Diefenthaeler, F., Bini, R. R., Stefanyshyn, D. J., Faria, I. E., & Mota, C. B. (2011). Influence of leg preference on bilateral muscle activation during cycling. *Journal of Sports Sciences, 29,* 151–159.

Carpes, F. P., Rossato, M., Faria, I. E., & Mota, C. B. (2007). Bilateral pedaling asymmetry during a simulated 40-km cycling time-trial. *Journal of Sports Medicine and Physical Fitness, 47,* 51–57.

Carpes, F. P., Rossato, M., Faria, I. E., & Mota, C. B. (2008). During an incremental exercise cyclists improve bilateral pedaling symmetry. *Brazilian Journal of Biomotricity, 2,* 155–159.

Carson, P. A. (1999). The rehabilitation of a competitive swimmer with an asymmetrical breaststroke movement pattern. *Manual Therapy, 4,* 100–106.

Carter-Saltzman, L. (1980). Biological and sociocultural effects on handedness: comparison between biological and adoptive families. *Science, 209*(4462), 1263–1265.

Cavanagh, P. R., & Lafortune, M. A. (1980). Ground reaction forces in distance running. *Journal of Biomechanics, 13,* 397–406.

Cavanagh, P. R. (1990). *Biomechanics of distance running.* Champaign, IL: Human Kinetics.

Chow, J. Y., Davids, K., Button, C., & Koh, M. (2007). Variation in coordination of a discrete multiarticular action as a function of skill level. *Journal of Motor Behavior, 39,* 463–479.

Ciacci, S., Di Michele, R., Fantozzi, S., & Merni, F. (2013). Assessment of kinematic asymmetry for reduction of hamstring injury risk. *International Journal of Athletic Therapy & Training, 18,* 18–23.

Daly, D. J., & Cavanagh, P. R. (1976). Asymmetry in bicycle ergometer pedalling. *Medicine and Science in Sports, 8,* 204–208.

Dufek, J. S., & Bates, B. T. (1991). Biomechanical factors associated with injury during landing in jump sports. *Sports Medicine, 12,* 326–337.

Dörge, H. C., Bull-Andersen, T., Sørensen, H., & Simonsen, E. B. (2002). Biomechanical differences in soccer kicking with the preferred and the non-preferred leg. *Journal of Sports Sciences, 20,* 293–299.

Exell, T. A., Gittoes, M. J., Irwin, G., & Kerwin, D. G. (2012). Gait asymmetry: composite scores for mechanical analyses of sprint running. *Journal of Biomechanics, 45,* 1108–1111.

Falloon, J., Ball, K., Taylor, S., & MacMahon, C. (2010). Coordination profiles of preferred and non-preferred foot kicking in Australian Football. In R. Jensen, W. Ebben, E. Petushek, C. Richter, & K. Roemer (Eds.), *Proceedings of the 28th international conference on biomechanics in sports* (pp. 466–469). Marquette, USA: Northern Michigan University.

Farrow, D., & Ball, K. (2011). *Preferred and non-preferred leg kicking in junior players* (Technical report for the AFL research board, Melbourne Australia).

Fousekis, K., Tsepis, E., Poulmedis, P., Athanasopoulos, S., & Vagenas, G. (2010). Intrinsic risk factors of non-contact quadriceps and hamstring strains in soccer: a prospective study of 100 professional players. *British Journal of Sports Medicine, 45,* 709–714.

Functional Movement Systems [FMS]. (March 02, 2015). *Functional movement screening.* Retrieved from: http://www.functionalmovement.com.

Grouios, G., Kollias, N., Koidou, I., & Poderi, A. (2002). Excess of mixed-footedness among professional soccer players. *Perceptual and Motor Skills, 94,* 695–699.

Gundersen, L. A., Valle, D. R., Barr, A. E., Danoff, J. V., Stanhope, S. J., & Snyder-Mackler, L. (1989). Bilateral analysis of the knee and ankle during gait: an examination of the relationship between lateral dominance and symmetry. *Physical Therapy, 69,* 640–650.

Hagerman, P. S. (2002). Training the non-dominant side. *Strength & Conditioning Journal, 24,* 61–62.

Hamill, J., Gruber, A. H., & Derrick, T. R. (2014). Lower extremity joint stiffness characteristics during running with different footfall patterns. *European Journal of Sport Science, 14,* 130–136.

Hancock, A., & Ball, K. (2008). Comparison of preferred and non-preferred foot kicking in Australian Football. In A. Burnett (Ed.), *Proceedings of the Australian association of exercise and sports science conference.* Melbourne: Australian Catholic University.

Herzog, W., Nigg, B. M., Read, L. J., & Olsson, E. (1989). Asymmetries in ground reaction force patterns in normal human gait. *Medicine and Science in Sports and Exercise, 21,* 110–114.

Hore, J., Watts, S., Tweed, D., & Miller, B. (1996). Overarm throws with the non-dominant arm: kinematics of accuracy. *Journal of Neurophysiology, 76,* 3693–3704.

Hreljac, A. (2004). Impact and overuse injuries in runners. *Medicine and Science in Sports and Exercise, 36,* 845–849.

Hreljac, A., Marshall, R. N., & Hume, P. A. (2000). Evaluation of lower extremity overuse injury potential in runners. *Medicine and Science in Sports and Exercise, 32,* 1635–1641.

Impellizzeri, F. M., Rampinini, E., Maffiuletti, N., & Marcora, S. M. (2007). A vertical jump force test for assessing bilateral strength asymmetry in athletes. *Medicine and Science in Sports and Exercise, 39,* 2044–2050.

James, S. L., Bates, B. T., & Osternig, L. R. (1978). Injuries to runners. *American Journal of Sports Medicine, 6,* 40–50.

Karamanidis, K., Arampatzis, A., & Brüggmann, G. P. (2003). Symmetry and reproducibility of kinematic parameters during various running techniques. *Medicine and Science in Sports and Exercise, 35,* 1009–1016.

Kiesel, K., Plisky, P. J., & Voight, M. L. (2007). Can serious injury in professional football be predicted by a preseason functional movement screen? *North American Journal of Sports Physical Therapy, 2,* 147.

Knapik, J. J., Bauman, C. L., Jones, B. H., Harris, J. M., & Vaughan, L. (1991). Preseason strength and flexibility imbalances associated with athletic injuries in female collegiate athletes. *The American Journal of Sports Medicine, 19,* 76–81.

Llaurens, V., Raymond, M., & Faurie, C. (2009). Why are some people left-handed? An evolutionary perspective. *Philosophical Transactions of the Royal Society B: Biological Sciences, 364*, 881–894.

McLean, B. D., & Tumilty, D. M. (1993). Left-right asymmetry in two types of soccer kick. *British Journal of Sports Medicine, 27*, 260–262.

van Mechelen, W. (1992). Running injuries. *Sports Medicine, 14*, 320–335.

Nadler, S. F., Malanga, G. A., Feinberg, J. H., Prybicien, M., Stitik, T. P., & DePrince, M. (2001). Relationship between hip muscle imbalance and occurrence of low back pain in collegiate athletes: a prospective study. *American Journal of Physical Medicine & Rehabilitation, 80*, 572–577.

Nielsen, R. O., Buist, I., Parner, E. T., Nohr, E. A., Sørensen, H., Lind, M., & Rasmussen, S. (2014). Foot pronation is not associated with increased injury risk in novice runners wearing a neutral shoe: a 1-year prospective cohort study. *British Journal of Sports Medicine, 48*, 440–447.

Nigg, B. M. (2001). The role of impact forces and foot pronation: a new paradigm. *Clinical Journal of Sport Medicine, 11*, 2–9.

Ning, Z., Faro, A., Sue, D., & Hamilton, N. (1999). Kinesiological analysis of overarm throwing for accuracy with dominant and non-dominant arms. In R. H. Sanders, & B. J. Gibson (Eds.), *Proceedings from the 17th international conference on biomechanics in sports* (pp. 37–40) (Perth, Australia).

Novacheck, T. F. (1998). The biomechanics of running. *Gait & Posture, 7*, 77–95.

Nunome, H., Ikegami, Y., Kozakai, R., Apriantono, T., & Sano, S. (2006). Segmental dynamics of soccer instep kicking with the preferred and non-preferred leg. *Journal of Sports Sciences, 24*, 529–541.

Pappas, E., & Carpes, F. P. (2012). Lower extremity kinematic asymmetry in male and female athletes performing jump-landing tasks. *Journal of Science and Medicine in Sport, 15*, 87–92.

Pappas, P., Paradisis, G., & Vagenas, G. (2015). Leg and vertical stiffness (a)symmetry between dominant and non-dominant legs in young male runners. *Human Movement Science, 40*, 273–283.

Parrington, L., Ball, K., & MacMahon, C. (2015). Kinematics of preferred and non-preferred handballing in Australian football. *Journal of Sports Sciences., 33*, 20–28.

Paterno, M. V., Schmitt, L. C., Ford, K. R., Rauh, M. J., Myer, G. D., Huang, B., & Hewett, T. E. (2010). Biomechanical measures during landing and postural stability predict second anterior cruciate ligament injury after anterior cruciate ligament reconstruction and return to sport. *The American Journal of Sports Medicine, 38*, 1968–1978.

Plisky, P. J., Rauh, M. J., Kaminski, T. W., & Underwood, F. B. (2006). Star excursion balance test as a predictor of lower extremity injury in high school basketball players. *Journal of Orthopaedic & Sports Physical Therapy, 36*, 911–919.

Potts, A. D., Charlton, J. E., & Smith, H. M. (2002). Bilateral arm power imbalance in swim bench exercise to exhaustion. *Journal of Sports Sciences, 20*, 975–979.

Psycharakis, S. G., & Sanders, R. H. (2008). Shoulder and hip roll changes during 200-m front crawl swimming. *Medicine and Science in Sports and Exercise, 40*, 2129–2136.

Running USA. (June 15, 2014). *2014 state of the sport – Part II: Running Industry report*. Retrieved from: http://www.runningusa.org/2014-running-industry-report?returnTo= annual-reports.

Sachlikidis, A., & Salter, C. (2007). A biomechanical comparison of dominant and non-dominant arm throws for speed and accuracy. *Sports Biomechanics, 6*, 334–344.

Sanders, R. H., Thow, J., & Fairweather, M. (2011). Asymmetries in swimming: where do they come from? *Journal of Swimming Science, 18*, 1–11. Retrieved from: http://swimmingcoach.org/journal/manuscript-sanders-vol18.pdf.

Sanders, R., McCabe, C., Alcock, A., Wright, L., Donald, N., Riach, I., & Fairweather, M. (2013). Case studies of asymmetries in swimming. In T. Shiang, W. Ho, P. Huang, & C. Tsai

(Eds.), *Proceedings of the 31st international conference on biomechanics in sports. Taipei, Taiwan* Retrieved from: https://ojs.ub.uni-konstanz.de/cpa/article/download/5523/5017.

Sanders, R. H. (2013). How do asymmetries affect swimming performance? *Journal of Swimming Research, 21*, 1–17. Retrieved from http://swimmingcoach.org/journal/manuscript-sanders-vol21.pdf.

Sanderson, D. J. (1990). The influence of cadence and power output on asymmetry of force application during steady-rate cycling. *Journal of Human Movement Studies, 19*, 1–9.

Schieb, D. A. (1987). Bilateral characteristics of running mechanics. In L. Tsarouchas, J. Terauds, B. A. Gowitzke, & L. E. Holt (Eds.), *Proceedings of the 5th international symposium on biomechanics in sports* (pp. 414–421) (Athens, Greece).

Seifert, L., Chollet, D., & Allard, P. (2005). Arm coordination symmetry and breathing effect in front crawl. *Human Movement Science, 24*, 234–256.

Seifert, L., Chehensse, A., Tourny-Chollet, C., Lemaitre, F., & Chollet, D. (2008). Effect of breathing pattern on arm coordination symmetry in front crawl. *The Journal of Strength & Conditioning Research, 22*, 1670–1676.

Smak, W., Neptune, R. R., & Hull, M. L. (1999). The influence of pedaling rate on bilateral asymmetry in cycling. *Journal of Biomechanics, 32*, 899–906.

Smith, C. A., Chimera, N. J., & Warren, M. (2014). Association of Y balance test reach asymmetry and injury in division I athletes. *Medicine and Science in Sports and Exercise, 47*, 136–141.

Smith, J., Ball, K., & MacMahon, C. (2009). Foot to ball interaction in preferred and non-preferred leg Australian Rules kicking. In R. Anderson, D. Harrison, & I. Kenny (Eds.), *Proceedings of the 27th international conference on biomechanics in sports* (pp. 650–653). Ireland: University of Limerick.

Söderman, K., Alfredson, H., Pietilä, T., & Werner, S. (2001). Risk factors for leg injuries in female soccer players: a prospective investigation during one out-door season. *Knee Surgery, Sports Traumatology, Arthroscopy, 9*, 313–321.

Starosta, W. (1988). Symmetry and asymmetry in shooting demonstrated by elite soccer players. In T. Reilly, A. Lees, K. Davids, & W. Murphy (Eds.), *Science and football* (pp. 346–355). London, UK: E and F N Spon.

Teixeira, L. A., De Oliveira, D. L., Romano, R. G., & Correa, S. C. (2011). Leg preference and interlateral asymmetry of balance stability in soccer players. *Research Quarterly for Exercise and Sport, 82*, 21–27.

Teixeira, L. A., Silva, M. V., & Carvalho, M. (2003). Reduction of lateral asymmetries in dribbling: the role of bilateral practice. *Laterality: Asymmetries of Body, Brain and Cognition, 8*, 53–65.

van den Tillaar, R., & Ettema, G. (2006). A comparison of performance and kinematics in throwing with the dominant and non-dominant arm in handball players. In H. Schwameder, G. Strutzenberger, V. Fastenbauer, S. Lindinger, & E. Müller (Eds.), *Proceedings of the 24th international conference on biomechanics in sports* (pp. 1–4) (Salzburg, Austria).

van den Tillaar, R., & Ettema, G. (2009). A comparison of overarm throwing with the dominant and non-dominant arm in experiences team handball players. *Perceptual and Motor Skills, 109*, 315–326.

Tourny-Chollet, C., Seifert, L., & Chollet, D. (2009). Effect of force symmetry on coordination in crawl. *International Journal of Sports Medicine, 30*, 182–187.

Vagenas, G., & Hoshizaki, B. (1988). Evaluation of rearfoot asymmetries in running with worn and new running shoes. *International Journal of Sport Biomechanics, 4*, 220–230.

Vagenas, G., & Hoshizaki, B. (1991). Functional asymmetries and lateral dominance in the lower limbs of distance runners. *International Journal of Sport Biomechanics, 7*, 311–329.

Vagenas, G., & Hoshizaki, B. (1992). A multivariable analysis of lower extremity kinematic analysis in running. *Journal of Applied Biomechanics, 8*, 11–29.

Vagenas, G., & Hoshizaki, T. B. (1986). Optimization of an asymmetrical motor skill: sprint start. *International Journal of Sport Biomechanics, 2*, 29–40.

Williams, K., Haywood, K. M., & Painter, M. A. (1996). Environmental versus biological influences on gender difference in the overarm throw for force: dominant and non-dominant arm throws. *Women in Sport and Physical Activity Journal, 5*, 29–48.

Zadpoor, A. A., & Nikooyan, A. A. (2011). The relationship between lower-extremity stress fractures and the ground reaction force: a systematic review. *Clinical Biomechanics, 26*, 23–28.

Zifchock, R. A., Davis, I., & Hamill, J. (2006). Kinetic asymmetry in female runners with and without retrospective tibial stress fractures. *Journal of Biomechanics, 39*, 2792–2797.

Zifchock, R. A., Davis, I., Higginson, J., McCaw, S., & Royer, T. (2008). Side-to-side differences in overuse running injury susceptibility: a retrospective study. *Human Movement Science, 27*, 888–902.

Laterality Effects on Performance in Team Sports: Insights From Soccer and Basketball

Tino Stöckel

University of Rostock, Rostock, Germany

David P. Carey

Bangor University, Bangor, United Kingdom

INTRODUCTION

In team sports like soccer or basketball, athletes are frequently confronted with situations demanding the flexible adjustment of their actions to fast changes of competitive play. Often, these situations require players to execute skills with their nonpreferred hand or foot. The degree to which a player is able to successfully perform with the nonpreferred side reflects his/her level of "bilateral competence" (Stöckel & Weigelt, 2012a, p. 1038). Players' individual level of bilateral competence was assumed to pose a constraint for the advancement to higher levels of competitive play (e.g., Bale & Scholes, 1986; Grouios, Kollias, Tsorbatzoudis, & Alexandris, 2002). For example, attackers in soccer who are able to shoot on goal or defenders who are able to clear the ball or tackle with either foot should be faster and more efficient than strongly lateralized athletes who need to radically adjust their position in order to use their dominant foot, running the risk that an opponent's reaction is faster. Similarly, basketball players who are unable to handle the ball with equal efficiency on both sides may not be able to adjust their play sufficiently to new situations and are (therefore) constrained to perform a particular skill with the dominant hand, even when the situation requires the use of the other hand. In that regard, it can be assumed that being as proficient with the nondominant hand/foot as with the dominant hand/foot is an advantage in team sports like soccer or basketball. Moreover, it has been argued that such two-sided proficiency, requiring athletes to overcome a strong inborn tendency to prefer one side, is important or even crucial for success in team sports like soccer (e.g., Grouios, 2004). Consequently, strong one-foot bias in professional players was often thought to be a consequence of poor coaching and insufficient practice (Carey et al., 2001). In that regard, it is not really surprising that a study found evidence for significantly higher salaries of allegedly two-footed European soccer players (Bryson, Frick, & Simmons, 2013) as compared to right- or left-footed players. But do less lateralized players actually have an advantage over players with a strong one-side preference, helping them to advance to higher competitive levels? Is there any evidence to support the notion of a plasticity of hand/foot preference and proficiency in response to increasing amounts of soccer- or basketball-specific practice?

The present chapter reviews some of the literature in the field to shed some light on these issues and to reexamine entrenched beliefs in sport, which actually have little empirical support. In order to get answers on the questions raised above, the chapter will focus on research from which footedness/handedness distributions among soccer and basketball players can be deduced, and studies that report training or expertise effects on foot/hand preference and/or proficiency in soccer and basketball. First, footedness/handedness distributions among soccer/basketball players from different competitive levels are analyzed to explore whether the bias in foot/hand preference is reduced in these athletes as compared to the general population. Second, we will establish if any of the sport-specific behaviors are more or less lateralized than any others. Third, we review the influence of soccer- and basketball-specific training on the proficiency and use of both feet/hands, in order to examine whether increasing amounts of bilateral practice can change skill and choice of both sides. Last, potential implications for practitioners in team sports as well as for future research are inferred from the literature reviewed in this chapter.

INSIGHTS FROM SOCCER

Although footedness in soccer players seems to be an important topic for coaches and athletes (cf. Bryson et al., 2013), we identified only four studies from which footedness distributions among soccer players can be inferred.

Grouios et al. (2002) examined foot preference in a large sample of professional ($n = 368$), semiprofessional ($n = 389$), and amateur soccer players ($n = 357$), as well as nonsporting university students ($n = 305$). Respondents were asked to complete a standardized foot preference inventory, the Waterloo Footedness Questionnaire-Revised (WFQ-R; Elias, Bryden, & Bulman-Fleming, 1998), which comprises questions on foot preference for standard active (e.g., kicking a ball or grasping a marble with the toes) and stabilizing tasks (e.g., one-leg stance or balancing a bar with one foot). They computed a trichotomous scale to identify right-, left-, and mixed-footed individuals. Surprisingly, the proportion of individuals who claimed to be mixed-footed increased dramatically, from 9.1% in nonsporting controls, to 12.6% in amateur soccer players, to 30.3% in semiprofessional players, and to 45.9% in professional soccer players. They concluded that being equally skilled with both feet is a prerequisite to be successful in professional soccer. Moreover, their data suggest that increased amounts of soccer-specific practice reduced one-foot preference.

Carey et al. (2001) investigated actual foot use of professional soccer players in regular games, rather than responses on paper-and-pencil questionnaires. They analyzed 19,295 individual behaviors of 236 players from nine videotaped games (16 teams) of the FIFA World Cup 1998 in France. They found that the sample of elite soccer players was as right-footed (79.2%) as the general population. Dominant foot use only slightly differed between skills, with clearance and tackle showing weakest lateralization (72.5% dominant foot use) and set-pieces (e.g., corner kick, penalty kick) being strongest lateralized (up to 96.2% dominant foot use). However, players were, on average, as proficient with their dominant as with their nondominant foot (at least when assessed using a simple success–fail set of rules). Consequently, the authors questioned the assumptions that: (1) extensive amounts of soccer-specific practice can modulate foot preference/choice in actual gameplay and (2) two-footed players have an advantage for the advancement to higher competitive levels.

In another study, Carey et al. (2009) examined foot preference in two large samples of amateur (Exp. 1) and professional soccer players (Exp. 2). In Experiment 1, they asked 400 amateur soccer players to self-report their standard foot preference for 10 items from standardized inventories and their foot preference for soccer-related behaviors within the Aberdeen Football Laterality Questionnaire (AFLQ). Their data indicated that amateur soccer players are as right-footed as the general population for both standard foot preference (79.7%) and soccer-specific foot preference (83.7%). Moreover, their data suggested that amateurs *believe* that there is an association between deliberate practice and foot preference. For Experiment 2, they analyzed actual foot use in regular games of another 226 players from the English Premier League and added these data to the Carey et al. (2001) sample, resulting in a combined sample of 426 elite soccer players for which a total of 43,938 individual behaviors were coded. Again, with 77.2% right-footed and 22.8% left-footed players, foot preference of elite soccer players (based on the foot with the majority of touches) was found to be similar to the distribution in the general population. Dominant foot use was highest for set-pieces, dribbling, and passing (up to 86.2% dominant foot use). For the remaining behaviors the dominant foot was used for around 70% of all contacts. Moreover, soccer players were as successful with their dominant as with their nondominant foot (first touch, dribbling, and passing included), assessed in a slightly more rigorous way than in their earlier study. With regard to their results, they concluded that professional soccer players use one foot most of the time (~85%), in spite of affordances to use either foot over many different soccer situations. Further, they assumed that skill, but not choice, of foot is affected by extensive amounts of soccer-specific practice.

Bryson et al. (2013) investigated the influence of elite soccer players' footedness on their salary. Therefore they used archival data on players' footedness and salary of two large samples (data set 1: 1991 players from first division teams in England, France, Germany, Italy, and Spain; data set 2: 1314 players from the German Bundesliga) provided by two sources (www.transfermarkt.de and Kicker magazine). A surprising minority of the players (18.4% of the European cross section, and 24.9% of the German Bundesliga) were classified as mixed-footed players. Most important, they found statistically higher salaries for mixed-footed (between 13.2% and 18.6% higher) as compared to right- or left-footed athletes, in particular for forwards and midfielders. They argue that the salary premium for mixed-footed players results from their responsibilities and tasks on the field. However, based on their analyses, they also argue against an implementation of more mixed-footed players in the teams as this would not add significantly to team performance. Note the fine print of the www.transfermarkt.de website does reveal that such ratings of individual footedness depend on expert opinion, however, it does not provide the specific criteria used to classify footedness. The significant minorities judged as two-footed in the Bryson et al. (2013) study are considerably higher than what is suggested by Carey and colleagues' data deduced from regular games, which suggests that only a very small number of players achieve anything approaching two-footed play. It is conceivable that even expert raters are biased by a belief in an association between skill and two-footedness, as is believed by amateur soccer players (Carey et al., 2009).

Soccer Players' Footedness

The dichotomous distributions of footedness among soccer players (Carey et al., 2009, 2001) are, with around 80% right-footed players (see Table 14.1), similar between amateur and professional soccer players and the distribution in the general population (e.g., Gabbard & Iteya, 1996; Porac & Coren, 1981). Considering a trichotomous distribution of footedness in soccer players, some differences between the studies

TABLE 14.1 Studies From Which Footedness Distributions Among Soccer Players Can Be Inferred

Study	Method	N	Competitive Level	%RF/LF	%RF/LF/MF
Carey et al. (2001)	Video analysis[a]	236	World Cup	79.2/20.8	n/a
Grouios et al. (2002)	WFQ-R	368	Professionals	n/a	36.1/17.9/45.9
		389	Semiprofessionals		56.0/13.6/30.3
		357	Amateurs		78.0/9.0/12.6
		395	Nonsport controls		83.3/7.6/9.1
Carey et al. (2009)	Footedness scale[b]	400	Amateurs	79.7/20.3	70.5/12.5/17.0
	AFLQ			83.7/16.3	68.9/13.0/18.5
	Video analysis[a]	426	World Cup + Nat. League	77.2/22.8	n/a
Bryson et al. (2013)	Archival data[c]	1991	Nat. Leagues (EU)	n/a	58.9/22.7/18.4
		1314	Nat. League (GER)		51.3/23.8/24.9

RF, right-footed; LF, left-footed; MF, mixed-footed; N, sample size; AFLQ, Aberdeen Football Laterality Questionnaire; WFQ-R, Waterloo Footedness Questionnaire-Revised.
[a] *Foot with the majority of touches.*
[b] *10 footedness items used in standard inventories (e.g., Chapman et al., 1987).*
[c] *www.transfermarkt.de that base footedness decisions on expert opinion.*

appear. While Grouios et al. (2002) found an increase in mixed-footedness with an increasing competitive level (up to 45.9% in professional players) using a standard foot preference inventory, Bryson et al. (2013) found only up to 24.9% mixed-footed professional soccer players in a large sample of European soccer players based on performance data of these players (judged by experts from www.transfermarkt.de). The figures presented by Carey et al. (2009) for amateur soccer players, assessed by their beliefs, not their actual play, however, are similar to the footedness distribution for amateurs in the Grouios et al. (2002) study. That said, it is likely that the questionnaire data of at least the semiprofessional and professional soccer players may at least partially reflect a type of social desirability, as it is a common belief in coaches and athletes that mixed-footed soccer players are more successful, and that two-footedness is highly desirable in skilled players (Carey et al., 2009). Another possibility is that players just claimed to be less lateralized for certain behaviors as soccer-specific practice increased proficiency of both feet, failing to notice that such improvements do not translate to *use* on the pitch. Although data of the Bryson et al. (2013) study would suggest a reduction of right-foot bias in professional soccer players, without knowing the criteria (as well as inter-rater reliabilities, number of raters, and so on) the expert raters at www.transfermarkt.de used to determine players' footedness, their data should be treated with caution. It is conceivable that such expert decisions are biased by factors like players' identity, skill level, or team, or that just all players who do not possess a strong one-foot bias are classified as mixed-footed by these experts.

Soccer-Specific Foot Preference

Actual foot use of professional soccer players in regular games (Carey et al., 2009, 2001) reveals a strong bias toward the use of the right foot in right-footed players and toward the use of the left foot in left-footed players across all soccer-related behaviors. Dominant foot use was highest for set-pieces (i.e., free kicks, penalty kicks, and corner kicks), dribbling, and passing (~85%), and somewhat lower for first touch, shots, clearance, and tackles (~70%). Hence, players seem to revert to their "weaker," nondominant foot only when facing high pressure by opponents, i.e., when there is no time to change to the other foot. That said, on the one hand, the strong bias toward the use of one foot across the soccer-specific skills suggests that even extensive amounts of soccer-specific training do not affect the inborn tendency to prefer one leg in actual game play. On the other hand, it could simply reflect training regimes (e.g., instructions, drills, practical examples) as well as game play that, apart from some brief drills exclusively dedicated to the nondominant foot, favor the dominant foot (i.e., getting about 80% of the practice). Data also indicate that left-footed players may be less lateralized than right-footers for dribbling, passing, clearance, and tackling. Of course, given the relative rarity of left-footed players, estimates of their biases for different behaviors are made with less confidence than in the right-footed majority of the Carey and colleagues' samples. Therefore, more data is needed to establish potential differences in actual foot use between right- and left-footed athletes in professional soccer.

Influence of Training on Performance and Preference

Carey et al. (2009, 2001) have shown that for the rare occasions the nondominant foot was used, professional soccer players were almost as proficient with their nondominant foot as with their dominant foot for the first touch, dribbling, and passing actions (see Table 14.2), indicating a high bilateral competence of these athletes, i.e., being equally skilled with both feet. A study by Haaland and Hoff (2003) confirmed the high plasticity of nondominant foot performance in an experiment with 39 competitive soccer players between 15 and 21 years of age assigned to either a training ($n = 18$) or a control group ($n = 21$). After eight weeks of extensive practice

TABLE 14.2   Percentage (%) Success Rates for First Touch, Dribbling, and Passing With the Dominant (d) and Nondominant Foot (nd) for Right- and Left-Footed Players (Carey et al., 2009)

	First Touch		Dribbling		Passing	
	d-Foot	nd-Foot	d-Foot	nd-Foot	d-Foot	nd-Foot
Right-footers	92	94	94	91	77	75
Left-footers	96	95	93	95	81	81

(except full play) with the nondominant foot, performance of the non-dominant foot significantly improved in two standardized foot-tapping tests (7.6–11.9%) and three soccer-specific tests (10.3–25.4%), while performance of a control group that continued with their normal practice did not improve. However, whether these improvements in performance have the potential to modulate nondominant foot *use* on the pitch remains elusive.

Other research indicates that high-level soccer players possess almost no differences between the two legs for segmental dynamics in kicking (Nunome, Ikegami, Kozakai, Apriantono, & Sano, 2006), muscle strength and Hamstring/Quadriceps ratio (Zakas, 2006), and balance stability (Gstoettner et al., 2009; Matsuda, Demura, & Uchiyama, 2008; Teixeira, de Oliveira, Romano, & Correa, 2011), while young soccer players show asymmetries for both, dynamics and accuracy measures (McLean & Tumilty, 1993). These findings suggest that both feet of high-level soccer players adapt to soccer-specific demands similarly, allowing players to perform equally with both feet. Bennet, O'Donohoe, Young, and Bennet (2005), however, suggested that the two feet adapt to *different* tasks and demands (e.g., right foot kicking vs. left foot stabilizing) as thigh circumference has been shown to be higher in the nondominant than in the dominant leg in professional soccer players, in particular in right-footed athletes. In support of this notion, it has been shown that experienced soccer players possess differences in leg preference for mobilization and stabilization tasks (Teixeira et al., 2011). In contrast, the absence of any asymmetries between dominant and nondominant foot proficiency for passing, first touch, and dribbling (see Table 14.2) would argue against the notion that the two feet adapt to different tasks and demands. That said, although there is evidence indicating that extensive soccer-specific training can reduce asymmetries between the two legs, the findings to date are not sufficient to clearly evaluate how this translates to use on the pitch.

Although the claim of higher proportions of mixed-footed players at higher competitive levels (Grouios et al., 2002) would imply that extensive soccer-specific practice decreases the incidence of right-foot bias, to date there is no direct evidence for modulations of (soccer-specific) foot preference in response to extensive amounts of soccer-specific practice. The high proportion of mixed-footed individuals among professional soccer players could not be confirmed when footedness was determined via performance measures (Bryson et al., 2013; Carey et al., 2009, 2001).

Taken together, both feet seem to adapt in response to extensive amounts of soccer-specific practice resulting in similar proficiency, but each develop different responsibilities (e.g., stabilizing vs. kicking). However, based on the present findings, it is very unlikely that soccer-specific training attenuates the inborn foot preference.

Summary and Implications

In sum, current data on laterality in soccer indicate that substantial amounts of soccer-specific practice and play can affect skill in both legs/ feet, but not choice. Although dominant and nondominant leg skills largely seem to be similar (and improved) in professional soccer players, most likely as a result of substantial amounts of bilateral practice (and play), this similarity does not result in a higher use of the nondominant foot on the pitch. Soccer professionals' foot use under competition (across all skills) is as biased to the right side as is foot preference in the general population. However, it is likely that the strong right-foot bias is a result of different responsibilities of both legs (i.e., left-foot stabilizing vs. right-foot kicking) that hardly allow players to easily change between both feet during fast game play. That means the nondominant leg in soccer players seems to be specialized for stabilizing the body during dominant leg actions (e.g., kicking for goal, passing, dribbling), hence, both legs are involved in a complex way in each action but with different tasks. That said, although soccer players possess a high proficiency with both feet for many soccer-related behaviors, they will preferably use their dominant foot for touching the ball, even on occasions where the conditions afford nondominant foot use. Consequently, we hypothesize that the dominant leg is less practiced in controlling stability for the complex interaction of both legs, so that touching the ball with the nondominant foot seems to be only done on *some* of the occasions when the situation does not allow for dominant foot use (e.g., due to high pressure by opponents). In that regard, we assume that the dominant foot of soccer players becomes a universal tool (i.e., being able to touch, dribble, pass, and shoot the ball with all parts of the foot, enabling the player to receive/kick the ball from/in any direction with only the dominant foot), for which degrees of freedom are increased with increasing amounts of soccer-specific training, thus being able to compensate for possible nondominant foot actions.

Theoretically, the "affordances" (opportunities for a particular motor response) over many players and matches should be crudely equivalent in a sport where all areas of the playing surface are used and opposing sides are arranged in an adversarial fashion (e.g., are literally opposing one another). Clearly there are occasions when players use the dominant foot where conditions afforded a nondominant foot action, and these are likely to be more frequent than those that come to conscious attention of players or spectators via the commentaries of expert commentary of live matches. The differences between these "missed" nondominant foot actions and the ~15% of actual nondominant foot actions remain unexplored. In any case, for at least these latter instances, nondominant foot skilled executions are crucial at a high level, for all of the soccer-specific actions we have examined to date. Hence, it is important to systematically involve the nondominant foot for all behaviors in soccer training from early on.

Whether mixed-footed soccer players actually have an advantage in soccer that would justify higher salaries (cf. Bryson et al., 2013) has not been shown to date. Although the surprising number of around 20% mixed-footed players in the best European soccer leagues presented by Bryson et al. (2013) would support such a view (as this estimate would be higher than in the general population, depending on chosen threshold for inclusion), to date there are no systematic investigations that compared performance measures in soccer as a function of players' footedness (Carey et al., 2001 found no relationship between overall success rate for passes, dribbles, shots and tackles, and degree of foot bias). In fact, objective data from actual on-the-field behavior of a large sample of professional soccer players (Carey et al., 2009) raise doubts that mixed-footedness prevalence is that high in soccer, as they only found a few players who actually used their two feet with a similar frequency.

That said, the field would definitely benefit from more research on how performance on the pitch differs between right-, left-, and mixed-footed soccer players (especially with regard to their responsibilities on the field, their expertise, and better measures of success), and also from longitudinal (experimental) approaches to explore changes in (soccer-specific) foot preference in response to increasing amounts of soccer-specific practice. In fact, as acknowledged by Carey et al. (2009), frequency-based measures of foot use could prove extremely useful in examining the efficacy of "two-footed" interventions designed for young players, insofar as a critical period for the emergence of one-footed play could be established scientifically.

INSIGHTS FROM BASKETBALL

Although the sport of basketball is very popular and bilateral demands are present very frequently during a game, only four studies could be identified that dealt more or less specifically with the question of laterality in basketball players, and from which handedness distributions among basketball players can be inferred.

In an early study, Bale and Scholes (1986) asked a sample of English National League players (33 male, 36 female) and players who trained as regularly but had not reached national-level standard (32 male, 35 female) to self-report their hand preference for 12 everyday life activities using the Edinburgh Handedness Inventory (EHI; Oldfield, 1971). Their data suggest that National League players are less lateralized than nonleague players. Moreover, mixed-handed individuals were overrepresented among National League basketball players (30.4%) as compared to the general population (about 10%) and lower leagues (13.4%). They assumed that being as proficient with both hands is crucial for success in elite basketball, resulting in either an advantage of mixed-handed individuals to advance to higher levels or training-induced adaptations of hand preference to meet the bilateral demands of the sport. However, as the exceptional high proportion of mixed-handed individuals deduced from this questionnaire study gets no support from actual on-the-court behavior (about 18% mixed-handed individuals among professional basketball players, Stöckel & Weigelt, 2012a), it is likely that athletes self-reported to be less lateralized just because they thought they should be mixed-handed.

Lawler and Lawler (2011) examined the relation between handedness and performance in a large sample of professional basketball players from the NBA. They analyzed archival data on players' handedness and game statistics from a web source (www.apbr.com) of 3647 players (all athletes who participated in at least five games between 1946 and 2009). Although handedness played a prominent role in their study, from both the Lawler and Lawler (2011) paper and the referenced internet source of the Association of Professional Basketball Researchers, it remains unclear how it was assessed. Ignoring the rather low incidence of 5.1% left-handers ($n = 186$) in their sample, which was probably caused by a very restrictive measure of handedness (i.e., handedness deduced from a single task like shooting or writing) or incomplete data (e.g., the web source only reports players' handedness when being left-handed), they found that left-handed individuals outperformed right-handed individuals for some important performance measures including rebounding, assists, points per game, and field-goal percentage. Based on their results, they assumed that left-handed players may have a frequency-dependent advantage over right-handed players. Although the study provides interesting insights in performance differences between right- and left-handed basketball players, the fact that, neither from the Lawler and Lawler (2011) paper nor from the web source itself (www.apbr.com), objective criteria on how handedness was determined can be inferred raises doubts at least regarding the low incidence of left-handed players, especially when having advantages over right-handers as suggested.

Stöckel and Vater (2014) asked expert basketball players from the three highest German leagues about their hand preference for 10 everyday life activities using the EHI. Higher prevalence of mixed-handed individuals (18% based on the EHI) was found, similar (although not to the same extent) to the results reported by Bale and Scholes (1986). Additionally, Stöckel and Vater (2014) asked the players to report their basketball-specific hand preference for various skills and details about their basketball-specific history via the Basketball Laterality Questionnaire (BLQ). They found that everyday life and basketball-specific hand preference are strongly interrelated; however, both measures were poorly related to self-reported measures of basketball-specific practice. They argued that the bias in hand preference seems to be robust against extensive amounts of bilateral practice, which would suggest that an advanced selection process accounts for the higher prevalence of mixed-handed individuals among professional basketball players.

In another study, Stöckel and Weigelt (2012a) examined the influence of basketball-specific expertise on nondominant and dominant hand use and proficiency in regular basketball games using video analysis. All ball contacts of a total of 206 male athletes playing on three competitive levels (professional, semiprofessional, amateur) were recorded and analyzed with respect to the used hand (right, left, both), the executed skill (dribbling, passing, catching, shooting), and proficiency (passing and shooting success). They found that professional basketball players use their nondominant hand more frequently (for 26.3% of all ball contacts in a game as compared to 21.4% in semiprofessionals and 11.5% in amateurs) and with greater success (95.8% for passing as compared to 97.3% in semiprofessionals and 78.8% in amateurs; 57.8% for shooting as compared to 35.4% in semiprofessionals and 35.8% in amateurs) than players from lower competitive levels. Likewise, the use of the dominant hand was reduced to 48.9% in professional players as compared to amateurs (59.2%). When only considering one-handed ball contacts (i.e., two-handed catching and passing excluded), a 60:40 and a 62:38 ratio of dominant compared to nondominant hand ball contacts appeared in professional and semiprofessional players respectively, while the ratio was 80:20 in amateurs. In particular, the higher nondominant hand use of professional players compared to amateurs appeared for dribbling actions (47.0% vs. 19.9%) and to a much lesser extent for passing (12.0% vs. 4.4%) and catching actions (8.0% vs. 2.0%). The authors assumed that the extensive basketball-specific practice (i.e., training of the dominant and nondominant hand) accounts for the reduced one-hand bias (i.e., the strong tendency to prefer either the right or the left hand) in professional basketball players (i.e., in terms of a training-induced plasticity of handedness).

Basketball Players' Handedness

Although the previously reported studies on laterality in basketball players used different methods to deduce players' everyday life handedness, the dichotomous distributions of handedness across all the studies are quite similar (see Table 14.3). The proportion of left-handed players is from about 4% (i.e., based on shooting hand of amateurs; Stöckel & Weigelt, 2012a) to around 15% (i.e., based on preference for activities of daily living in 2nd National League players; Stöckel & Vater, 2014) similar to the handedness distribution in the general population (7–15% LH people, Raymond & Pontier, 2004). The lower proportion of left-handed players in the studies by Lawler and Lawler (2011) and by Stöckel and Weigelt (2012a) might be explained with more restrictive methods to assess handedness (e.g., shooting or writing hand), as opposed to the Edinburgh Handedness Inventory used in the other two studies, which determines handedness based on at least 10 activities of daily living. That said, although performance data of Lawler and Lawler (2011) would indicate an advantage of left-handed over right-handed athletes,

TABLE 14.3 Studies From Which Handedness Distributions Among Basketball Players Can Be Inferred

Study	Method	N	Competitive Level	|LQ|	%RH/LH	%RH/LH/MH
Bale and Scholes (1986)[a]	EHI	69	1st Nat. League	57.9	88.4/11.6	62.3/7.2/30.4
		67	Lower leagues	74.2	88.1/11.9	76.1/10.4/13.4
Lawler and Lawler (2011)	Archival data[b]	3647	1st Nat. League (NBA or equal)	n/a	94.9/5.1	n/a
Stöckel and Weigelt (2012a)	Video analysis[c]	63	Professionals	n/a	92.1/7.9	n/a
		43	Semiprofessionals		90.7/9.3	
		100	Amateurs		96.0/4.0	
Stöckel and Vater (2014)	EHI	46	1st Nat. League	70.1	88.9/11.1	73.3/8.9/17.8
		61	2nd Nat. League A	65.1	85.2/14.8	70.5/11.5/18.0
		69	2nd Nat. League B	73.6	89.9/10.1	75.4/10.1/14.5

EHI, Edinburgh Handedness Inventory; *RH*, right-handed; *LH*, left-handed; *MH*, mixed-handed; *LQ*, Lateral Quotient; *N*, sample size.
[a] *Data was reanalyzed using the values provided in the original paper.*
[b] *www.apbr.com (no indication how handedness is determined).*
[c] *Hand used for free throws.*

the expected or below-expected incidence of left-handedness in the studies reviewed here argues against any frequency-dependent advantages of left-handed players in basketball.

Considering a trichotomous distribution of handedness (i.e., identifying mixed-handed athletes with lateral quotients in the EHI between −40 and +40; see Stöckel & Vater, 2014), the percentage of right-handed individuals (62–76%, based on hand preference for activities of daily living) is reduced among expert basketball players as compared to the general population with about 84% right-handed individuals (cf. Gabbard & Iteya, 1996). Notably, mixed-handed individuals seem to be overrepresented with 13–30% as compared to about 10% in the general population (Bale & Scholes, 1986; Stöckel & Vater, 2014). The laterality quotients (LQ) based on EHI confirmed lower league players to be stronger lateralized than players from 1st National League in the Bale and Scholes' study (1986). However, Stöckel and Vater (2014) found LQs to be consistent across high competitive levels.

In sum, data yield a reduced right-hand bias in high-level basketball players, along with a higher prevalence of mixed-handed individuals.

Basketball-Specific Hand Preference

In the study by Stöckel and Vater (2014), players were asked to self-report the hand preference for 12 basketball-specific behaviors on a seven-point Likert scale ranging from "always left" over "equal use" to "always right." First, they found no difference in basketball-specific hand preference (i.e., dominant vs. nondominant) between right- and left-handed players. Mixed-handed individuals (as deduced from the EHI) also reported a higher equal-hand use (as compared to right- and left-handed players) across the basketball-specific skills, which was further supported by a strong positive relation between everyday life and basketball-specific handedness. Therefore, the authors used deviation scores from equal-hand use for further analyses and did not further differentiate between right- and left-hand preferences. Their data revealed three subscales that received similar hand preference ratings within the 12 basketball-specific skills. Specifically, for layup and dribbling skills (plus short passes), players reported lowest deviations from equal-hand use, followed by catching and passing skills (plus steals). For all shots from larger distances, players reported to strongly prefer their dominant hand (as lead hand behind the ball).

Analyzing actual hand use during regular games, Stöckel and Weigelt (2012a) found that professional basketball players use their nondominant hand for 27.7% of all ball contacts. More specifically, they use the nondominant hand for 47.0% of all dribbling, 17.6% of all shooting, 12.0% of all passing, and 8.0% of all catching action (see Table 14.4). Nondominant hand contacts were lower for all skills in athletes from lower competitive levels. The high proportion of nondominant hand ball contacts in dribbling and shooting seem to reflect common training approaches in basketball, in which the nondominant hand is involved in practice systematically from early on, especially for dribbling and layups (i.e., shots made from close to the basket). However, with regard to these training approaches, one might expect the nondominant hand shooting actions close to the basket to be much higher, but it seems that even professional players preferably revert to their dominant hand skills, even for the less demanding conditions of layups, which on many occasions may include defenders pressuring the use of the dominant hand of the shooter. The lower proportion of nondominant hand ball contacts in catching can be explained by the high number of two-handed contacts (82.4%); however, rates of one-handed catching are quite similar between the dominant (9.6%) and nondominant hands (8.0%). Two-handed catching is much safer than one-handed catching, the latter of which will typically have higher risk, even among the skilled players at the highest competitive levels. Therefore coaches call for the use of both hands from early on.

The data of both studies indicate that hand preference/use in professional basketball players greatly varies between tasks, with the dominant hand used for virtually all shots from longer distances, whereas the lowest deviations from equal-hand use are reported for dribbling. The self-report of reduced one-hand preference for shooting directly at the basket (i.e., layups), catching, and passing skills as reported in Stöckel and Vater (2014), gets no clear support from actual on-the-court behavior (Stöckel & Weigelt, 2012a). However, it appears that when the choice of effector can be made independently (i.e., without being pressed by time, opponents, or tactics, e.g., free throws) and/or the task implies high dynamic demands

TABLE 14.4   Proportion (%) of Dominant, Nondominant, and Two-Handed Ball Contacts for the Main Skills in Professional Basketball Players (n = 63)

	Dribbling	Shooting[a]	Passing	Catching	Total
Dominant hand	53	82	54	10	49
Nondominant hand	47	18	12	8	28
Two-handed	n/a	n/a	34	82	23

[a] *Only shots from a distance less than 1 m to the rim are included. For all other shots, no nondominant hand ball contacts were recorded.*

Reanalyzed data from Stöckel, T., & Weigelt, M. (2012a). Plasticity of human handedness: decreased one-hand bias and inter-manual performance asymmetry in expert basketball players. Journal of Sports Sciences, 30, 1037–1045.

(e.g., generation and execution of force for three-point shots and long distance passes), people revert to their more skilled, dominant hand. But when skills have to be performed in interaction with others and/or under high pressure (e.g., layups, dribbling, and short passes), where the choice of effector most often depends on the situation on the court (i.e., interaction with others), then the hand used is the one that is most proficient in the given situation (cf. Stöckel & Vater, 2014; Stöckel & Weigelt, 2012a). It is noteworthy that patterns of hand preference/use did not differ between playing positions (i.e., guard, forward, center), although previous work assumed a differential involvement of both hands based on the tasks and responsibilities of the players on the court (Bale & Scholes, 1986).

Influence of Training on Performance and Preference

Stöckel and Weigelt (2012a) have shown that professional basketball players were as proficient with their nondominant hand as with their dominant hand for shooting and passing actions (see Table 14.5), indicating a high bilateral competence of these athletes, i.e., being equally skilled with both hands. As proficiency increased with an increasing competitive level, they hypothesized that this high bilateral competence of professional basketball players is a result of extensive amounts of bilateral practice. However, in contrast to Bishop (1989), who stated that hand preference is determined by hand skill, in basketball a higher proficiency was not associated to a more frequent use of the nondominant hand for passing and shooting. Also, other studies found evidence for a high plasticity of nondominant hand skills in response to basketball-specific training, especially when the nondominant hand is involved in practice systematically from early on (i.e., during skill acquisition at young ages; cf. Stöckel & Weigelt, 2012b; Stöckel, Weigelt, & Krug, 2011).

A causal link between basketball-specific practice and hand preference, however, lacks direct evidence. Although it has been assumed that extensive amounts of bilateral (or lateralized) practice lead to

TABLE 14.5 Success Rates (%) for Passing and Shooting (Close to the Rim) With the Dominant (d) and Nondominant Hand (nd) (Stöckel & Weigelt, 2012a)

	Passing		Shooting[a]	
	d-Hand	nd-Hand	d-Hand	nd-Hand
Professionals	96	96	56	58
Semiprofessionals	94	97	48	35
Amateurs	89	79	55	36

[a] *Only shots from a distance less than 1 m to the rim are included. For all other shots, no nondominant hand ball contacts were recorded.*

modulations of lateral preference (e.g., Mikheev, Mohrb, Afanasiev, Landis, & Thut, 2002; Stöckel & Weigelt, 2012a; Teixeira & Okazaki, 2007; Teixeira et al., 2011), to date there is no direct evidence for training-induced adaptations of (basketball-specific) hand preference in basketball players. Stöckel and Weigelt (2012a) primarily based their assumption on the fact that professional basketball players used their nondominant hand more frequently across all skills as compared to semiprofessionals that in turn used their nondominant hand more often than amateurs. However, in the absence of measures on how much practice with the nondominant hand individual's had experienced in their own coached career and more sensitive measures of players' everyday life handedness (determined by shooting hand in their study), it is hard to speculate about any causal relationships. For instance, it is very likely that nondominant hand use is biased by a higher prevalence of mixed-handed individuals on the highest levels in basketball in particular (cf. Bale & Scholes, 1986; Stöckel & Vater, 2014).

Stöckel and Vater (2014) approached the link between basketball-specific training and hand preference patterns by correlating measures of basketball-specific practice (i.e., years of coached practice, rough estimate of ever-achieved nondominant hand practice) and measures of basketball-specific and everyday life hand preference. As only preference scores for layup and dribbling skills were significantly related to measures of basketball-specific practice, they argued that training-induced modulations of lateral preference seem to be very specific to only a few basketball-specific skills and do not generalize to other skills within the domain of basketball nor do they extend into everyday life handedness. This finding was supported by a strong relation between basketball-specific and everyday life hand preference. They concluded that the bias in hand preference, which has been shown to be an innate trait (Annett, 2002; Corballis, 1997; McManus, 2002), seems to be robust against even extensive amounts of bilateral practice.

That said, it seems that extensive amounts of basketball-specific practice (i.e., training on both the dominant and nondominant hand) affect skill (i.e., proficiency of both hands), but hardly choice of hand.

Summary and Implications

Playing at the highest levels in basketball may be facilitated by the proficiency to use both hands, particularly in dribbling (cf. Stöckel & Weigelt, 2012a). Nevertheless, professionals should be able to use their nondominant hand more often than lower league players for the other activities like catching, passing, and shooting actions as well. From that, practitioners in basketball are well advised to practice these skills with the nondominant hand systematically from early on. For distance shots, basketball players from all levels use their dominant hand exclusively. That said, shooting is actually a two-handed activity in which the dominant hand applies force and spin to the ball while the nondominant hand stabilizes the ball and the intended shooting trajectory. Hence, it is likely that the different, but very specific responsibilities of both hands in shooting tasks prevent changing hands for shooting actions.

Most important, to date there is no evidence for training-induced modulations of lateral preference, except for dribbling (Stöckel & Weigelt, 2012a). That said, basketball-specific bilateral practice improves proficiency of both hands but influences hand preference less dramatically (only preference for layup and dribbling skills). The higher prevalence of mixed-handed individuals among professional basketball players (as compared to the general population) seems to be more likely to account for the more frequent use of the nondominant hand as reported by Stöckel and Weigelt (2012a), than basketball-specific training regimes (cf. Stöckel & Vater, 2014). In turn, this finding suggests that strongly lateralized individuals may be at a disadvantage in basketball, as it is very likely that these players will use their dominant hand most of the time even in situations in which the nondominant hand is most proficient. However, for those occasions in which players use their nondominant hand, they have been shown to be as proficient as they are with their dominant hand. Therefore, hand preference screenings could be useful for talent identification in basketball. Moreover, practitioners and researchers should try and develop practice regimes that allow strongly lateralized players to "overcome" their inborn hand preference at least for basketball-specific skills. For example, the choice of hand could be restricted to the nondominant hand in game-like play for a while, or the nondominant hand could be exclusively used for predefined parts of the training session for a couple of weeks (e.g., during preseason). That said, it is tempting to suggest more nondominant hand drills etc. to try and ameliorate hand preference biases that persist in basketball. We suggest using a more considered approach where specific training interventions are properly evaluated by recording actual hand use in regular games or game-like play using techniques like those we have developed for measuring actual use on the pitch/court.

CONCLUSION

In summary, it appears that in high-level basketball players the right-hand bias is reduced (along with a higher prevalence of mixed-handed individuals), while soccer players' footedness is as biased to the right side as in the general population, even on the highest levels. However, a remaining set of questions have to do with differences in estimates of lateral "preference" when measuring behavior on the pitch versus self-reported behavior by questionnaire. The latter suggests that there are some selection biases etc. for top-level soccer and basketball—the former suggests footedness at least is roughly representative of that found in the general population. Demand characteristics in the questionnaire studies may play some role of course in a way that elite players think they should be two-sided (perhaps compared to other groups, they could be quite aware of why they are being asked questions about their sidedness). We have little doubt that players (and expert raters such as those used by www.transfermarkt.de) have some knowledge of foot or hand bias in themselves or individual players that they observe, but consistent and accurate monitoring of use of one side or the other really is not done, except in the frequency count studies mentioned above. We suspect salient events are noted, including missed opportunities to use the nondominant side, that probably do reveal something approximate about side bias in individual players. Studies which contrast self-report and actual use on the pitch/court *in the same players* need to be done to resolve this interesting issue.

The studies reviewed here suggest another intriguing finding in soccer- and basketball-specific lateral skill development and expression. In both sports, there is now good reason to believe that practice and training improves the execution of some of the one-sided skills necessary for proficiency in these sports; what is less clear is whether or not improvements in skill in the less preferred side results in increased use of that side. In soccer the behavioral evidence for this dissociation between skill and use is pretty unequivocal to date, although there are power issues here when nonpreferred foot use is rare, and issues of accuracy given the simple success–fail measure used to evaluate skill. In basketball, dribbling (and to some extent layups) is the exception to this skill-use dissociation. These findings suggest that dribbling in basketball is distinct in some motor learning and control sense relative to dribbling in soccer. Obviously, in spite of sharing the same label in English, dribbling in soccer, in a bipedal species like us, requires a considerable degree of bilateral control; in a way that one-handed dribbling in basketball does not. Professional basketball players are often doing things with the nonused arm/hand while dribbling (like signaling to teammates, holding off opponents, and so on), but those activities do not have to be coordinated with the dribbling limb in quite the same way as the two legs do when shooting, passing, or dribbling in soccer.

These outstanding issues suggest further research efforts, in both sidedness-related questions in neuropsychology and cognitive neuroscience, as well as in motor skill expression and development in sports science and motor control.

References

Annett, M. (2002). *Handedness and brain asymmetry. The right shift theory.* Hove, East Sussex, UK: Psychology Press.

Bale, P., & Scholes, S. (1986). Lateral dominance and basketball performance. *Journal of Human Movement Studies, 12,* 145–151.

Bennet, S., O'Donohoe, P., Young, D., & Bennet, G. (2005). Quadriceps assessment in professional soccer players. *British Journal of Sports Medicine, 39,* 182.

Bishop, D. V. M. (1989). Does hand proficiency determine hand preference? *British Journal of Psychology, 80,* 191–199.

Bryson, A., Frick, B., & Simmons, R. (2013). The returns to scarce talent: footedness and player remuneration in European soccer. *Journal of Sports Economics, 14,* 606–628.

Carey, D. P., Smith, D. T., Martin, D., Smith, G., Skriver, J., Rutland, A., & Shepherd, J. W. (2009). The bi-pedal ape: plasticity and asymmetry in footedness. *Cortex, 45,* 650–661.

Carey, D. P., Smith, G., Smith, D. T., Shepherd, J. W., Skriver, J., Ord, L., & Rutland, A. (2001). Footedness in world soccer: an analysis of France '98. *Journal of Sport Science, 19,* 855–864.

Chapman, J. P., Chapman, L. J., & Allen, J. J. (1987). The measurement of foot preference. *Neuropsychologia, 25*(3), 579–584.

Corballis, M. C. (1997). The genetics and evolution of handedness. *Psychological Review, 104,* 714–727.

Elias, L. J., Bryden, M. P., & Bulman-Fleming, M. B. (1998). Footedness is a better predictor than is handedness of emotional lateralization. *Neuropsychologia, 36,* 37–43.

Gabbard, C., & Iteya, M. (1996). Foot laterality in children, adolescents, and adults. *Laterality: Asymmetries of Body, Brain and Cognition, 1,* 199–205.

Grouios, G. (2004). Motoric dominance and sporting excellence: training versus heredity. *Perceptual and Motor Skills, 98,* 53–66.

Grouios, G., Kollias, N., Tsorbatzoudis, H., & Alexandris, K. (2002). Overrepresentation of mixed-footedness among professional and semi-professional soccer players: an innate superiority or a strategic advantage? *Journal of Human Movement Studies, 42,* 19–29.

Gstoettner, M., Neher, A., Scholtz, A., Milloning, M., Lembert, S., & Raschner, C. (2009). Balance ability and muscle response of the preferred and nonpreferred leg in soccer players. *Motor Control, 13,* 218–231.

Haaland, E., & Hoff, J. (2003). Non-dominant leg training improves the bilateral motor performance of soccer players. *Scandinavian Journal of Medicine and Science in Sports, 13,* 179–184.

Lawler, T. P., & Lawler, F. H. (2011). Left-handedness in professional basketball: prevalence, performance, and survival. *Perceptual and Motor Skills, 113,* 815–824.

Matsuda, S., Demura, S., & Uchiyama, M. (2008). Centre of pressure sway characteristics during static one-legged stance of athletes from different sports. *Journal of Sports Sciences, 26,* 775–779.

McLean, B. D., & Tumilty, D. M. (1993). Left-right asymmetry in 2 types of soccer kick. *British Journal of Sports Medicine, 27,* 260–262.

McManus, I. C. (2002). *Right hand, left hand: The origins of asymmetry in brains, bodies, atoms and cultures.* London, UK: Weidenfeld and Nicolson.

Mikheev, M., Mohrb, C., Afanasiev, S., Landis, T., & Thut, G. (2002). Motor control and cerebral hemispheric specialization in highly qualified judo wrestlers. *Neuropsychologia, 40,* 1209–1219.

Nunome, H., Ikegami, Y., Kozakai, R., Apriantono, T., & Sano, S. (2006). Segmental dynamics of soccer instep kicking with the preferred and non-preferred leg. *Journal of Sports Sciences, 24,* 529–541.

Oldfield, R. C. (1971). The assessment and analysis of handedness: the Edinburgh inventory. *Neuropsychologia, 9,* 97–113.

Porac, C., & Coren, S. (1981). *Lateral preferences and human behavior*. New York: Springer.

Raymond, M., & Pontier, D. (2004). Is there geographical variation in human handedness? *Laterality: Asymmetries of Body, Brain and Cognition, 9*, 35–51.

Stöckel, T., & Vater, C. (2014). Hand preference patterns in expert basketball players: interrelations between basketball-specific and everyday life behavior. *Human Movement Science, 38*, 143–151.

Stöckel, T., & Weigelt, M. (2012a). Plasticity of human handedness: decreased one-hand bias and inter-manual performance asymmetry in expert basketball players. *Journal of Sports Sciences, 30*, 1037–1045.

Stöckel, T., & Weigelt, M. (2012b). Brain lateralisation and motor learning: selective effects of dominant and non-dominant hand practice on the early acquisition of throwing skills. *Laterality: Asymmetries of Body, Brain and Cognition, 17*, 18–37.

Stöckel, T., Weigelt, M., & Krug, J. (2011). Acquisition of a complex basketball-dribbling task in school children as a function of bilateral practice order. *Research Quarterly for Exercise and Sport, 82*, 188–197.

Teixeira, L. A., & Okazaki, V. H. A. (2007). Shift of manual preference by lateralized practice generalizes to related motor tasks. *Experimental Brain Research, 183*, 417–423.

Teixeira, L. A., de Oliveira, D. L., Romano, R. G., & Correa, S. C. (2011). Leg preference and interlateral asymmetry of balance stability in soccer players. *Research Quarterly for Exercise and Sport, 82*, 21–27.

Zakas, A. (2006). Bilateral isokinetic peak torque of quadriceps and harmstring muscles in professional soccer players with dominance on one or both two sides. *Journal of Sports Medicine & Physical Fitness, 46*, 28–35.

15

Skill Acquisition in Left- and Right-Dominant Athletes: Insights From Elite Coaching

Dave Whiteside, Tim Buszard

Innovation and Insights Group, Tennis Australia, Melbourne, VIC, Australia; Victoria University, Footscray, VIC, Australia

Georgia Giblin

Innovation and Insights Group, Tennis Australia, Melbourne, VIC, Australia; Queensland Academy of Sport, Brisbane, QLD, Australia

Machar Reid

Innovation and Insights Group, Tennis Australia, Melbourne, VIC, Australia; University of Western Australia, Crawley, WA, Australia

INTRODUCTION

Understanding how experts learn the skills necessary to excel in domains such as sport, medicine, or music has been a primary focus of skill acquisition research since 1975. Traditionally, skill acquisition is defined as the internal processes that bring about relatively permanent changes in a learner's movement capabilities (Schmidt & Wrisberg, 2000). In particular, skill acquisition researchers are concerned with the mechanisms underpinning learning and how these processes facilitate the acquisition of new skills. With sports performance in mind, skill acquisition considers how the dynamics of practice and instruction influence how athletes acquire the perceptual, cognitive, and motor skills required to perform their sport-specific movements. For coaches and/or skill acquisition specialists, the prevailing goal is to facilitate performance improvements by creating a practice environment that optimizes learning and expedites the acquisition of new skills.

Recently, the concept of laterality, specifically motoric dominance in sport, has been a fertile area for research, with particular focus on the purported benefits that left-handed/footed athletes possess in specific sports. While left-handers account for approximately 10–12% of the general population (Gilbert & Wysocki, 1992), they are often overrepresented in high-level sports. For example, left-handed overrepresentation has been documented in baseball (Goldstein & Young, 1996), fencing (Harris, 2010), cricket (Brooks, Bussiere, Jennions, & Hunt, 2004), and tennis (Holtzen, 2000; Loffing, Hagemann, & Strauss, 2012). In such sports, left-handers often demonstrate a tactical or strategic advantage over their right-handed counterparts, which poses a concurrent challenge and opportunity for coaches. Indeed, the Hawthorn Football Club, arguably the most successful contemporary team in Australia's premier football code, even laud the relatively higher technical skill (kicking efficiency) of left-footed players (compared to right-footed players) and recruit accordingly (Stevens, 2010). The left-handed advantage is also evident among cricket batsmen, where left-handers demonstrate higher batting averages and bat for longer before being dismissed than their right-handed counterparts (Brooks et al., 2004). That 85% of the opening batsmen for the Australian cricket team since 2005 have been left-handed offers an insight into how motor dominance is being used to shape team strategy in elite sport. While the bulk of research investigating the left-handed advantage has explored two main theories, "the innate superiority hypothesis" and the "strategic advantage hypothesis" (Grouios, Tsorbatzoudis, Alexandris, & Barkoukis, 2000; Loffing & Hagemann, 2012; see also Chapter 12: Performance Differences Between Left- and Right-Sided Athletes in One-on-One Interactive Sports), there is a lack of investigative rigor around the relationship between motor dominance and skill acquisition. Correspondingly, it is difficult for practitioners to design evidence-based training environments that cater to laterality, thereby exposing this aspect of athlete development to the less resolute coaching anecdote.

With an overarching emphasis on elite sport, in this chapter, we focus on (1) the athlete's learning process and the effects of different coaching styles thereon; (2) learning by observing model demonstrations; (3) how the provision of feedback influences the acquisition of motor skills; and (4) how coaches can structure practice to facilitate the acquisition of perceptual and motor skills. These sections are presented alongside practical examples that help to operationalize the relationship between motor dominance and coaching philosophies in elite sport.

Explicit Motor Learning and Prescriptive Coaching Strategies

Explicit motor learning is a conscious process, whereby an individual acquires specific knowledge about a skill and is, therefore, aware of the learning process (Berry & Broadbent, 1988). Typically, this occurs when a coach provides information about the mechanics involved in the skill. For example, an individual learning to play tennis may be provided with a set of explicit verbal instructions by the coach that pertain to certain aspects of performance (e.g., "Don't flick your wrist when you toss the ball up to serve," "Transfer your weight to your front foot when hitting through the ball," "Rotate your shoulders away from the net during the backswing of the forehand stroke," etc.). A coaching style that involves the propagation of explicit instructions to the athlete is termed "prescriptive." Explicit motor learning can also occur without any involvement from a coach. If an athlete attempts to "solve" a movement skill by consciously experimenting with different movement patterns and contemplating how they affect the performance outcome, explicit learning can ensue (e.g., Hardy, Mullen, & Jones, 1996; Masters, 1992; Maxwell, Masters, & Eves, 2003). For example, a basketball player may intentionally engage her legs more when shooting in an effort to improve the arc of her jump shot. If the desired effect is realized, she would be cognizant of this relationship and could verbalize the acquired knowledge (i.e., "If I push off harder with my legs, I achieve a better arc on my shot").

Whether a consequence of prescriptive instruction from a coach or deliberate movement experimentation, explicit learning leads the athlete to develop a body of declarative knowledge about the skill to which he/she can consult during subsequent performances thereof.

Implicit Motor Learning and Less Prescriptive Coaching Strategies

Berry (1997, p. 1) describes implicit learning as a process "where a person learns about the structure of a fairly complex stimuli environment, without necessarily intending to do so, and in such way that the resulting knowledge is difficult to express". Contrary to explicit learning, there is no development of explicit knowledge about the skill by virtue of external instruction or conscious attention to performance (e.g., Green & Flowers, 1991; Hardy et al., 1996; Masters, 1992; Maxwell et al., 2003). Professional golfer and two-time US Masters winner Bubba Watson offers a working example of this phenomenon in maintaining that he has never received explicit coaching instructions and, not surprisingly, prefers to discuss his swing in terms of "feel," rather than biomechanics. He describes:

> As a kid, you don't think of the mechanics and I have to get my grip this way or be stronger or weaker. You just think, 'I did this and it went that way.' So that's how I did it, by practicing feel. So now my shots are all feel. *Michaux (2013)*

Thus he has seemingly acquired his golf skills in an implicit manner. Since implicit learning reduces the accumulation of explicit knowledge about the skill, the learner's propensity to draw upon such information during performance is also diminished.

Implicit and Explicit Learning in Practice

Numerous studies have compared the efficacy of implicit and explicit motor learning, consistently showing that skills acquired implicitly (as opposed to explicitly) are less susceptible to breakdown in situations of high psychological stress or anxiety (Hardy et al., 1996; Liao & Masters, 2001; Masters, 1992; Pijpers, Oudejans, & Bakker, 2005) or physiological fatigue (Masters, Poolton, Maxwell, & Raab, 2008; Poolton, Masters, & Maxwell, 2007). Additionally, performance does not decline when a cognitively demanding secondary task is simultaneously included (e.g., Lam, Maxwell, & Masters, 2009; Maxwell, Masters, Kerr, & Weedon, 2001). In professional sport, it is not uncommon to see players "choke" or fail under pressure, and this is often attributed to athletes directing their attention inwards toward their mechanics and the explicit rules/knowledge they developed through explicit learning (e.g., the theory of reinvestment; Masters & Maxwell, 2008). Thus, it appears that coaches should generally refrain from providing explicit instructions about performance and discourage athletes from consciously attending to their mechanics.

Since 1995, Masters and colleagues have identified several practice strategies that lead to the implicit acquisition of motor skills. These include: dual-task practice (Hardy et al., 1996; Masters, 1992; Maxwell, Masters, & Eves, 2000), removing feedback (Maxwell et al., 2003), providing "subliminal" feedback (Maxwell, Masters, & Eves, 2009), using analogies as instructions (Lam et al., 2009; Liao & Masters, 2001; Poolton, Masters, & Maxwell, 2006), limiting errors during practice (Masters, Lo, Maxwell, & Patil, 2008; Masters, Poolton, et al., 2008; Maxwell et al., 2001; Poolton, Masters, & Maxwell, 2005; Poolton et al., 2007), and directing attention to external cues as opposed to internal movements (Poolton, Maxwell, Masters, & Raab, 2006).

For coaches in elite sport, these practice techniques are advantageous for developing automaticity: the point at which an athlete can perform a motor skill devoid of conscious attention to their mechanics (Anderson, 1983; Fitts & Posner, 1967). As an example, let's imagine a scenario in which a skilled right-handed cricket batsman has developed a tendency to "overthink" the mechanics of his batting technique when facing left-arm bowlers, leading him to "choke." Given that the batsman already possesses the necessary technical proficiency to perform the skill, it may be advantageous for a coach to utilize the dual-task strategy, which requires the batsman to perform a concurrent secondary task (e.g., saying "yes" every time the coach claps their hands) while batting against left-arm bowlers. In doing so, the batsman's attention resources are preoccupied with the secondary task, thereby preventing him from directing his attention to the mechanical intricacies of the task. Alternatively, as evidenced by the work of Liao and Masters (2001) in teaching the topspin table-tennis forehand, coaches may guide the mechanics of learners through analogies (e.g., rather than explicitly describe the requisite shoulder joint kinematics that precede the forwardswing phase of the tennis serve, a coach may employ the analogy "use your racket to scratch your back"). Here, task relevant knowledge is acquired passively, usually at a subconscious level, and cannot be easily verbalized by the learner.

Practice that minimizes errors also encourages implicit processing during performance of the movement skill. For instance, an expert golfer who has developed the "putting yips" (i.e., uncharacteristically missing putts from a close distance) would begin putting from very close to the hole and gradually move further away. By minimizing errors, the athlete is less likely to engage in error-correction strategies—the very strategies that typically lead to the agglomeration of explicit rules about the skill. Instructions that direct athletes' attention to external sources (e.g., the ball, the racket, or the ground) have also been shown to promote implicit learning. An external—as opposed to internal—focus has further been shown to place a lower load on attentional resources, thereby allowing learners to perform better under secondary task conditions (Poolton, Maxwell, et al., 2006). As a case in point, soccer players practicing the penalty kick may be instructed to focus on the desired target within the goals, thus not interfering with implicit learning as they are not being provided any knowledge about their mechanics.

Although implicit learning approaches may appear preferable, effectively all coaches employ some degree of explicit instruction when developing athletes. Indeed, in situations that require athletes to inhibit their automatic or implicit tendencies, explicit instructions are seemingly more effective. For example, the manager of a baseball team may want his batters to refrain from swinging at pitches when the count is 3–0. Accordingly, the batter would need to restrain their inclination to swing at the ball, even if it may appear to be traveling toward the strike zone. In this sense, prescriptive coaching may be most effective when athletes are required to inhibit their automatic (implicit) processes during competition in order to achieve a desired tactical outcome. Contrastingly, more fundamental aspects of performance, such as the development of correct batting mechanics, should be promoted using subtle practice techniques that encourage an implicit mode of learning.

DELIVERING INFORMATION VIA DEMONSTRATIONS

One of the many problems faced by coaches concerns how they instruct an athlete to perform a new skill. Coaches may choose to verbally describe the skill, although it has been established that this is more likely to lead to an explicit mode of learning. Alternatively, the coach could provide the athlete with a visual demonstration, which is more conducive to implicit learning.

Learning From Observation and Imitation

Observing and imitating an "expert" model performer (e.g., footage of a professional athlete) has significant benefits for skill acquisition. Indeed, research has demonstrated that the combination of physical practice with observational learning is more advantageous to skill learning than physical practice alone, particularly in mature performers (i.e., over 16years; Ashford, Davids, & Bennett, 2007). It is theorized that the observation of a model performer provides the learner with the opportunity to detect important and often subtle information regarding the coordinative movement patterns that are required to perform the task (Shea, Wulf, Whitacre, & Wright, 2000). Additionally, there is evidence implying that the information acquired through observation of an expert is stored passively via implicit processes (Vinter & Perruchet, 2002), particularly if the observer's attention is directed to the key cues of the task (Masters, Lo, et al., 2008). With this in mind, it is plausible that a coach could communicate desired instructions subconsciously through a model, rather than explicitly directing the athlete.

In elite sport, the concept of *learning by observation* is common practice. For instance, a coach could demonstrate a skill with the intention of improving the player's awareness of a particular movement. Alternatively, the coach may provide the player with video footage of an expert performer, as is commonly implemented in research studies. In each instance however, the notion of *laterality* presents a distinct challenge to the coach. Namely, are the benefits associated with observing a model performer apparent for a left-handed tennis player observing a right-handed model? It is possible that observing a model of opposite handedness or footedness would reduce the athlete's familiarity with the task, thereby limiting the efficacy of the demonstration (e.g., de Nooijer, van Gog, Paas, & Zwaan, 2013). Australian baseball coach, John Deeble, explains how this has presented a challenge when teaching players how to field the ball:

> Demonstrating how to pick up the ball and throw to young children of opposite handedness has caused me a few problems, particularly with regards to teaching correct footwork. When coaching right-handers, I use the correct footwork for a left-hander (John is left-handed) and tell them that they need to use the other foot. I then show them using a right-handed technique with the correct footwork but the delivery isn't as smooth. *J. Deeble, personal communication (October 8, 2014)*

From this example, it is clear that demonstrations involving opposite handedness or footedness can limit the effectiveness of demonstrations. Evidence from neuroscience demonstrates that a set of common neural structures is activated during both action production and action observation (referred to as *the Mirror Neuron Network* or *the Action Observation Network*), and this neural response is stronger when observing tasks that are familiar to the performers (Calvo-Merino, Glaser, Grezes, Passingham, & Haggard, 2005; Cross, Kraemer, Hamilton, Kelley, & Grafton, 2009). Thus if the observer has difficulty familiarizing with the task, the benefits associated with observational learning are likely to diminish.

To our knowledge, no study has directly assessed whether observational learning is affected by handedness or footedness; however, the extent to which the *familiarity effect* exists among tasks that are similar for both left and right handers (e.g., a tennis serve or an overarm throw) would be instructive. Indeed, one study reported differences in neural activations among the Mirror Neuron Network of right- and left-handers when observing simple hand movements (Rocca, Falini, Comi, Scotti, & Filippi, 2008). However, whether or not these different neural activations influence the efficacy of observational learning is unknown. Notwithstanding this, advances in technology allow sports coaches to address this issue using video-editing programs (e.g., Dartfish, Siliconcoach Ltd), whereby the footage is inverted such that a right-handed performer appears as left-handed on the screen. Presumably, this would afford athletes greater familiarity with the movement, thereby facilitating the concomitant benefits associated with observing an expert model. Indeed, the advantages of being familiar with the observed model were highlighted by English footballer Kyle Walker, who attributed his success as a right-back to studying video footage of fellow right-backs Dani Alves and Gary Neville (Jones, 2012).

Our understanding of observational learning has been enhanced by researchers utilizing point-light displays (e.g., Hayes, Hodges, Scott, Horn, & Williams, 2007; Scully & Carnegie, 1998). In point-light displays, biological motion is reduced to and represented using a selection of dots (which, for example, are representative of the joint locations). By manipulating which dots (i.e., biological features) are visible in a point-light display, a researcher can isolate components of a movement and identify those biomechanical features that provide meaningful information to an observer. For example, it appears that observation of the skill end points, such as the motions of the wrist and toes in lawn bowling, provides the most critical information to assist skill learning (Hayes, Hodges, Huys, & Williams, 2007). Following this logic, coaches should ensure (i.e., though vantage points, video resolution, etc.) that athletes are provided unhindered access to such information during demonstrations. With these endeffectors (i.e., hands and feet) the very segments that we associate with motor dominance, there is a logical necessity that the representations provided to an athlete. Furthermore, coaches can assist athletes to assimilate crucial information by guiding their attention to key cues. For example, Masters, Lo, et al. (2008) and Masters, Poolton, et al. (2008) guided the attention of trainee surgeons during a surgery task by placing markers on the simulated patients' skin. After every five trials, one marker was removed, and the surgeons progressively began to rely more on their own intuition to perform the task. It is plausible that sequentially reducing the available information would be equally useful for sports coaches, though an emphasis on the perception of skill end points and maximizing the athletes' familiarity with the model performer appears critical.

Another potential dilemma, particularly in elite sport, is the application of "observational learning" as a practice technique for elite junior athletes.

Specifically, it has been demonstrated that physical attributes (i.e., organismic constraints) effectively determine an individual's potential solutions to a motor task (Newell, 1986). That being the case, there are questions surrounding the suitability of using adult performance models as educational tools in junior sport (e.g., showing a pubescent sprinter footage of Usain Bolt), as younger athletes likely lack the strength, anthropometry, cognitive ability, and so on to replicate the movement patterns of professionals. This is evident in practice where, for example, elite female junior tennis players utilize significantly different movement patterns (due to strength differences) and projection angles (due to stature differences) compared with professional female players (Whiteside, Elliott, Lay, & Reid, 2013). Likewise, strength and muscle mass disparities are postulated to be responsible for the developmental differences in joint loading and velocity generation in elite baseball pitchers (Fleisig, Barrentine, Zheng, Escamilla, & Andrews, 1999). For this reason, when learning complex or maximal effort sporting skills, observations of professional athletes seem most useful for athletes who have physically matured to adolescence. The efficacy of observational learning strategies also appears to asymptote as athletes develop expertise. That is, research suggests that once a learner is a proficient performer of the skill, the "model example" no longer contributes to learning and may even hamper the process (i.e., the "expertise-reversal effect"; Kalyuga, Ayres, Chandler, & Sweller, 2003). Seemingly, this issue would be compounded if the skilled athlete observes a model of opposite motor dominance.

PROVIDING FEEDBACK TO FACILITATE LEARNING AND PERFORMANCE

Feedback is essential for the continual development of sports skills. Typically feedback falls into two broad categories: intrinsic and extrinsic. Intrinsic feedback is available from the performer's sensory systems such as the kinesthetic feedback arising from the sensory receptors in muscles, tendons, and joints. Extrinsic or augmented feedback provided to the learner or athlete from an external source such as a coach. This section will focus on augmented feedback and how coaches can use feedback to enhance both learning and performance in sports.

Types of Feedback

Augmented feedback can generally be placed into one of two categories: knowledge of results (KR) or knowledge of performance (KP). KR refers to feedback concerning the outcome of a movement (i.e., whether a free throw in basketball was successful or not), while KP relates to specific aspects of the movement pattern (i.e., wrist posture at ball release).

Historically, the majority of research in this domain focused on KR, revealing how KR feedback is crucial for learning (Bennett & Simmons, 1984; Bilodeau, Bilodeau, & Schumsky, 1959). However, the value of such feedback in a sports setting, where KR is almost always readily available, is questionable. As a result, contemporary investigative interest has transitioned toward the efficacy of KP, which can be provided using various methods such as verbal feedback, visual feedback via video displays, and kinematic and biofeedback. Given the variety of options available to coaches and the disparate effects each may elicit, one of the major considerations when providing feedback is its content.

Content of Feedback

For coaches, deciding the most appropriate information to provide an athlete, and the precision with which to do so can be challenging. With recent advances in technology, the mediums through which feedback can be provided have grown in both number and sophistication. Although this affords coaches numerous avenues through which they can convey feedback to their athletes, these advances can also present unique challenges to the learning process.

Currently, motion analysis technologies enable practitioners to deliver incredibly precise and highly detailed kinematic information about almost any aspect of their movement. While such technology can be beneficial in many instances, it is critical that coaches consider whether the content of their feedback is valuable for the athlete. It has been suggested that feedback provided to an athlete should match what the performer can control (Schmidt & Wrisberg, 2008) and needs to control (Whiting & Vereijken, 1993). Of specific interest are the parameters, or biomechanical variables that should serve as the subject of feedback. Again, advances in technology allow for a multitude of variables to be measured, analyzed, and potentially relayed to the athlete, yet communicating this information is necessarily consistent with an explicit learning process. It follows that the provision of augmented feedback must not only be accurate, but also relevant for improving skill execution (Phillips, Farrow, Ball, & Helmer, 2013). Phillips et al. (2013) suggested that parameter selection should be based on three criteria. First, the parameter must be integral to performance improvement. For example, if a coach were trying to improve a baseball pitcher's throwing speed, it would not make sense to provide the athlete with information about the speed of his nonthrowing hand. Second, the athlete must be capable of modifying the parameter. The height of a tennis player's impact point in the serve, for example, is effectively constrained by their stature (Whiteside et al., 2013), thereby rendering it unreasonable for a coach for demand that a player markedly adjust this feature of their service action. Third, the system or device must be able to accurately and reliably measure the parameter(s) in question. This pertains to the criterion validity of measurement tools whereby invalid measures do not provide useful information for the athlete or coach. As an example, it would be critical for a coach to confirm that a newly developed sensor or tablet application can accurately quantify what it is purported to measure prior to using those data for instructional purposes.

When providing feedback on technical execution, coaches must carefully consider the content thereof. To this point, addressing motoric dominance would logically serve to effect more specific feedback for the athlete. In sports such as tennis, cricket, and baseball—where left-handers demonstrate a tactical and/or perceptual advantage—it is logical that technical instructions should differ according to handedness. For example, it has been reported that a tennis player's set-up position and stroke characteristics when returning serve are dependent on the handedness of the server (Loffing, Hagemann, & Strauss, 2009). Likewise, an ice hockey goaltender will necessarily possess bilateral differences in their upper limb mechanics when saving to the left and right (as they hold the stick and wear a blocker on one hand and wear a glove on the other). In team sports, an athlete's laterality (and corresponding playing position) can also dictate the tactical feedback that they should receive. As an example, a footballer playing on the left side of midfield may oppose a particularly proficient right fullback during a crucial game. Accordingly, the coach may discourage the player from trying to attack the fullback and instead instruct his team to focus on creating attacking opportunities down the right flank. In this sense, coaches must be aware that the provision of feedback should be athlete- and situation-specific.

Scheduling of Feedback

A further consideration for coaches concerns the timing and frequency of feedback. This is particularly critical as the consequences of incorrectly scheduling feedback are well established. There is considerable evidence to suggest that providing feedback after every trial is detrimental to learning (Young & Schmidt, 1992). The guidance hypothesis was proposed by Salmoni, Schmidt, and Walter (1984) and insinuates that while feedback provides an essential role in the learning process, learners can develop a dependence there on, producing adverse repercussions when feedback is withdrawn (e.g., during competition). Dependence may occur if feedback is provided too frequently, immediately after the trial before the learner has the ability to process task intrinsic feedback, or if it is provided concurrently during performance (Salmoni et al., 1984). To overcome this, research has used various feedback schedules such as delaying feedback (Anderson, Magill, Sekiya, & Ryan, 2005), presenting feedback as a summary (Schmidt,

Young, Swinnen, & Shapiro, 1989), or allowing the learner to self-select when they receive feedback (Patterson & Carter, 2010). However, the guidance hypothesis theory has been criticized for failing to consider how augmented feedback is interpreted when learning complex skills common in sports. Using a complex ski simulator task, Wulf, Shea, and Matschiner (1998) showed that frequent feedback (100%) was more beneficial for performance compared to a faded feedback schedule (50%). While such findings seem to run contrary to the guidance hypothesis, it has been reported that highly salient task intrinsic feedback can prevent dependence on augmented feedback (Wulf & Shea, 2004). In summary, the likelihood of dependence on augmented feedback can be reduced by ensuring task intrinsic feedback is both meaningful (relevant to the task) and easy for the athlete to use and interpret. Conversely, an athlete will be less likely to develop a reliance on augmented feedback if it is inhibited by the coach, instead deferring to intrinsic sources (Williams & Hodges, 2004).

STRUCTURING PRACTICE

As recently as 2005, sports practice was described as repetitive, prescriptive, and grounded in tradition (Williams & Hodges, 2005). Although this ideology may persist in some circles, the majority of professional sporting organizations have largely begun to embrace an evidence-based approach to practice. Empirical data have engendered more deliberate training regimes that target even the most intricate facets of performance (e.g., strength, conditioning, tactics, cognition). With effectively all sports involving some degree of unilateral performance, the concept of laterality is relevant in effectively all sports. The current body of evidence in this area highlights how structuring practice can influence learning and is, therefore, a crucial part of the coaching process.

Contextual Interference

From a coaching perspective, contextual interference may be thought of as the degree of variety in the movement skills that are rehearsed in a given practice session. A session that is structured to involve repeated (i.e., "blocked") performance of a single skill contains low contextual interference. For example, if a basketball player were to shoot 20 three-point jump shots in succession, from the same location on court. On the contrary, a session wherein an athlete performs a variety of movement skills in a randomized sequence contains high contextual interference. This would be the case if the basketball player's 20 three-point attempts were randomly interspersed with layups, fadeaway jump shots, free throws and contested hook shots. Contextual interference is a vital aspect for coaches to consider when structuring practice as it can have a considerable effect on how athletes acquire skills.

The seminal work of Shea and Morgan (1979) showed that practicing motor tasks in a setting that contained high levels of contextual interference promoted long-term retention of the skill. These results have since been replicated in numerous movement scenarios, and there is now a large body of evidence that advocates structuring practice to involve high levels of contextual interference (Gabbett, 2006; Li & Lima, 2002; Naimo et al., 2013; Porter, Landin, Hebert, & Baum, 2007; Porter & Magill, 2010). Perhaps the best evidence of its effectiveness in elite sport lies in Brazilian football, where junior players are renowned for spending their formative years devoid of coaches or structured practice (Fonseca & Garganta, 2008; Koslowsky & Botelho, 2010; Salema & Morales, 2004). Instead, these young players engage in informal football games that contain variations in playing numbers, playing surfaces, and even objects to serve as the football. In spite of this, Brazilian players are heralded for developing exceptional levels of technical prowess. Brazilian footballer Oscar, also of Chelsea FC, recalls growing up in his homeland:

> I learned how to play football as a kid through trial and error, playing every day in the street or in the park. When you start kicking a ball about in Brazil, there are no tactics. Whoever can dribble the ball and score just does it. And that's what I learned to do. *Bernstein (2014)*

In this sense, contextual interference is seemingly greatest during unstructured practice where athletes participate in scenarios that mimic competition and foster intrinsic learning. Although contextual interference may be greatest during game play, coaches in elite sport can structure practice to take advantage of this learning effect.

From a laterality perspective, the concept of contextual interference is relevant to numerous aspects of training and competition in elite sport. While several sports require a degree of bilateral proficiency at the elite level, laterality ensures that athletes will generally display a preference or dominance when executing a unilateral skill (i.e., kicking in the football codes, dribbling a basketball, passing in rugby). To maximize an athlete's effectiveness, a coach may assign the athlete's playing position according to their handedness or footedness. As an example, footballers who play wide positions will generally play on the side of the field that corresponds to their preferred kicking foot (where they will both be required and also afforded greater opportunities to utilise their preferred foot). Practice drills for these athletes would intuitively involve their preferred foot, as this is what they will be utilizing during a game, yet this leaves less room to exploit the contextual interference effect. Contrastingly, incorporating bilateral performance allows the coach to create a more varied practice environment and increase contextual interference. For example, instead of practicing crossing from the left flank using her preferred left foot, a footballer may variously shape to cross with her left before cutting back on to her weaker right foot to cross the ball. This way she is afforded opportunities to practice crossing the ball using both feet. The potential applications of this approach are further endorsed by the notion of bilateral transfer (or "cross education"), wherein unilateral performance is improved after practice with the contralateral limb (Lee & Carroll, 2007; Ruddy & Carson, 2013; Teixeira, 2000; Teixeira, Silva, & Carvalho, 2003). In the example above, crossing the ball with the right foot would not only introduce greater contextual interference to promote the acquisition of skilled right-footed kicking, but may also present some benefits to the player's natural left-footed kicking through the cross-education effect. Equally, the coach could move the footballer to the right flank and have her continue the drill from that side of the pitch. Therein, the higher volume of crosses with her nonpreferred right foot would be expected to yield improvements in both kicking legs. Thus, in sports where ambidexterity is required, accentuating performance with the nonpreferred limb is seemingly beneficial for enhancing performance bilaterally, while also curbing the development of morphological asymmetries.

More recently, it has been postulated that the effectiveness of learning a particular movement skill is dependent on (1) which side is initially used to practice the skill and (2) the nature of the skill (e.g., precision/accuracy-based or strength-based) (Stöckel & Weigelt, 2012a, 2012b; Stöckel, Weigelt, & Krug, 2011). More specifically, children who practiced accuracy-based tasks with their nonpreferred hand before their preferred hand have exhibited enhanced skill acquisition compared with those who practiced in the opposite order (Stöckel & Weigelt, 2012a, 2012b; Stöckel et al., 2011). In strength-based tasks, however, skill acquisition was enhanced when the children practiced using their preferred limb first, followed by their nonpreferred limb (Stöckel & Weigelt, 2012a, 2012b). It is, therefore, critical for the coach to consider the complexion of the motor task (e.g., precision-based fine motor task or maximal effort task) when designing training programs.

In the majority of sports, it is not feasible to alter the hand/foot when executing sport-specific movement skills (e.g., hitting in racket sports, golf, baseball, and cricket). However, contextual variations of the same skill can still promote learning of unilateral skills. For example, tennis players can alter the type of groundstrokes being performed (e.g., shots hit crosscourt and down-the-line with topspin and/or slice). An ice hockey player could practice shooting from various locations in the attacking zone while the puck is delivered to him from a variety of angles and speeds. Likewise, baseball pitchers—agents of a particularly constrained skill—may incorporate long tosses, fielding bunts, or picking off runners while alternating between different pitch variations during practice. In this way, these athletes are able to increase contextual interference and promote long-term retention of unilateral movement skills.

Constraints

Prior to the 1980s, the motor learning landscape was dominated by information-processing models: namely, Adams' (1971) closed-loop theory and Schmidt's (1975) schema theory. Both emphasized the role of the central nervous system, memory, and information feedback in the learning of motor skills but could not account for the dynamism of the perceptual-motor landscape. In 1986, Karl Newell developed an alternative theoretical framework to describe how movement skills emerge. His work proposed that motor performance was effectively a product of organismic, environmental and task constraints. In sporting contexts, Newell's constraints model describes how athletes' individual characteristics (e.g., height, mass, strength, intelligence) help to govern how they will execute a movement skill. Similarly, the manner in which athletes perform a movement will be influenced by environmental factors (e.g., temperature, humidity, lighting, wind, altitude) and the specific nature of the task (e.g., the way in which an ice hockey player shoots the puck will differ according his distance from the goal, whether he is aiming into an open net, shooting past opponents, stationary, skating, shooting a one-timer, shooting backhand, etc.). Perhaps unintentionally, elite coaches have utilized this framework to structure practice sessions and elicit performance improvements for several decades.

Manipulating the Practice Context (Task) to Elicit Performance Improvements

In contemporary sport, practice is often underpinned by the principle of specificity through the rehearsal of game-like scenarios that prepare athletes for competition. However, while replicating competition scenarios (e.g., playing an actual game) maximizes specificity (and contextual interference as we have learned), it may not always offer the most effective method for developing expertise in practice settings. For example, when a particular athlete requires precise refinements to a specific aspect of her game/technique, it is not reasonable to design an unstructured training drill and expect the desired outcome to manifest of its own accord. It is more practical for the coach to make strategic alterations to the practice context that will expose the athlete to the desired scenario(s). Indeed, Heiko Vogel—former under 19 coach at the famed Bayern Munich FC youth academy—indicates that:

> Specially conceived skills training (especially ball control exercises) is quickest and best at developing technique. However, it is essential to ensure that the skill is embedded in the situational context of a game. *H. Vogel, personal communication (August 14, 2014)*

In a rudimentary sense, imagine you are a football coach who wants to improve the shooting ability of your forwards... Would you administer a full match at training in the hope that it produces several shooting opportunities for the forwards? Or would you rather design a practice drill that retains a high degree of specificity while providing these players with ample shooting practice (e.g., three forwards vs. two defenders, played in the front third)? Employing a constrained practice task seems like the obvious choice. Environmentally, the notion of constraining the training environment forms the basis for practices such as altitude training, which can elicit performance improvements that would not otherwise manifest (Levine & Stray-Gundersen, 1997; Lorenzo, Halliwill, Sawka, & Minson, 2010; Stray-Gundersen, Chapman, & Levine, 2001).

With laterality in mind, a coach can also methodically alter practice tasks to promote the learning of particular unilateral motor skills. Previous research has demonstrated that actions by left dominant players are more difficult to anticipate (Hagemann, 2009; McMorris & Colenso, 1996), so let us take the example of a right-handed batter in baseball who consistently strikes out when facing left-handed pitchers. The coach may deliberately structure practice such that he faces more left-handed pitchers than the other batters on the team. By exposing the batter to a higher volume of pitches in this practice context, the coach is able to "direct" his athlete's learning, without relying on prescriptive methods. Indeed, the recent work of Schorer, Loffing, Hagemann, and Baker (2012) highlighted the value of this approach among novice handball players, where improvements in their ability to predict the outcome of left- or right-handed penalty shots was contingent on the nature (handedness) of the penalty shots that they observed in practice. Accordingly, a boxer with a tendency to under-utilize her left hook may be forced to spar with a partner who has been told, surreptitiously, to leave herself exposed to this particular punch. It is clear that creating specific practice contexts can expose athletes to critical performance scenarios and encourage them to create current event profiles and action plans therefor (McPherson, 1999; McPherson

& Kernodle, 2007). Thereafter, the athlete can draw on these profiles/ plans to enhance performance during competition. The other obvious advantage of structured practice is that it need not involve explicit instruction.

Elite sport is replete with examples of athletes learning fundamentals in a highly constrained practice environment: footballer George Best dribbling with a tennis ball (George Best: Victim of stardom, March 10, 2000); cricketer Don Bradman hitting a golf ball with a cricket stump (Bradman, 1950); Joe Frazier punching beef carcasses (Goldstein, 2011); Bruce Lee "fighting" his "wooden man" (McCafferty, 2013); and so on. These examples provide rather intriguing insights into the potential benefits of representative tasks in the acquisition of motor skills. On this basis, coaches should be open to the idea of designing representative tasks that target specific, technical aspects of performance.

While athletes will tend to use their dominant side to execute movement skills, ambidexterity is advantageous in many sports. Heiko Vogel (Bayern Munich FC), notes that:

> The ability to use both feet is an important skill and plays a significant role when we scout for talent. At the highest level of football being two-footed is a basic requirement.
> H. Vogel, personal communication (August 14, 2014)

In these cases, it is essential to not only nurture the preferred side, but to promote ambidexterity. To develop the nondominant side, coaches must design drills that force athletes out of their comfort zone. That is, constrain the practice task such that the athlete inevitably begins to experiment with their nondominant limb (i.e., Stöckel & Weigelt, 2012a, 2012b; Teixeira et al., 2003). Examples include games where athletes are only permitted to kick/throw/handball/catch with their nonpreferred side or reassigning player positions (e.g., assigning a right-footed footballer to play on the left side of the field). Aside from encouraging players to develop ambidexterity, these activities also reduce the extent to which strength, flexibility, and morphological asymmetries naturally develop when athletes favor one side of their body. This is particularly important as, in some cases—as detailed in Chapter 6: Perspectives From Sports Medicine—asymmetries have been linked to sporting injuries (Croisier, Ganteaume, Binet, Genty, & Ferret, 2008; Fousekis, Tsepis, Poulmedis, Athanasopoulos, & Vagenas, 2010; Paterno et al., 2010).

In many sports, it is not possible nor practical to balance the training loads between the preferred and nonpreferred sides (e.g., a tennis player cannot switch and play with his nondominant hand). In these sports, it may be customary for an athlete to perform all of his/her movements using their preferred limb (e.g., baseball pitcher, American football punter, golfer). Consequently, these activities obligate asymmetrical biomechanics. Over time, these repetitive movements can induce the aforesaid strength or morphological asymmetries as athletes engage muscles on one side of their body while neglecting those on the other side. To combat the likelihood of injury in these cases, strength and/or conditioning programs are integral to maintaining musculoskeletal symmetry.

While it is obvious that constraining practice scenarios provides coaches with a valuable training tool, it is important to note this approach is not unequivocally guaranteed to enhance performance. This seems to be related to the apparent trade-off that exists between constraining practice contexts and retaining task specificity. Put simply, when a coach alters the practice context, it often acts to decrease the specificity of the training exercise. This is particularly evident in the "whole-part" approach to training, wherein coaches attempt to simplify movement skills by breaking them down into their component parts and having athletes perform each part in isolation (e.g., in the tennis serve: practicing the ball toss and swinging motion separately; in swimming: practicing kicking without arm movements, using a kickboard). However, research conducted since the turn of the century suggests that if training drills are too far removed from the competition context, they can actually have a detrimental effect on performance. For example, Renshaw, Oldham, Davids, and Golds (2007) reported that elite cricket batsmen performed differently when facing a ball machine as compared to an actual bowler. Likewise, the height and spin of elite junior tennis players' ball toss has been shown to differ when they practice the ball toss (i.e., without hitting the ball) independent of the actual serve (Reid, Whiteside, & Elliott, 2010). For this reason, where possible, practice should be structured in a context that is analogous with that of competition to promote learning of complex motor skills.

It is also important to note that specially designed drills can elicit desired improvements while having unintended consequences on other aspects of performance. For example, to promote a more vertical racket trajectory, it is not uncommon for tennis coaches to have players serve from their knees. Recent research confirmed that players did indeed employ a vertical racket trajectory when performing this drill but significantly decreased the dynamism of their trunk rotations when doing so (Reid, Whiteside, Gilbin, & Elliott, 2013). Thus if the improved racquet trajectory subsequently transferred to competition, so too may the undesirable trunk mechanics, thereby producing a performance outcome contrary to that intended. Similarly, modifying the mass and inertial properties of the racket can significantly reduce tennis players' ability to wield it effectively (Whiteside, Elliott, Lay, & Reid, 2014) and/or increase injury risk (Creveaux et al., 2013) when serving. Pursuant to these data, coaches should consider the holistic effects of training drills that alter the context of the task. In other words, coaches should contemplate not only the purported benefits of a drill, but also the detrimental effects it could have. Where unsure, it is important for coaches to employ an evidence-based approach to instruction. Without contesting the value of anecdotal training drills, it is worth taking note of the shortcomings of subjective human perception! Ultimately, the notion of constrained practice provides a theoretical underpinning that, when used correctly, can develop almost all aspects of performance be they physical, cognitive, biomechanical, or otherwise, and is limited only by the imagination of the coach.

Accounting for Athletes' Individual Traits and Flair

Manipulating organismic (i.e., athlete) characteristics forms the basis for effectively all strength and/or conditioning programs in elite sport. In these cases, coaches hope to modify an athlete's physical capacities (e.g., a high-jumper's lower limb power) to alter how they will perform their sport-specific motor task (e.g., jump higher).

Although manipulating characteristics (i.e., core strength, explosiveness, perception) presents obvious benefits for the athlete, developing these attributes is often a time-intensive process. In some cases, it is even necessary to break "bad habits" (e.g., poor coordination or perceptual ineptitude) and have athletes relearn skills entirely. Equally, coaches may place a premium on identifying and cultivating anomalous attributes, such that these individual traits afford the athlete a competitive advantage (a primary component of talent identification).

It is well established that athletes' genetic composition and anthropometry makes them more suited to specific sports (Clarkson, Kroll, & McBride, 1980; Costill et al., 1976; Krawczyk, Sklad, & Jackiewicz, 1997; Mathews & Wagner, 2008; Thorland, Johnson, Fagot, Tharp, & Hammer, 1980). Famously, Michael Jordan was not deemed tall enough to warrant selection on his high school's varsity basketball team (McGrath, 2009) before a growth spurt the following summer allowed him to revolutionize his playing style and become a high school all-American only two seasons later (Clemons, 2014). This concept also applies from a tactical standpoint, where certain athletes are better suited to specific strategies (e.g., counter-puncher vs. serve-and-volleyer in tennis) or playing positions (e.g., linebacker vs. wide receiver in American football) (Carter, Ackland, Kerr, & Stapff, 2005; Duncan, Woodfield, & Al-Nakeeb, 2006; Gil, Gil, Ruiz, Irazusta, & Irazusta, 2007; Malousaris et al., 2008). For example, at the time of writing, an astonishing 59 of Major League Baseball's top 100 career leaders in batting average are left-handed (Baseball-Reference.com), while 29 of the top 100 batting averages in test cricket belong to left-handers (ESPNcricinfo.com). As discussed in our introduction, given that left-handedness comprise≈10% of the general population, it would seem difficult to argue that left-handers do not hold some form of advantage in these elite hitting skills. In this sense, it is crucial that coaches are aware of the innate capacities of their athletes, and coach to those strengths. This may include such things as designating playing positions (e.g., playing right-footers on the right side of the football field), match-ups (e.g., calling up a left-handed pinch-hitter to face a right-handed baseball pitcher), or tactics (e.g., left-handed tennis player working angles to a right-handed opponent's backhand), according to an athlete's laterality. Offering a working example is Lionel Messi, who scored 83% of his first 400 goals for club and country with his left foot, 13% with his right foot, and 4% with his head (Conn, 2014). Based on these numbers, it would seem advantageous for his coaches to promote attacking scenarios that place the ball at Messi's left foot.

Akin to other organismic factors, laterality may be considered a quality that coaches/players can leverage to gain a competitive advantage. For example, it was noted earlier in this section that football coaches often select left-footed players to play in left-sided positions of the field. In response, that player's opponent may deliberately coerce him to kick with his right foot so as to negate any advantage he may hold. Similarly, a team sport coach (or captain) may alter the batting or pitching/bowling order midmatch to counter the effectiveness of a certain opponent depending on their handedness, as has been recommended through the work of Hirotsu and Wright (2005). Indeed, Simon Helmot, former coach of the Melbourne Renegades T20 cricket team, discusses a working example of how laterality can dictate team strategy in T20 cricket:

> I think it's imperative to try and manipulate match-ups between batsmen and bowlers. For example, if a left handed orthodox spinner is bowling well, I will try and send a left-handed batsman in next to counter this, and vice versa if a right-handed off-spinner is bowling well. Also, often particular batsmen have weaknesses against bowling of a certain handedness and we always try to exploit these weaknesses by dictating who bowls each over. S. Helmot, personal communication (October 10, 2014)

These are intuitive methods of exploiting athletes' laterality to enhance or counter their performance. However, it is important to acknowledge that the notion of laterality extends across the entire body. For example, lateral dominance is not only true in the hand and foot, but also the eye and ear. Likewise, lateral preferences are displayed in athletes' preferred movement strategies (e.g., whether they prefer to rotate to their right or left when turning around). This information can also prove informative for coaches when developing athletes.

Determining the different aspects of an athlete's laterality can uncover his/her strengths and weaknesses and help to direct appropriate training programs. Garipuy (2001) proposed a laterality test for tennis players that was intended to inform athlete-specific playing styles and training regimes. The test appraised laterality in the hands, eyes, trunk, and pelvis, with a view to revealing the playing styles and strokes (i.e., the strengths and weaknesses) that are best suited to his/her laterality profile. For example, a right-handed player whose preferred direction of pelvis rotation is rightward possesses a laterality pattern consistent with a strong forehand. In this case, it would be in the coach's best interest to develop and encourage tactics around this stroke. On the other hand, a right-eye, right-hand dominant player whose preferred direction of pelvis rotation is leftward possesses a laterality pattern that is unfavorable for the serve. It would then be the coach's responsibility to dedicate more time to refining aspects of the service action to combat this organismic constraint.

While the above example pertains specifically to tennis, laterality has implications for all whole body sporting movements that involve multisegment coordination. In these movements, it is important to acknowledge the laterality of not only the end-effector (i.e., the hand in throwing or foot in kicking), but also the other segments in the kinetic chain. Obtaining this information allows coaches to both exploit the innate coordinative advantages of the player and rectify weaknesses in specific movement patterns.

SUMMARY

In this chapter, we discussed how athletes learn and how this may shape the instructional approach that is delivered by their coaches. Fundamentally, coaches must administer carefully curated training regimes that cultivate optimal learning for the athlete, irrespective of motor dominance.

With respect to learning processes, a comprehensive knowledge of mechanics can prove detrimental for athletes as they become susceptible to "overthinking" their movements when under pressure. Consequently, explicitly telling an athlete how to orient her nondominant arm during freestyle swimming or how to release a curveball from his fingers may not prove fruitful in the long-term. Preferably, more subtle methods can help athletes implicitly acquire motor expertise without subjecting them to prescriptive instruction.

One such option is to provide athletes with opportunities to observe model performers. Whether this involves real-time observation or video footage, it is critical for coaches to select a model with whom their athlete is familiar. Importantly, this involves matching the laterality of their athlete with that of the model (e.g., a left-footed rugby kicker should observe a left-footed model) in order to optimize learning. Likewise, positional athletes in team sports (e.g., a right-midfielder in football) should be exposed to footage of models who play the same position to better acquire an appreciation of specific positional tactics and roles, as they relate to laterality. This acts to maximize the neural response of the observing athlete and, in turn, promote learning.

The provision of feedback is also a crucial part of learning sports skills. Athletes benefit from accurate, clearly presented feedback about aspects of their performance that they have the ability to alter. With this in mind, objective measurement tools and feedback that is pertinent to the individual are most beneficial. In practice, this may necessitate the provision of different feedback for left- and right-dominant athletes. That is to say, coaches should acknowledge that dominance will influence how athletes perform (e.g., the angle at which they project the ball in baseball/tennis and their tactical inclinations in invasion sports) and provide feedback accordingly. However, excessive feedback can lead to an unhealthy and deleterious dependence on extraneous guidance, which is often unavailable during competition.

Finally, structuring practice is a time-honored method of promoting improvements in elite sport. Designing practice drills that encourage athletes to rehearse movement skills in a game-specific context can facilitate learning opportunities that may not otherwise manifest. Critically, this approach can help to combat athletes' natural tendency to rely on their dominant limb, thereby promoting ambidexterity in relevant sports. Likewise, practice drills or constraints can be designed to expose athletes to both left- and right-dominant opponents and develop counter strategies for both. It is equally relevant that coaches be aware of athletes' laterality as this information can be used to inform tactics that exploit athletes' motor dominance to gain a competitive advantage, such as set plays that result in shots on goal with the (stronger and more accurate) dominant foot.

Finally, it is important to acknowledge that left- and right-dominant athletes appear to possess disparate tactical advantages and will, therefore, benefit from instruction that is directly tailored to their laterality. For this reason, it is imperative that coaches are attuned to their athletes' laterality, as this information can be used to enhance the acquisition of motor and tactical expertise, within each of the domains presented in this chapter.

References

Adams, J. A. (1971). A closed-loop theory of motor learning. *Journal of Motor Behavior, 3*(2), 111–150.

Anderson, J. (1983). *The architecture of cognition.* Cambridge, MA: Harvard University Press.

Anderson, D. I., Magill, R. A., Sekiya, H., & Ryan, G. (2005). Support for an explanation of the guidance effect in motor skill learning. *Journal of Motor Behavior, 37*, 231–238.

Ashford, D., Davids, K., & Bennett, S. J. (2007). Developmental effects influencing observational modeling: a meta-analysis. *Journal of Sports Sciences, 25*, 547–558.

Baseball-Reference.com. (December 30, 2015). *Career leaders & records for batting average. Baseball-reference.com.* Retreived from http://www.baseball-reference.com/leaders/batting_avg_career.shtml.

Bennett, D., & Simmons, R. (1984). Effects of precision of knowledge of results on acquisition and retention of a simple motor skill. *Perceptual and Motor Skills, 58,* 785–786.

Bernstein, J. (May 24, 2014). *Oscar – The secret of our samba success: When you're a kid in Brazil you don't worry about tactics and coaching... You just dribble the ball and score.* The Daily Mail. Retrieved from http://www.dailymail.co.uk/sport/worldcup2014/article-2638246/Brazil-Chelsea-star-Oscar-The-secret-samba-success.html.

Berry, D. C. (1997). *How implicit is implicit learning?* Oxford, UK: University Press.

Berry, D. C., & Broadbent, D. E. (1988). Interactive tasks and the implicit–explicit distinction. *British Journal of Psychology, 79,* 251–272.

Bilodeau, E. A., Bilodeau, I. M., & Schumsky, D. A. (1959). Some effects of introducing and withdrawing knowledge of results early and late in practice. *Journal of Experimental Psychology, 58,* 142–144.

Bradman, S. D. (1950). *Farewell to cricket.* London: Hodder & Stoughton.

Brooks, R., Bussiere, L. F., Jennions, M. D., & Hunt, J. (2004). Sinister strategies succeed at the cricket world cup. *Proceedings of the Royal Society of London B, 271*(Suppl. 3), S64–S66.

Calvo-Merino, B., Glaser, D. E., Grezes, J., Passingham, R. E., & Haggard, P. (2005). Action observation and acquired motor skills: an fMRI study with expert dancers. *Cerebral Cortex, 15,* 1243–1249.

Carter, J. E. L., Ackland, T. R., Kerr, D. A., & Stapff, A. B. (2005). Somatotype and size of elite female basketball players. *Journal of Sports Sciences, 23,* 1057–1063.

Clarkson, P. M., Kroll, W., & McBride, T. C. (1980). Maximal isometric strength and fiber type composition in power and endurance athletes. *European Journal of Applied Physiology and Occupational Physiology, 44,* 35–42.

Clemons, J. (January 10, 2014). *UNC recruiting letters to Michael Jordan hit the auction circuit.* Fox Sports. Retrieved from http://www.foxsports.com/south/story/unc-recruiting-letters-to-michael-jordan-hit-the-auction-circuit-011014.

Conn, T. (September 27, 2014). *Leo Messi scores 400th career goal.* Inside Spanish Football. Retrieved from http://www.insidespanishfootball.com/126992/leo-messi-scores-400th-career-goal/.

Costill, D. L., Daniels, J., Evans, W., Fink, W., Krahenbuhl, G., & Saltin, B. (1976). Skeletal muscle enzymes and fiber composition in male and female track athletes. *Journal of Applied Physiology, 40,* 149–154.

Creveaux, T., Dumas, R., Hautier, C., Macé, P., Chèze, L., & Rogowski, I. (2013). Joint kinetics to assess the influence of the racket on a tennis player's shoulder. *Journal of Sports Science & Medicine, 12,* 259–266.

Croisier, J. L., Ganteaume, S., Binet, J., Genty, M., & Ferret, J. M. (2008). Strength imbalances and prevention of hamstring injury in professional soccer players: a prospective study. *American Journal of Sports Medicine, 36,* 1469–1475.

Cross, E. S., Kraemer, D. J. M., Hamilton, A. F., Kelley, W. M., & Grafton, S. T. (2009). Sensitivity of the action observation network to physical and observational learning. *Cerebral Cortex, 19,* 315–326.

Duncan, M. J., Woodfield, L., & Al-Nakeeb, Y. (2006). Anthropometric and physiological characteristics of junior elite volleyball players. *British Journal of Sports Medicine, 40,* 649–651.

ESPNcricinfo.com (December 30, 2015). *Batting Records | Test Matches. ESPNcricinfo.* Retrieved from http://stats.espncricinfo.com/ci/engine/stats/index.html?class=1;filter=advanced;orderby=batting_average;qualmin1=20;qualval1=innings;template=results;type=batting.

Fitts, P. M., & Posner, M. I. (1967). *Human performance.* Belmont, CA: Brooks/Cole.

Fleisig, G. S., Barrentine, S. W., Zheng, N., Escamilla, R. F., & Andrews, J. R. (1999). Kinematic and kinetic comparison of baseball pitching among various levels of development. *Journal of Biomechanics, 32*, 1371–1375.

Fonseca, H., & Garganta, J. (2008). *Futebol de rua, um beco com saída. Jogo espontâneo e prática deliberada [Football on the street, an alley with escape. Spontaneous game and deliberate practice].* Lisboa: Visão e Contextos.

Fousekis, K., Tsepis, E., Poulmedis, P., Athanasopoulos, S., & Vagenas, G. (2010). Intrinsic risk factors of non-contact quadriceps and hamstring strains in soccer: a prospective study of 100 professional players. *British Journal of Sports Medicine, 45*, 709–714.

Gabbett, T. J. (2006). Skill-based conditioning games as an alternative to traditional conditioning for rugby league players. *Journal of Strength and Conditioning Research, 20*, 309–315.

Garipuy, C. (2001). The use of laterality in tennis training. *ITF Coaching and Sport Science Review, 23*, 3–5.

George Best: Victim of stardom (March 10, 2000). Retrieved from http://news.bbc.co.uk/2/hi/sport/football/672732.stm.

Gil, S. M., Gil, J., Ruiz, F., Irazusta, A., & Irazusta, J. (2007). Physiological and anthropometric characteristics of young soccer players according to their playing position: relevance for the selection process. *The Journal of Strength and Conditioning Research, 21*, 438–445.

Gilbert, A. N., & Wysocki, C. J. (1992). Hand preference and age in the United States. *Neuropsychologica, 30*, 601–608.

Goldstein, R. (November 7, 2011). *Joe Frazier, ex-heavyweight champ, dies at 67.* The New York Times. Retrieved from http://www.nytimes.com/2011/11/08/sports/joe-frazier-ex-heavyweight-champ-dies-at-67.html?pagewanted=all&_r=1&.

Goldstein, S., & Young, C. (1996). Evolutionary stable strategy of handedness in major league baseball. *Journal of Comparative Psychology, 110*, 164–169.

Green, T. D., & Flowers, J. H. (1991). Implicit versus explicit learning processes in a probabilistic, continuous fine-motor catching task. *Journal of Motor Behavior, 23*, 293–300.

Grouios, G., Tsorbatzoudis, H., Alexandris, K., & Barkoukis, V. (2000). Do left-handed competitors have an innate superiority in sports? *Perceptual and Motor Skills, 90*, 1273–1282.

Hagemann, N. (2009). The advantage of being left-handed in interactive sports. *Attention, Perception, & Psychophysics, 71*, 1641–1648.

Hardy, L., Mullen, R., & Jones, G. (1996). Knowledge and conscious control of motor actions under stress. *British Journal of Psychology, 87*, 621–636.

Harris, L. J. (2010). In fencing, what gives left-handers the edge? Views from the present and distant past. *Laterality: Asymmetries of Body, Brain and Cognition, 15*, 15–55.

Hayes, S. J., Hodges, N. J., Huys, R., & Williams, A. M. (2007). End-point focus manipulations to determine what information is used during observational learning. *Acta Psychologica, 126*, 120–137.

Hayes, S. J., Hodges, N. J., Scott, M. A., Horn, R. R., & Williams, A. M. (2007). The efficacy of demonstrations in teaching children an unfamiliar movement skill: the effects of object-orientated actions and point-light demonstrations. *Journal of Sports Sciences, 25*, 559–575.

Hirotsu, N., & Wright, M. (2005). Modelling a baseball game to optimise pitcher substitution strategies incorporating handedness of players. *IMA Journal of Management Mathematics, 16*, 179–194.

Holtzen, D. W. (2000). Handedness and professional tennis. *International Journal of Neuroscience, 105*, 101–119.

Jones, D. (April 15, 2012). *Kyle Walker inspired by YouTube videos of Alves and Neville.* Sunday Mirror. Retrieved from http://www.mirror.co.uk/sport/football/kyle-walker-inspired-by-youtube-videos-1676934.

Kalyuga, S., Ayres, P., Chandler, P., & Sweller, J. (2003). The expertise reversal effect. *Educational Psychologist, 38*, 23–31.

Koslowsky, M., & Botelho, M. F. C. (2010). Domains in the practice of the football learning: comparative study among football athletes of junior category in Portugal and Brazil. *Journal of Human Sport and Exercise, 5*.

Krawczyk, B., Sklad, M., & Jackiewicz, A. (1997). Heath-Carter somatotypes of athletes representing various sports. *Biology of Sport, 14*, 305–310.

Lam, W. K., Maxwell, J. P., & Masters, R. S. W. (2009). Analogy versus explicit learning of a modified basketball shooting task: performance and kinematic outcomes. *Journal of Sports Sciences, 27*, 179–191.

Lee, M., & Carroll, T. J. (2007). Cross education. *Sports Medicine, 37*, 1–14.

Levine, B. D., & Stray-Gundersen, J. (1997). "Living high-training low": effect of moderate-altitude acclimatization with low-altitude training on performance. *Journal of Applied Physiology, 83*, 102–112.

Li, Y., & Lima, R. P. (2002). Rehearsal of task variations and contextual interference effect in a field setting. *Perceptual and Motor Skills, 94*, 750–752.

Liao, C.-M., & Masters, R. S. (2001). Analogy learning: a means to implicit motor learning. *Journal of Sports Sciences, 19*, 307–319.

Loffing, F., & Hagemann, N. (2012). Side bias in human performance: a review on the left-handers' advantage in sports. In T. Dutta, M. Mandal, & S. Kumar (Eds.), *Bias in human behaviour* (pp. 163–182). Hauppauge, NY: Nova Science.

Loffing, F., Hagemann, N., & Strauss, B. (2009). The serve in professional men's tennis: effects of players' handedness. *International Journal of Performance Analysis in Sport, 9*(2), 255–274.

Loffing, F., Hagemann, N., & Strauss, B. (2012). Left-handedness in professional and amateur tennis. *PLoS One, 7*(11), e49325.

Lorenzo, S., Halliwill, J. R., Sawka, M. N., & Minson, C. T. (2010). Heat acclimation improves exercise performance. *Journal of Applied Physiology, 109*, 1140–1147.

Malousaris, G. G., Bergeles, N. K., Barzouka, K. G., Bayios, I. A., Nassis, G. P., & Koskolou, M. D. (2008). Somatotype, size and body composition of competitive female volleyball players. *Journal of Science and Medicine in Sport, 11*, 337–344.

Masters, R. S. W. (1992). Knowledge, knerves and know-how: the role of explicit versus implicit knowledge in the breakdown of a complex motor skill under pressure. *British Journal of Psychology, 83*, 343–358.

Masters, R. S. W., Lo, C. Y., Maxwell, J. P., & Patil, N. G. (2008). *Surgery, 143*, 140–143.

Masters, R. S. W., & Maxwell, J. P. (2008). The theory of reinvestment. *International Review of Sport and Exercise Psychology, 1*, 160–183.

Masters, R. S. W., Poolton, J. M., Maxwell, J. P., & Raab, M. (2008). Implicit motor learning and complex decision making in time-constrained environments. *Journal of Motor Behavior, 40*, 71–79.

Mathews, E. M., & Wagner, D. R. (2008). Prevalence of overweight and obesity in collegiate American football players, by position. *Journal of American College Health, 57*, 33–38.

Maxwell, J. P., Masters, R. S. W., & Eves, F. F. (2000). From novice to no know-how: a longitudinal study of implicit motor learning. *Journal of Sports Sciences, 18*, 111–120.

Maxwell, J. P., Masters, R. S. W., & Eves, F. F. (2003). The role of working memory in motor learning and performance. *Consciousness and Cognition, 12*, 376–402.

Maxwell, J. P., Masters, R. S. W., & Eves, F. F. (2009). Marginally perceptible outcome feedback, motor learning and implicit processes. *Consciousness and Cognition, 18*, 639–645.

Maxwell, J. P., Masters, R. S. W., Kerr, E., & Weedon, E. (2001). The implicit benefit of learning without errors. *The Quarterly Journal of Experimental Psychology, 54*, 1049–1068.

McCafferty, H. (September 14, 2013). *Run with the dragon: The Bruce Lee workout.* Swide. Retrieved from http://www.swide.com/sport-man/fitness/bruce-lee-workout-and-diet-routine/2013/09/14.

McGrath, D. (September 10, 2009). *Chapter 2: Wilmington.* Chicago Tribune. Retrieved from http://www.chicagotribune.com/sports/basketball/bulls/michaeljordan/chi-michael-jordan-chicago-bulls-chapter-2-story.html#page=1.

McMorris, T., & Colenso, S. (1996). Anticipation of professional soccer goalkeepers when facing right-and left-footed penalty kicks. *Perceptual and Motor Skills, 82,* 931–934.

McPherson, S. L. (1999). Tactical differences in problem representations and solutions in collegiate varsity and beginner female tennis players. *Research Quarterly for Exercise and Sport, 70,* 369–384.

McPherson, S. L., & Kernodle, M. (2007). Mapping two new points on the tennis expertise continuum: tactical skills of adult advanced beginners and entry-level professionals during competition. *Journal of Sports Sciences, 25,* 945–959.

Michaux, S. (April 9, 2013). *Bubba's way.* The Augusta Chronicle. Retrieved from http://www.augusta.com/masters/bubba/.

Naimo, M. A., Zourdos, M. C., Wilson, J. M., Kim, J. S., Ward, E. G., Eccles, D. W., & Panton, L. B. (2013). Contextual interference effects on the acquisition of skill and strength of the bench press. *Human Movement Science, 32,* 472–484.

Newell, K. M. (1986). Constraints on the development of coordination. *Motor Development in Children: Aspects of Coordination and Control, 34,* 341–360.

de Nooijer, J. A., van Gog, T., Paas, F., & Zwaan, R. A. (2013). When left is not right: handedness effects on learning object-manipulation words using pictures with left- or right-handed first-person perspectives. *Psychological Science, 24*(12), 2515–2521.

Paterno, M. V., Schmitt, L. C., Ford, K. R., Rauh, M. J., Myer, G. D., Huang, B., & Hewett, T. E. (2010). Biomechanical measures during landing and postural stability predict second anterior cruciate ligament injury after anterior cruciate ligament reconstruction and return to sport. *American Journal of Sports Medicine, 38,* 1968–1978.

Patterson, J. T., & Carter, M. (2010). Learner regulated knowledge of results during the acquisition of multiple timing goals. *Human Movement Science, 29,* 214–227.

Phillips, E., Farrow, D., Ball, K., & Helmer, R. (2013). Harnessing and understanding feedback technology in applied settings. *Sport Medicine, 43,* 919–925.

Pijpers, J. R., Oudejans, R. R., & Bakker, F. C. (2005). Anxiety-induced changes in movement behaviour during the execution of a complex whole-body task. *The Quarterly Journal of Experimental Psychology, 58,* 421–445.

Poolton, J. M., Masters, R. S. W., & Maxwell, J. P. (2005). The relationship between initial errorless learning conditions and subsequent performance. *Human Movement Science, 24,* 362–378.

Poolton, J. M., Masters, R. S. W., & Maxwell, J. P. (2006). The influence of analogy learning on decision making in table tennis: evidence from behavioral data. *Psychology of Sport and Exercise, 7,* 677–688.

Poolton, J. M., Masters, R. S. W., & Maxwell, J. P. (2007). Passing thoughts on the evolutionary stability of implicit motor behavior: performance retention under physiological fatigue. *Consciousness and Cognition, 16,* 456–468.

Poolton, J., Maxwell, J., Masters, R., & Raab, M. (2006). Benefits of an external focus of attention: common coding or conscious processing? *Journal of Sports Sciences, 24,* 89–99.

Porter, J. M., Landin, D., Hebert, E. P., & Baum, B. (2007). The effects of three levels of contextual interference on performance outcomes and movement patterns in golf skills. *International Journal of Sports Science and Coaching, 2,* 243–255.

Porter, J. M., & Magill, R. A. (2010). Systematically increasing contextual interference is beneficial for learning sport skills. *Journal of Sports Sciences, 28,* 1277–1285.

Reid, M., Whiteside, D., & Elliott, B. (2010). Effect of skill decomposition on racket and ball kinematics of the elite junior tennis serve. *Sports Biomechanics, 9,* 296–303.

Reid, M., Whiteside, D., Gilbin, G., & Elliott, B. (2013). Effect of a common task constraint on the body, racket, and ball kinematics of the elite junior tennis serve. *Sports Biomechanics, 12,* 15–22.

Renshaw, I., Oldham, A. R., Davids, K., & Golds, T. (2007). Changing ecological constraints of practice alters coordination of dynamic interceptive actions. *European Journal of Sport Science, 7,* 157–167.

Rocca, M. A., Falini, A., Comi, G., Scotti, G., & Filippi, M. (2008). The mirror-neuron system and handedness: a "right" world? *Human Brain Mapping, 29,* 1243–1254.

Ruddy, K. L., & Carson, R. G. (2013). Neural pathways mediating cross education of motor function. *Frontiers in Human Neuroscience, 7,* 1–22.

Salema, J. H., & Morales, L. C. (2004). Coaching families and learning in Brazilian youth football players. *Insight, 2,* 36–37.

Salmoni, A. W., Schmidt, R. A., & Walter, C. B. (1984). Knowledge of results and motor learning: a review and critical appraisal. *Psychological Bulletin, 95,* 355–386.

Schmidt, R. A. (1975). A schema theory of discrete motor skill learning. *Psychological Review, 82,* 225–260.

Schmidt, R. A., & Wrisberg, C. A. (2000). *Motor learning and performance: A situation-based learning approach.* Champaign, IL: Human Kinetics.

Schmidt, R. A., & Wrisberg, C. A. (2008). *Motor learning and performance* (Vol. 3). Champaign, IL: Human Kinetics.

Schmidt, R. A., Young, D. E., Swinnen, S., & Shapiro, D. C. (1989). Summary knowledge of results for skill acquisition: support for the guidance hypothesis. *Journal of Experimental Psychology: Learning, Memory, and Cognition, 15,* 352–359.

Scully, D., & Carnegie, E. (1998). Observational learning in motor skill acquisition. *Irish Journal of Psychology, 19,* 472–485.

Shea, J. B., & Morgan, R. L. (1979). Contextual interference effects on the acquisition, retention, and transfer of a motor skill. *Journal of Experimental Psychology: Human Learning and Memory, 5,* 179–187.

Shea, C. H., Wulf, G., Whitacre, C., & Wright, D. L. (2000). Physical and observational practice afford unique learning opportunities. *Journal of Motor Behaviour, 32,* 27–36.

Stevens, M. (March 31, 2010). *Foot fetish that won Hawks a flag.* Herald Sun. Retrieved from http://www.heraldsun.com.au/sport/afl/foot-fetish-that-won-hawks-a-flag/story-e6frf9jf-1225847711369.

Stöckel, T., & Weigelt, M. (2012a). Plasticity of human handedness: decreased one-hand bias and inter-manual performance asymmetry in expert basketball players. *Journal of Sports Sciences, 30,* 1037–1045.

Stöckel, T., & Weigelt, M. (2012b). Brain lateralisation and motor learning: selective effects of dominant and non-dominant hand practice on the early acquisition of throwing skills. *Laterality: Asymmetries of Body, Brain and Cognition, 17,* 18–37.

Stöckel, T., Weigelt, M., & Krug, J. (2011). Acquisition of a complex basketball-dribbling task in school children as a function of bilateral practice order. *Research Quarterly for Exercise and Sport, 82,* 188–197.

Stray-Gundersen, J., Chapman, R. F., & Levine, B. D. (2001). "Living high-training low" altitude training improves sea level performance in male and female elite runners. *Journal of Applied Physiology, 91,* 1113–1120.

Teixeira, L. A. (2000). Timing and force components in bilateral transfer of learning. *Brain and Cognition, 44,* 455–469.

Teixeira, L. A., Silva, M. V., & Carvalho, M. (2003). Reduction of lateral asymmetries in dribbling: the role of bilateral practice. *Laterality: Asymmetries of Body, Brain and Cognition, 8,* 53–65.

Thorland, W. G., Johnson, G. O., Fagot, T. G., Tharp, G. D., & Hammer, R. W. (1980). Body composition and somatotype characteristics of junior olympic athletes. *Medicine and Science in Sports and Exercise, 13,* 332–338.

Vinter, A., & Perruchet, P. (2002). Implicit motor learning through observational training in adults and children. *Memory & Cognition, 30,* 256–261.

Whiteside, D., Elliott, B., Lay, B., & Reid, M. (2013). The effect of age on discrete kinematics of the elite female tennis serve. *Journal of Applied Biomechanics, 29,* 573–582.

Whiteside, D., Elliott, B., Lay, B., & Reid, M. (2014). The effect of racquet swing weight on serve kinematics in elite adolescent female tennis players. *Journal of Science and Medicine in Sport, 17,* 124–128.

Whiting, H. T. A., & Vereijken, B. (1993). The acquisition of coordination in skill learning. *International Journal of Sport Psychology, 24,* 343–357.

Williams, A. M., & Hodges, N. J. (2004). *Skill acquisition in sport: Research, theory and practice.* London: Routledge.

Williams, A. M., & Hodges, N. J. (2005). Practice, instruction and skill acquisition in soccer: challenging tradition. *Journal of Sports Sciences, 23*(6), 637–650.

Wulf, G., & Shea, C. H. (2004). Understanding the role of augmented feedback. In A. M. Williams, & N. J. Hodges (Eds.), *Skill acquisition in sport: Research, theory and practice* (pp. 121–144). London: Routledge.

Wulf, G., Shea, C. H., & Matschiner, S. (1998). Frequent feedback enhances complex motor skill learning. *Journal of Motor Behavior, 30,* 180–192.

Young, D. E., & Schmidt, R. (1992). Augmented feedback for enhanced skill acquisition. *Journal of Motor Behaviour, 24,* 261–273.

Index